T0275843

Cambridge History of Medicine
EDITORS: CHARLES WEBSTER AND
CHARLES ROSENBERG

Morbid Appearances

OTHER BOOKS IN THIS SERIES

Charles Webster, ed.   *Health, medicine and mortality in the sixteenth century*
Ian Maclean   *The Renaissance notion of woman*
Michael MacDonald   *Mystical Bedlam*
Robert E. Kohler   *From medical chemistry to biochemistry*
Walter Pagel   *Joan Baptista Van Helmont*
Nancy Tomes   *A generous confidence*
Roger Cooter   *The cultural meaning of popular science*
Anne Digby   *Madness, morality and medicine*
Guenter B. Risse   *Hospital life in Enlightenment Scotland*
Roy Porter, ed.   *Patients and practitioners*
Ann G. Carmichael   *Plague and the poor in early Renaissance Florence*
S.E.D. Shortt   *Victorian lunacy*
Hilary Marland   *Medicine and society in Wakefield and Huddersfield, 1780–1870*
Susan Reverby   *Ordered to care*

Morbid Appearances

THE ANATOMY OF PATHOLOGY
IN THE EARLY NINETEENTH CENTURY

Russell C. Maulitz

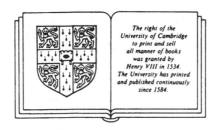

The right of the
University of Cambridge
to print and sell
all manner of books
was granted by
Henry VIII in 1534.
The University has printed
and published continuously
since 1584.

CAMBRIDGE UNIVERSITY PRESS

CAMBRIDGE

NEW YORK   NEW ROCHELLE   MELBOURNE   SYDNEY

PUBLISHED BY THE PRESS SYNDICATE OF THE UNIVERSITY OF CAMBRIDGE
The Pitt Building, Trumpington Street, Cambridge, United Kingdom

CAMBRIDGE UNIVERSITY PRESS
The Edinburgh Building, Cambridge CB2 2RU, UK
40 West 20th Street, New York NY 10011-4211, USA
477 Williamstown Road, Port Melbourne, VIC 3207, Australia
Ruiz de Alarcón 13, 28014 Madrid, Spain
Dock House, The Waterfront, Cape Town 8001, South Africa

http://www.cambridge.org

© Cambridge University Press 1987

This book is in copyright. Subject to statutory exception
and to the provisions of relevant collective licensing agreements,
no reproduction of any part may take place without
the written permission of Cambridge University Press.

First published 1987
First paperback edition 2002

A catalogue record for this book is available from the British Library

Library of Congress Cataloguing in Publication data
Maulitz, Russell Charles, 1944–
Morbid appearances.
(Cambridge history of medicine).
Includes index.
1. Anatomy, Pathological – France – History – 19th
century. 2. Anatomy, Pathological – Great Britain –
History – 19th century. I. Title. II. Series.
[DNLM: 1. Pathology – history – France. 2. Pathology –
history – Great Britain. QZ 11 GF7 M44m]
RB25.M36 1987 616.07'09034 86-34347

ISBN 0 521 32828 4 hardback
ISBN 0 521 52453 9 paperback

A portion of Chapter 6 is based on an article entitled "Channel crossing: the
lure of French pathology for English medical students, 1816–36," pp. 475–496
in Bulletin of the History of Medicine, vol 55 (1981)

Contents

To Joy Eva Fellheimer and Herbert Russell Maulitz

Preface

To begin, a word of explanation and several words of thanks.

I cannot remember reading a book with an exposition based on selection principles quite like those I ended up using in this work. While the central account of the monograph is of persons who will be well known in at least bare outline to most readers, I have moved off (especially in the second half of the monograph) into territory that is considerably more arcane. Why, after sketching the evolution of pathological anatomy in its fullest development in France, should one allow the story to veer off on paths that seem to fall short of the traditional "important" feat of progress?

The answer, as the reader might expect, lies in my reasons for writing the book in the first place. I have not intended to provide a symmetrical comparison of French and British pathology in the era before the microscope, but sought rather to look at the reception of a suite of medical ideas in one culture after examining how they unfolded in another. My intention was to study the development of pathological anatomy and, in particular, tissue pathology in France and then scrutinize various attempts to implant it in England.

Readers familiar with my work will know that I have studied German pathology in the nineteenth century, and that I am aware of the contributions of important figures from Johannes Meckel to Julius Cohnheim. Those developments, however, are not part of the story, for one very simple reason: the Anglo–French medical relationship was a special one. It was a connection not dissimilar, in intent if not in scale or precise content, to the links forged in the final quarter of the century between Germany and the United States, or between Germany and Japan.

It is *connections* (not merely analogy, contrast, and comparision); and *innovation* (not isolated individual creation), therefore, that most deserve close historical attention, even at the expense of certain omissions. I have said next to nothing, for example, about Meckel in Germany, about Richard Bright in England, or about François Broussais in France. I have chosen this tack in part for the intrinsic interest of the approach itself. I have done so as well because of the inherent interest of the figures and episodes that I do cover, and for what my account of them says about the forces that move medical ideas and techniques across national boundaries.

★　★　★　★　★

I see it now. Authors accumulate a considerable store of intellectual debt when they attempt to treat a historical subject systematically and at some length. I think they accumulate a lot more debts in developing a sustained work than in tripping about ten essays of one–tenth the length. In any event, that is what happened to me, and I therefore owe a debt of gratitude to a sizeable number of individuals in France, Britain, and the United States. Many of them I am unable to thank by name. I hope they will understand.

I first make mention of the public and private agencies who, through the provision of research leave and summer support, made the investigation possible. Between 1972 and 1982 I was the recipient of grants from the Josiah Macy, Jr., Foundation; the National Institutes of Health; the Wellcome Trust; the Faculty Research Fund of the University of Pennsylvania; and the American Philosophical Society. The support of each proved invaluable and I gratefully acknowledge it here.

I also acknowledge the help I received from the staffs of the libraries and archives of the following institutions: in France, the Medical Faculties of Paris and Nantes; the Archives Nationales and Assistance Publique in Paris; the Collège de France and the Paris Academy of Medicine. In Britain I was graciously assisted by the librarians at the Royal Colleges of Physicians and Surgeons of both London and Edinburgh, as well as the University of Edinburgh, the University of London (University College), and Guys Hospital Medical School. In London, year in and year out, I received unflagging attention and support, most particularly, from the Wellcome Institute for the History of Medicine. I would be remiss if I were to fail to single out William Bynum and Christopher Lawrence in the academic unit, and Robin Price and Eric Freeman in the library, for special thanks.

In the United States I thank the librarians at the National Library of Medicine; early on, the Duke University Medical Center (especially G. S. T. and Susan Cavanagh); and most recently the College of Physicians of Philadelphia; all provided tireless aid. The former Curator of Historical Collections, Christine Ruggere, at the last named institution, was the source of sustained wisdom and assistance over several years.

A number of people provided intellectual support. At Duke, Gert Brieger, with insuperable patience, oversaw the writing of a dissertation that was the distant ancestor of the present work. Seymour Mauskopf read that version as well and watched it evolve in the dozen years since. The late Joseph Schiller discovered me muttering and thrashing in the belly of the Paris Faculty one day in 1972, and gradually thereafter assumed the important role of a continent-side mentor. He is missed. In Boston, Edward and Amalie Kass aided in my understanding of Thomas Hodgkin. At a crucial moment, George Weisz of Montreal directed my attention to an all-important, newly opened archive in Paris. Also in Paris, Mirko D. Grmek was of great and gracious assistance. And in Philadelphia, critically, Rosemary Stevens, Charles Rosenberg, and Steven Peitzman all read and materially helped improve the manuscript. So, too, did an anonymous reader for Cambridge University Press.

Finally I acknowledge the assistance and support of those who furnished that other key ingredient, survivability. In bits and pieces, Sandra Paschale typed all of the manuscript at least once over the years. Dr. Bonnie Blustein supplied invaluable research assistance on Chapter 8. Donna Evleth provided imaginative research assistance in the preparation of virtually all those parts of Parts I and II requiring what the French call *dépouillement*. And finally, Kristine Billmyer patiently awaited the end. To all of them, my heartfelt gratitude.

Introduction: *Ouverture:* Bichat's head

The Père Lachaise cemetery in Paris is known to much of the world as one of the most remarkable monumental legacies of Napoleonic France. Opened in 1804, it is a grand baroque gesture made solid in granite and marble. Its monuments, massed and massive, embody the homage of an entire society to its famous and notorious. Nearly overgrown in a corner of the cemetery rests an unprepossessing stub of a monolith bearing the name "Bichat." Only the most deliberate of wanderers in Père Lachaise would remark it.

Today medical historians revere the name of Marie-François-Xavier Bichat (1771–1802) as a founder of French scientific medicine. He is seen as a pioneer in the study of tissues and the father of dual medical traditions that came to include such luminaries as François Magendie and Claude Bernard in physiology and Théophile Laennec and Thomas Hodgkin in pathology. Thus it seems only natural that Bichat should be immortalized in the stone of Père Lachaise. But it was not always so. An odd tale looms behind the arrival of Bichat's remains, some forty years after his death, in this final place of rest.

By 1802, at the age of thirty, when today's physicians are often still in training, Bichat was already a respected, if not very elevated, member of the Parisian medical community. He died on July 22 of that year. The same day, following custom, one of his prize students, Philibert-Joseph Roux (1780–1854) dissected his preceptor's body. He noted certain pathological changes including some abnormalities of dentition and an occipital skull fracture, the latter perhaps related to the tuberculous meningitis to which he is thought to have succumbed. Bichat's remains were then laid to rest in the Cemetery of Saint-Catherine.

Forty years later the Saint-Catherine cemetery had become overcrowded and decayed, a hazard to the public health. In 1845, authorities closed it and announced that it would soon be abandoned. As it happened, in November of that year thousands of physicians from across France convened in Paris to attend a national medical congress. The congress officers designated a special commission to arrange the transfer of Bichat's remains to a permanent grave in Père Lachaise. To the medical community this seemed altogether fitting: The cemetery was rapidly becoming a pantheon for French cultural heroes, from Abélard and Héloise to Molière. Just two years earlier, in 1843, Samuel Hahnemann had been buried here. Like the others, Bichat, too, was now hero and exemplar. His body could hardly be consigned to the anonymity of some near-forgotten ossuary. By 1845 Bichat had finally come to belong in the company of the demigods of Père Lachaise. In his own time Paris had been the foremost medical center of Europe, although it was now rapidly yielding its preeminence to the German states. Bichat had become part of the official iconology of French medicine just as its reputation faded to, at best, parity with other nations' medical cultures.

Thus it was that over two dozen family and friends convened in the early morning of November 16, 1845. The grave was found, badly decayed, next to the east wall of the Saint-Catherine cemetery. Among the assembled there was a small clutch of medical men, panjandrums of the Paris hospital scene, men like Bichat's student, Philibert-Joseph Roux, and the surgeon Joseph Malgaigne (1806–1865), who, though he had never known Bichat, was devoted to the hagiography of the Paris hospital.

The exhumation began. When the diggers reached a point five or six feet down, they hit a skeleton. When they finished unearthing it, the congregants were puzzled. The remains, otherwise well-preserved, lacked a head. Considerable further digging revealed no cranium. Only after some delay did Roux step forward with an explanation. Several years after his young master's death, in circumstances that he apparently never divulged, Bichat's head had come into his possession. Roux now produced a skull, demonstrating from the original autopsy findings that it was indeed Bichat's. He ceremoniously rejoined it to the skeleton. Eulogies were offered. A laurel wreath was laid beside the skeleton and the newly rejoined skull was adorned with a "crown of immortality."

* * * * *

My account of the growth of anatomical pathology begins with Bichat's career. But the tale need not begin there. The history of pathology in the century before him teems with major figures in the field of morbid anatomy, men like John Hunter (1728–1793) and Giovanni Battista Morgagni (1682–1771). In this discussion, however, I am by choice and convention using the phrase "pathological anatomy" to mean something more specific. By that phrase I wish to denote an approach to the theory and practice of pathology that, while not yet resorting to the microscope, relied nonetheless on emerging notions of histopathology. This approach, also known sometimes as tissue pathology, was first clearly systematized by Xavier Bichat.

Histopathology was characterized, in essence, by two key features. First, there was the recognition that a systemic, or medical theory of pathology could be elaborated around solid, rather than humoral, components of the body. Those components were variously designated by writers as the membranes, tissues, or serosal tunics of organs in the major body cavities. The tissues were recognized to react, for example, by inflammation and hydropsy (an outpouring of transudative fluid), according to stereotyped patterns independent of the location or the noxious stimulus initiating the reaction. This might be termed the general theory of histopathology. A second key component was the elaboration of a "special" histopathology that applied the general theory and underscored its utility: the description, for example, of the peritonitis accompanying puerperal fever.

But even in the context of this narrower construction of pathological anatomy, the story does not begin with Bichat, from the standpoint of intellectual history. He was not the first to expound either of these defining characteristics of histopathology. The genealogy of ideas about tissue pathology is confined neither to the early nineteenth century nor to Bichat, nor even to the French milieu. It is ironic, given the order of events as I present them below, that British authors contributed most significantly to the "prehistory" of histopathology. Between 1760 and 1790, men like James Carmichael Smyth, William Cullen, John Hunter and Edward Johnstone, some of them now wholly forgotten, others well remembered but for matters quite other than histopathology, contributed some of the earliest insights into the pathology of the tissues and membranes.[1]

But I am not so much concerned here with the genealogy of ideas. Rather I want to unravel the story of a tradition. The emergence of medical traditions depends upon a great deal more than the enunciation of key ideas. It depends upon even more than the sharing of those ideas among members of an elite, educated community given to reading memoirs of their peers. So defined, the medical community on both sides of the English Channel at the end of the eighteenth century was a well-knit one. Philippe Pinel (1745–1826) knew of Smyth's work and stimulated Bichat's; Laennec followed in Bichat's footsteps but knew of Johnstone's work; and so on.

Acknowledging antecedents and tracing intellectual lineages were and remain common habits of scientifically disposed physicians, not to mention historians of medicine. But minds thus drawn together do not in themselves form a tradition. Something very different, something in the nature of a conjunction of institutions, professional groups, and ideas is needed to effect such a change. This sort of juncture appeared in France at the end of the eighteenth century. After 1794, when medicine and surgery were fused by fiat of the Revolution, Bichat brought together their two pathologies, and called the resulting intellectual hybrid pathological anatomy. For the first time in modern Europe, there was a context, a set of structures and arrangements centered on the existence of a newly ecumenical faculty, within which a new theoretical canon could flourish. Under such circumstances, pathological anatomy could expand beyond a small elite and become a project, an enterprise with real practical and professional implications.

Two basic conditions made this possible. One was the creation of an institutional context for the reinforcement and dissemination of theoretical notions about tissue pathology. The second condition was a technical corollary of the first: theoretical notions were as nothing without the milieux within which they might be put into practice. In Paris, beginning with Bichat's teachers, pathological anatomy became a matter of workaday routine. For surgeon and physician alike, the everyday possibility of conducting large numbers of postmortem dissections was every bit as important in entrenching Bichatian pathology as was the "fit" between that pathology and the structure of the newly conjoined medical – surgical faculty. In the nineteenth century English-speaking students as well as Frenchmen began coming to Paris seeking this experience. It was an experience accessible in Paris on a scale without parallel elsewhere. For such reasons, the ideas that I describe in this book tended to flow westward, across the English Channel and at times even across the Atlantic.

⋆   ⋆   ⋆   ⋆   ⋆

Bichat's remains were transferred to a hearse and a cortege was formed. Some four thousand French physicians joined in the journey toward its next stop, the grand court on the Ile de la Cité. On one side stood the mammoth hospital, the Hôtel-Dieu, where Bichat had toiled fifty years before. On the other side stood the mother of cathedrals, Notre Dame de Paris. Here the cortege stopped for a service. The cathedral was full to overflowing. A two-hour procession followed, more festive than funereal, aiming for the eastern borders of the city and the new gravesite in Père Lachaise. Accompanied by an endless succession of *discours,* Bichat's remains were buried again.

Six years later, in 1851, a statue of Bichat, fashioned by David d'Angers, was erected in the central courtyard of the Paris Faculty. This too seemed altogether appropriate. Nearly half a century after his death, Bichat epitomized the Faculty's image of itself.[2]

During the young pathological anatomist's lifetime it had been otherwise. The documentary record makes it clear that on at least two occasions Bichat attempted in vain to join the Paris faculty. Though already a prestigious member of the community that Erwin Ackerknecht and others dub the Paris Hospital, Bichat evinced great interest but little success in gaining entrance to the innermost circle of state-supported teaching physicians.

It seems, then, that Bichat's fortunes shifted in intriguing ways, moving from the (at best) ambiguous success that he met officially in his own lifetime, to the talismanic role his figure had come to play four decades later. What was the source and the motive force of this shift in Bichat's official standing in the medical Pantheon? The evidence permits few ironclad conclusions. But some inferences are possible. First, the Paris medical faculty was indeed in some significant sense a central institution, perhaps even uniquely so, in spreading new medical knowledge to the borders of France and beyond. Bichat's failure to gain a foothold in that institution thus takes on added importance, for it sheds light on the distinction between those, like Bichat, who created medical traditions, and those, like the mandarins of the Paris faculty, who exploited and disseminated them.

Second, if Bichat's reputation had by 1845 become so mystified and mythicized that he was now ritually embraced by the Paris medical faculty, perhaps this curious turn of events can be put to historical use. In early nineteenth-century French medicine there were particular reasons for such an amplification of images and reputations. In this shift one may look for insight about the elaboration and embellishment of medical traditions like pathological anatomy.

My discussion resembles a diptych. In the four chapters of Part I that follow, I concern myself with the elaboration of Bichat's, and others', systems of morbid anatomy. In Part II I comment on the "hinge," the perception shared by at least some medical men across the English Channel that the new French tradition was attractive and worthy of adoption. Finally, in Part III, I examine the other panel of my diptych, the fate of that perception. To what extent was the Bichatian tradition successfully imported in Britain? Mutation, implantation, and adaptation are among the fates new ideas may encounter on foreign shores. I will discuss the destiny of pathological anatomy as its British proponents, and some of its detractors, tried to assign it a role in their own medical culture.

PART I

Paris

1

Genesis of a tradition

I believe only in French culture, and regard everything else in
Europe which calls itself "culture" as a misunderstanding. I do
not even take the German kind into consideration.
– Friedrich Nietzsche, *Ecce Homo* (1888)

Was the veneration of Bichat a matter of mere expediency, oc-
casioned by the need to move a few bones? How did this young
outsider's career come to assume, after his premature death, an
almost totemic value?[1] Much of the answer lies in the structure of
the French medical community in the postrevolutionary period.
In life, as we have seen on the one hand, Bichat was never a central
figure in that community. But he fashioned a career, on the other
hand, that embodied key features of an emerging professional culture. For decades to come, the image his life and work conjured
up was a tightly woven tapestry of the medical and surgical concerns knit together by the revolution. Bichat's memory bound
them together still further. The full extent of how it did so is the
central concern of this chapter and Chapters 2 through 4.

MEDICAL COMMUNITIES: THE PROFESSIONAL STAGE

Xavier Bichat arrived in Paris at an explosive time in the history
of French institutions. He came to the capital city on June 30, 1794.
Some five years had passed since the paroxysm of energy unleashed
in 1789 and now already partly spent. Only days remained before
the fall of Robespierre amidst the Thermidorean reaction. Thus
Bichat's arrival coincided with the waning of that first burst of
revolutionary fervor. Paris institutions were, at worst, immobilized
in a state of disarray. At best they were in a state of flux that

caused each to be pulled in several directions at once by the competing demands of other factions and interests.

Only nine months earlier, the National Convention had suppressed all of the nation's faculties and corporations as part of its systematic plan to abolish all bastions of privilege. The medical faculties, including that ancient and staid Parisian body on the Seine's left bank, were dissolved at a critical moment for military manpower. Experience on the battlefield was beginning to make clear the imminent need for the assured continuity, if not an absolute increase, in health care personnel.[2] The air of tumult and crisis that in varying degrees had pervaded the nation for five years thus had its medical dimension.

In the upheaval leading up to Thermidor, the tumult had been real enough. In people's minds the crisis of national life, however concrete, was also a perceived impetus for social change, as they viewed a rapidly changing society and shared the sense that it faced a multitude of needs. Health care for all was just one of those perceived needs, borne out of crisis.[3] The sense of crisis, and thus of opportunity, was most acute at precisely the time when many of the old means for meeting the needs of French society had been lost through the abolition of privilege.

This was the setting that Xavier Bichat confronted in mid-1794. Where the Revolution had pulled down the bastions of the old regime, new ones were to be erected in their place. The second half of 1794, as Bichat launched his own career, was a remarkably fecund period of renewal and reconstruction. Postthermidorean Paris was a seedbed of ideas and practical efforts directed toward the rational reconstitution of the national life along revolutionary democratic lines. Anything seemed possible. A significant amount of this energy focused on the issue of an appropriate design for reforming medical education. That reform stood squarely at the intersection of two other, broader lines of reform: one envisioned for medical care, and the other contemplated for higher education.[4]

Three men – Antoine Fourcroy (1775–1809), François Chaussier (1746–1828), and Michel Thouret (1748–1810) – physicians all, provided the central vision behind the new form of medical education set in place in December, 1794. According to their plan, as it was outlined in the celebrated law of 14 *Frimaire an III* (December 4, 1794), three new schools (not faculties) of health (not medicine) were to be created in Paris, Strasbourg, and Montpellier.

The plan reflected the character of French institutions and aspirations in the mid-1790s: centralization of control but nationalization of opportunity (e.g., for student posts, carefully parceled out to slight no *département*); social and economic democratization of student entry and faculty mobility (faculty posts were now to be selected by public *concours*); and a reallocation and rationalization of power, expertise, and elite status in the health professions.[5]

This last impulse toward rationalization accounts in part for the unification of medicine and surgery. It was the one reform that Napoleon and the bureaucracy he invented would never need to dismantle. That medicine and surgery were now perforce taught under one roof was probably the single most important measure taken by the leaders of turn-of-the-century Paris medicine. Other measures, including the newly increased emphasis on pathological anatomy, were important corollaries of this overarching impulse toward rationalization and unification.

But medicine and surgery could no more achieve complete and absolute fusion in the late eighteenth century than they could in the late twentieth. The impulse toward merger was just that: an impulsion, a salient, a direction toward which the two separate professional groups could point themselves, recognizing that their respective areas of expertise overlapped.

Bichat arrived at just that historical moment when the need arose for cognitive guideposts to show how such a symbiosis could work intellectually *for the practitioner*. By elaborating a system of pathological anatomy that was a roadmap of the human body decipherable by surgeon and physician alike, Bichat responded to this need. He did so by developing a pathology of tissues. It revolutionized medical thought and shored up the at first tenuous alliance between the two great branches of the profession.[6]

RESOURCES: THE INTELLECTUAL STAGE

Most historians now agree that the effect of the French Revolution on the medical world was in large measure a permissive rather than a creative one. The events of 1789 had uncorked impulses and ideas about professional reform that had been fermenting for half a century and more.[7] A wide range of concepts of body function and dysfunction, most already espoused by various eighteenth-century practitioners, found new champions.[8] When Xavier

Bichat arrived five years later, no single member of this bewildering array of systems was yet clearly dominant. In order to understand precisely how Bichat's histopathological system served to bind together different parts of this received wisdom, however, it will be necessary first to separate them and provide a brief sketch of each.[9]

The surgical mentality

Perhaps because it was more "academic" – that is to say, its members had more incentive to wax literary and to speculate on such matters as the nature of life and disease – the medical community evinced a far greater diversity of tradition in nosology and pathology than did the surgeons. The surgical viewpoint, though hardly monolithic, mainly revolved around a localistic notion of disease.[10] This seems natural enough when one considers the texture of eighteenth-century surgical practice. Though still far from ready to invade the major body cavities with scalpel and bistoury, surgeons shared an outlook on the body that was in many ways strikingly similar to that of their twentieth-century successors. Their nosology and their diagnosis were, in essence, anatomical. To locate the lesion was to be enabled to name it and, with luck, to treat it.

Questions of possibilities for therapeutic intervention in specific surgical problems gained perhaps even greater importance in attracting surgeons to hew to the localistic tradition. Within such a tradition the natural approach to surgical disorders – the abscessed tissue, the gangrenous limb, even the fistula – was either evacuative or extirpative. Find the lesion, then drain it, or cut it out. Healing could then proceed. Such a procedure was unambiguously localistic in approach. But even in more ambiguous circumstances, such as those presented by *erysipèle* – the commonly occurring inflammatory disorder, erysipelas – where systemic and local manifestations were not so obviously distinguishable, the surgeon was naturally drawn to seek the specific lesion.[11] Thus a leading surgical practitioner, Pierre Desault (1738–1795), could describe erysipelas as a disorder that, while not as well circumscribed as a foreign body, abscess, or cyst, was nonetheless best understood as a localized tumorous phenomenon.[12]

The medical mentality: Hippocratism

Medical men, by contrast, espoused a wide range of doctrines of health and illness. Some of those doctrines, such as those identified primarily with the old Faculty of Medicine in Montpellier, overlapped considerably. Thus the belief systems that have come to be labeled "vitalism" and "Hippocratism" had much in common, not only at the intellectual level, but also at the level of individual actors: Those who styled themselves as Hippocratics were more often than not proponents of the vitalistic synthesis.

Hippocratism entailed the whole range of implied notions and beliefs about the human body and its ills inherited from the ancients. Though no more (and possibly less) observational than its surgical analogue, the Hippocratic medical viewpoint was more natural-historical. That is to say, the physician inclined toward Hippocratic doctrine, placing considerable emphasis on the precise description of disease progression. Another overarching emphasis was that which, for lack of a better word, might be termed "holistic." A holistic approach had two prongs. Its advocates emphasized the discovery of constitutional signs and symptoms – the sort of generalized manifestations of disease that might be susceptible to therapeutic "action at a distance." Constitutionally-minded practitioners of "physic," that is the traditional physicians, tended to conceive of disease states, even local diseases, as distributed within the frame of the patient. In such a way pathological changes were conceived to be amenable to treatment by cures and potions that, like Galenic remedies, were themselves dispersed throughout the body by the bloodstream.

A holistic physiology exhibited the additional characteristic of deemphasizing the distinction between health and disease. Even if the two- or three-dimensional margins of the lesion were physically distinct, the cognitive margins were indistinct: The normal and the pathological blurred into one another. Humoral balance and imbalance depended on normal or aberrant states of the body fluids. But in most formulations, such alterations were more a matter of changes in degree than they were of changes in kind.[13]

Hippocratism meant something else as well, something closely linked to the observational and natural historical approach that had, since the classical age, periodically characterized clinical thinking. In addition to providing a body of methods and concepts, Hippocratic doctrine by the late eighteenth century had also become an ideological option. It was an option filled with contradictions, a two-edged sword with respect to medical orthodoxy. On the one hand, Hippocratic belief opposed observationalism to dogmatism and allowed its proponents to profess their aversion to hollow theorizing. On the other hand, those proponents were defeatist with respect to their ability to divine the ultimate causes of disease, and were indifferent when not overtly hostile in their view toward new conceptual tools such as microscopy, animal experimentation, or chemical analysis.

When threatened by those new forms of science, the most conservative elements in the medical community could soon be counted upon to invoke the shade of Hippocrates in order to shore up their own posture as archclinicians. Indeed, a group of those who opposed many of the reforms and new emphases embedded in the Paris scheme of medical education after 1794 coalesced around a symbolic rallying point, the erstwhile chair of Hippocratic Medicine in the Paris Faculty, appealing for its restitution.[14] It is clear that by the first decade of the new century, those styling themselves "Hippocratic" could range from a Théophile Laennec (1775–1826), who esteemed pathological anatomy but held fast to the natural historical clinical ideal, to a F.-C.-F. De Mercy (1775–1849), who eschewed the new science and sought with great vigor, if no great success, to reinstitute Hippocratic empirical doctrine as a formal course in the Paris curriculum.[15]

Vitalism

Through its link with the Montpellier nexus, the doctrine known as vitalism was often closely identified with Hippocratic traditionalism. This fusing of interests was only partly correct. By 1800 to be identified as a "vitalist" no longer specified the sort of Catholic traditionalism that permeated Montpellier during the eighteenth century, often under the banner of Hippocratism. The latter tradition had been characterized in its view of life by a sort of spiritualism, quick to repudiate the materialism perceived in Parisian efforts to extend the laws of inanimate nature to the living world. It is of less concern here to enter into the debates of the eighteenth and early nineteenth centuries on the question of whose vitalism was purest – certainly Bichat's was perceived by some not to be – than to find the participants' common denominator. What the vitalists of the eighteenth century had in common was their belief in a vital force or elan, distinctly separating living from inert matter and requiring that the physician apply different principles for studying each one.

Of the Montpellier vitalists, the clearest influence on Bichat was probably Théophile de Bordeu (1722–1776), whose widely disseminated writings on the vitalistic interpretation of life fell early into Bichat's hands. Claiming to infer the vital properties of living organisms through close observation of phenomena, and abjuring experimentation, Bordeu and his Montpellier colleagues received considerable exposure in forums ranging from the salons of Paris to Diderot's *Encyclopedia*. I will return to Bordeu's influence on Bichat's development as a physician, analogous to Desault's influence on the latter's surgical development. Recent scholarship has amply demonstrated this with respect to Bichat's approach to the study of living phenomena, that is to say, his physiology: While he was certainly a vitalist, Bichat was with equal certainty no anti-experimentalist. A long internalist tradition in the history of physiology has, indeed, obscured the subtleties of his real relationship with those, like François Magendie and Claude Bernard, who followed in the developmental sequence by which physiology ultimately became an experimental discipline. Since I am more interested here in another sequence in which Bichat's work was also a point of origin, namely the evolution of histopathology, I will rather quickly pass beyond the notion of vital forces, returning to it only tangentially in considering the pivotal ideas of sensibility and irritability.[16]

Bordeu

Undoubtedly Bichat's most influential nonsurgical predecessor was the Montpellier controversialist and physiological vitalist, Théophile de Bordeu. Bordeu's centrality in establishing the link between Bichat and a *medical* tradition stems from his own professional and intellectual location.[17] He was both a Hippocratist and a vitalist. He taught at Montpellier when Bichat's father was a medical student. Like Bichat he was the son of a physician. He was also the scion of one of the great dynasties, concentrated in the Pyrenees, of medical balneologists – advocates of the ultimate constitutional treatment, "taking the waters" to restore humoral imbalances and hence the ideal state of health.[18]

It is not possible to disentangle Bordeu's pathophysiology of the *tissus muqueux,* the precursor of Bichat's mucous and cellular or connective tissue membranes, from his hydrotherapeutics.[19] For Bordeu, the *tissu cellulaire* was the organizing principle that drew together and organized the body's disparate parts. Pleura, peritoneum, and other investing coats were all "portions of the *tissu cellulaire*," though they were neither distinguished from the underlying organ structures nor from one another. What was important to the Montpellier vitalist, however, was not anatomical verisimilitude, but rather the functional significance of the *tissu cellulaire* as an "atmosphere" through which the fluids of the organism could course. Thus it created a sympathetic bodily *département*:

The *département* of an organ is nothing other than its cellular atmosphere, if one may thus speak; or . . . that portion of the *tissu cellulaire* which is related to its action: such that when this part changes its position or its constitution, the entirety of the *tissu cellulaire* of that [part's] *département* also undergoes that particular modification.

Inflammation and suppuration were, in Bordeu's view, derangements of the solid – fluid balance in these sympathetic *départements* of the body, closely allied with the edema and swelling, the *tumor* or tumefaction of the ancients, that represented a "distension of the *tissu cellulaire*." Through a process of "sideration" the organs would, once inflamed, become engorged and invaded by a mucous substance of varying degrees of fluidity.[20]

Bordeu's system was thus one that dealt with "tissues" but, lacking anatomical specificity, emphasized instead the manner in which surfaces and departments of the organism were interconnected and acted upon one another. For this reason some have been tempted to locate Bordeu not only as a precursor of Bichat, which one infers from his frequent manuscript notes to himself ("refute here the account [*l'histoire*] provided by Bordeu"), but also as an antecedent of the modern endocrinologist.[21] But Bordeu's notion of the sympathies between *départements,* mediated by the *organe cellulaire,* is more appropriately located in the context of Bordeu's commitment to both the Montpellier Hippocratism of his colleagues and the balneology that was his family's livelihood – a doctrine of sympathies, a holistic system, resonated with the physician's belief in the unlocalized healing power of appropriate environment, of "airs, waters, and places." Indeed, appended to his 1787 work on pathophysiology and published between the same covers was a promotional essay on the salutary effects of the waters of Barèges.[22]

Idéologie

Traditional historiography locates Bichat's important eighteenth-century antecedents not only in the physiological ontology of Montpellier, but also in a form of biological and psychological epistemology most readily found in the *salons* of a more worldly and latitudinarian Paris. The *salon* was a heady place to be in the waning days of the *ancien régime*. Many salon habitués, men like Pierre Cabanis (1757–1808) and the Abbé de Condillac (1715–1780), espoused the phenomenalist and sensualist Enlightenment philosophy familiarly known as *idéologie*. The ideologues' notion of medical knowledge was for the most part compatible with both the surgeons' anatomical approach and the physicians' clinical ideals of natural historical observation and Hippocratic description-as-explanation. It was predicated upon the Enlightenment notion that natural knowledge – in this case knowledge about nosology and nosography, or knowledge about anatomy – could be obtained through the straightforward mental processing and classification of directly observed phenomena.[23]

Brunonianism

As the eighteenth century waned, an increasing number of medical systems, that is, ways of understanding the body in its functional and dysfunctional states, began to veer away from the purely humoral approach that for centuries had been the hallmark of the Galenic model. One such system was elaborated by John Brown (1735–1788) in Edinburgh. Abandoning the notion of health as a state of *crasis,* or balance of humors, Brown posited instead the states of "sthenia" (or "hypersthenia") and "asthenia," representing the antipodes of a scale of muscular and nervous excitability, and placing greater emphasis on the relative condition of solid parts of the body. An excess of nervous excitement (hypersthenia) thus required calmative medicines. Conversely, an asthenic state would require stimulants in order to restore the appropriate measure of force.[24]

Almost intuitively one can grasp the attractiveness, both philosophical and practical, of the Brunonian system. That it had wide appeal in France is not surprising: it smacked of modernity and a willingness to depart from Galenic dogma while remaining for the physician an essentially global, as opposed to local, approach to pathophysiology.[25] Brown's synthesis retained the notion of physiological checks and balances, which is to say the principle of restitution of appropriately middling levels of the several qualities, while departing from the fluidist doctrine of the ancients. Physicians on both sides of the English Channel could find such a system enticing.

Solidism and pathological anatomy

A long step away from the global approach of the Galenic model of the body, and toward a truly localizationist view of its ills, was taken by a series of pathological anatomists of the eighteenth century. Led by the Italian, Giovanni Battista Morgagni (1682–1771), Bichat's predecessors were concerned, as Morgagni's *Seats and Causes of Disease* (1761) suggested in its title, to find not only the antecedents but the actual anatomical seats, or locations, of disease. To localize disease in this way implied, in fact, an essentially surgical impulse to situate morbid appearances in the palpable, solid parts of the body. This was the simplest way of quite literally putting one's finger on that abstraction, "disease," at the postmortem table. It posed problems, however, in many affections such as phlebitis or septicemia where both systemic – that is, potentially humorally mediated – and local phenomena were observed in the patient. It is partly for this reason that there were probably few, if any, unalloyed localists during this period; rather, localization remained a goal, an additional value that came to be superadded to others medical men still harbored.

Thus it was possible to have an honest debate on the question of which structural elements of the body, its fluid *versus* its solid components, mainly determined the functional dimension of disease. By and large, to reiterate, surgeons, who could be expected to treat locally, took the localizationist viewpoint, while physicians, who would treat globally, took the opposite tack.[26] There were exceptions to this dictum in the eighteenth century among physicians; there were those, like Morgagni, who were especially disposed toward performing postmortem dissection. In the nineteenth century, their heirs were men who were trained in both medicine and surgery. Among the earliest exemplars of this last group, and the archetype for the breed, was Xavier Bichat.[27]

THE EPIDEMIOLOGIC STAGE: DISEASES AND DIAGNOSES

I ask the reader next to indulge me in a brief excursus on the relation between changing patterns of disease and the diagnostic categories that men form to accommodate them. Even in the best of circumstances, such as those in which twentieth-century morbidity and mortality records are available, it is difficult to infer the relationships between changing patterns of disease and the social or institutional structures devised to contend with them.[28] Few historians have circumvented the pitfalls of this sort of approach. The historiographic issue is an important one for the study of French medicine in the first quarter of the nineteenth century: when Marc-Antoine Petit and Etienne R. A. Serres published their *Traité de la fièvre entéromésentérique* in 1813, for example, hospital populations were much more likely to be segregated according to diagnostic categories, both physically and epidemiologically, than they had been just a decade and a half earlier.[29]

If one wishes to delineate the even more complex interrelationships between biological, social, and cognitive substrates – that is, between diseases, pathologies, and professions – then one proceeds doubly at one's own peril. Another element, that of intellectual or epistemic structures, human inventions, must be added. Such structures consist of those descriptions and conceptions of disease, such as "fever," that may mediate between the "reality" of disease and the institutional response to that "reality." The modern historian, medically expert or not, finds it difficult to "get behind" nosologies prevalent before, roughly, the final quarter of the nineteenth century. There is always the possibility of a masking phenomenon: While shifting disease patterns and shifting nosological categories no doubt bore some definite relationship to one another, it is notoriously difficult to separate out and sort one from the other in examining their impact on society, or *vice versa*.

Though the foregoing may seem excessively abstract, it bears directly on an important point about the milieu in which Xavier

Bichat found himself in the 1790s. Ideally one should like to specify the mechanisms by which disease patterns generated nosological categories and then in turn an institutional response. One should like to appraise Bichat's pathology of tissues, in particular, in terms of the disease that he or anyone else might have been able to see laid out on the postmortem table. This is possible only to a limited extent. What follows, therefore, is intended to be no more than an impressionistic view of the epidemiologic stage, based on autopsy records and hospital admission registers.[30]

A measure of the character and specificity of the diagnostic categories confronted by Bichat and his medical mentor, Philippe Pinel (1745–1826), whose own classificationist impulse yielded his magisterial *Nosographie Philosophique* of 1798, may be gleaned, for example, from a survey of the admission registers of the hospitals in which they worked. The archive of the *Assistance Publique,* the social welfare arm of the government under whose aegis the major hospitals came after 1849, preserves many of these records. It is instructive, for example, to look at the cases admitted to the hospital that Bichat (thanks to Desault) knew best, the Hôtel-Dieu itself, in the late spring and summer of 1802, a fairly representative period. From 24 *Germinal* to 25 *Fructidor* in revolutionary year X (Wednesday 14 April to Sunday 25 August) 100 patients were admitted. Bichat himself contracted a febrile and rapidly fatal illness during this time, dying on 22 July.

Tabulating the Hôtel-Dieu cases arrestingly demonstrates the dominance of the simple eighteenth-century diagnosis of "fever."[31] Of the 100 cases, 55 were admitted with this diagnosis alone. Another single case had fever and "internal cachexia." Three other categories contained four or more cases: "external" [*externe*] cases, almost assuredly the sort of surgical cases that represented Desault's stock-in-trade, numbering fifteen, and four cases each of wound trauma and "fluxion of the chest." The latter category probably represented a small series of cases of pleural effusion, gauged either by symptomatology or by physical signs elicited by maneuvers such as succussion and immediate (direct) auscultation. Such a finding in the chest, along with its peritoneal counterpart in the abdominal cavity, must have been particularly suggestive to Bichat when he set out to devise his own histopathological system.[32]

While inflammatory affections of one of the serous membranes lining the major body cavities, in this case the pleura that surrounds and protects the contents of the thorax, can be implicated directly in only four of the 100 cases surveyed, the great bulk of cases, well over half, were characterized simply as fever. That fever, now recognized as both a symptom and a pathophysiological final common pathway, should have appeared so frequently as a diagnosis at the turn of the nineteenth century will surprise no one familiar with nosology before Pinel and Bichat. For Paris medicine *circa* 1800, "fever" was a respectable diagnostic entity. The historical epidemiologist might now wish to break it down further. Did "fever" reflect a predominance of cases of septicemia, i.e., of widely disseminated infection from a multiplicity of pathogens? Or was there, rather, a predominance of the serositides – pleuritis, pericarditis, and peritonitis – by which medical men were becoming increasingly intrigued? Or, indeed, was there a mixture of the two on a spectrum whereon localized affections led to generalized fever, debility, and death?[33]

This last suggestion seems a reasonable and tempting hypothesis. To attempt to document it quantitatively would risk pseudoprecision, however, precisely for the reasons discussed already with respect to nosological "masking." The greater specificity of postmortem examinations performed in the same period, on the other hand, is illuminating. These *ouvertures de cadavres* clearly suggest that localized inflammatory disease, especially of the membranous structures, gave rise to global complaints such as "fever." Most instructive in examining this hypothesis are the autopsy reports actually compiled on Bichat's own service at the Hôtel-Dieu. At the turn of the nineteenth century he was at the threshold between the old nosology and the new, tissue-oriented pathological anatomy.[34]

The form in which these autopsy reports were recorded is itself significant. They followed a rigid and revealing protocol. Most in this series were written in the hands of Bichat or of his students, notably his cousin and protégé, Regis Buisson (1777–1804). They were prepared in large folio leaves of manuscript (Fig. 1.1) marked off in six or seven vertical columns. One column was reserved for general observations, the remainder distributed among the broadly conceived systems of the body. This was not the regional anatomy of the unfinished *Anatomie descriptive* but the systemic or "general" anatomy of the magisterial *Anatomie générale* of 1801.[35]

The bodily "systems," sometimes denoted "organs," to which

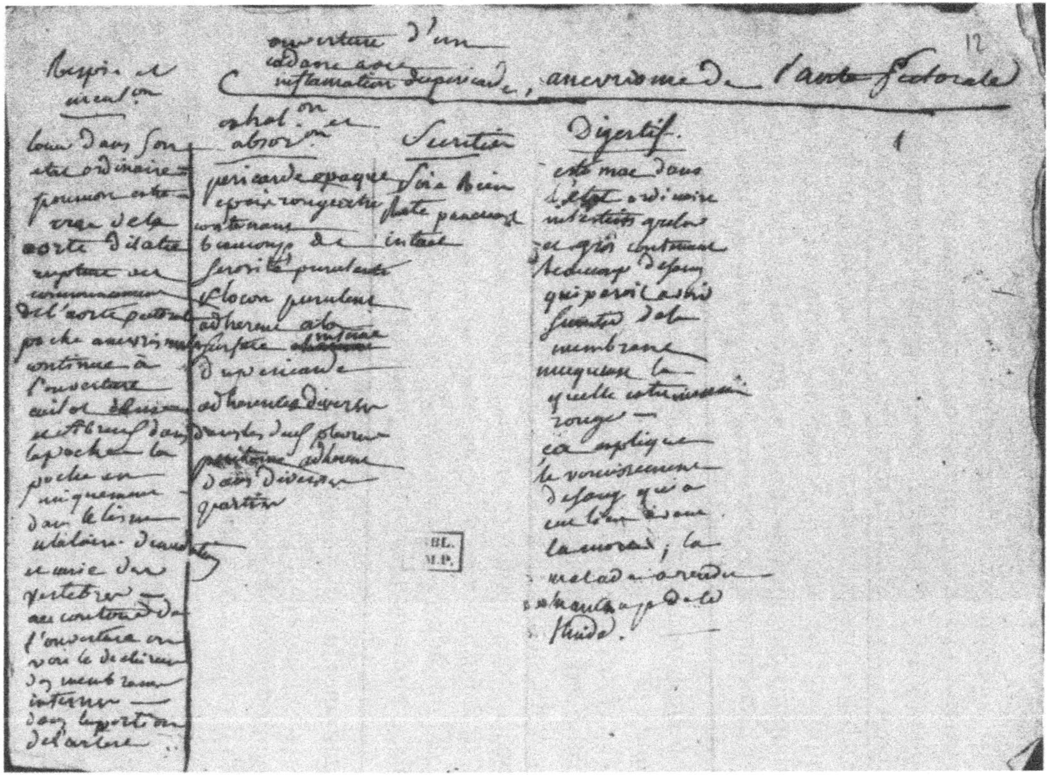

Figure 1.1. Specimen folio leaves in autopsy format of Bichat and Buisson. Note the emphasis on the "exhalant-absorbent" system linking serous membranes surrounding major viscera. In the figure to the right, the operator describes opacified pericardium, pus-filled serous fluid (sérosité) containing purulent flecks, possibly tubercle. In the above figure note description of "false membrane" (compare Fig. 3.2), and of inflammation. See Appendix on p. 230.

Bichat and company addressed themselves in seeking the morbid appearances of disease in its final stage were the circulatory and respiratory, the digestive, nervous, genital (omitted on occasion), secretory, and exhalant-absorbent. The last two, and especially the absorptive-exhalational systems, received particularly close scrutiny. This, too, is hardly surprising. The physiology and pathophysiology of the body's humoral – solid boundary would have preoccupied anyone who obeyed Bichat's admonition, "ouvrez des cadavres." And it was the exhalant-absorbent system, the membranes capable of producing effusions, that formed that boundary.[36]

The Hôtel-Dieu postmortems, blocked in and recorded on large broadsheets under the heading *"Ouverture de cadavres"* followed by diagnostic subheadings, bear out this notion. A preponderance of patients were victims of *maladies hydropiques* or hydropsy, or of *anasarca, inflammation de la péricarde,* or *inflammation du péritoine.* The common denominator was the presence of exudative affections of the membranous structures, particularly the serous coats of major viscera. Of primary importance was the state of these coats or membranes in the exhalant-absorbent system, and the presence or absence of serosity [sérosité] in the various cavities into which this ubiquitous (and, in disease, much augmented) fluid was "wept." Such findings were a source of fascination, evidenced by the many glosses and lengthy comments noted alongside by Bichat and his colleagues. Typical is the following, from *Messidor an VIII* (June/July 1800) in what is probably Bichat's hand:

Peritoneum intact[,] a liter of serosity discharged into the abdominal cavity[.] Pleura, pericardium whitish and opaque[,] containing a great deal of serosity – mesenteric and bronchial glands engorged – generalized infiltration of cellular tissue [*tissu cellulaire*] throughout the body.[37]

This was already a far cry from the "fever" of contemporary admission registers. Of especial importance was the manner in which Bichat and colleagues cut across traditional anatomical boundaries, across disparate structures, and regions of the body. If they found excessive quantities of serosity in the peritoneal cavity they would look in the chest and in the head, going into the cerebral ventricles in search of allied, or "sympathetic," changes.

With surprising regularity they found them. Another representative case, autopsied on 27 *Prairial an VIII* (27 May 1800) was presented by Buisson under his twenty-eight-year-old cousin's watchful eye. In the absorbent system Buisson noted:

serous membrane of the peritoneum reddish, studded its entire extent with whitish tubercle[;] abundant serosity in the cavity[,] whitish flakes floating in this serosity[.] Epiploon transformed into a hard mass consistently presenting an infinity of small whitish points – pleura and pericardium intact.[38]

Bichat added:

At present the disease has its reaction in the peritoneum, which has been augmented in thickness – and before the pleura offers this [?reaction] – the whitish flakes, were not copious but as though fibrous . . .

And he added the following further general commentary on the patient's antemortem course:

slow and generalized inflammation of the peritoneum – the patient had suffered for a long time a dolor of the abdomen following a peripneumonia – he had a chronic cough and purulent sputum – the belly had been tight and distended. . . .[39]

These findings supply no more than a glimpse seen through a hospital window at a particular, critical moment. How did Bichat arrive at this point, where he could speak with facility of irritated and inflamed tissues enmeshed in the exquisite interplay of solids and fluids, of local and systemic pathological events? I have referred briefly to the professional, intellectual, and epidemiological resources with which he had to work. To disentangle these strands further, I turn next to the path by which his career came to this pass.

THE MODEL UNFOLDS

Xavier Bichat arrived in the capital in the summer of 1794. He was twenty-three years old, the scion of a large provincial family of ample means, rooted since the seventeenth century in the town of Thoirette, in the Jura. His father, Jean-Baptiste Bichat, was a physician who bore the vitalistic stamp of a medical education in Montpellier, where P. J. Barthez and Théophile de Bordeu had held forth in the mid-eighteenth century. The young Bichat had been sent to Nantua and then to Lyons for his early education. Interested early in the classification and manual dissection of natural objects, he had presented himself in 1791 to the Lyons Hôtel-Dieu for medical training.[40]

The newly arrived Bichat was immediately taken under his wing by Pierre Desault, who, just five years before, had implemented his own proposals to revamp practical teaching of surgery as Chief Surgeon at the Hôtel-Dieu.[41] Desault became the younger man's physical as well as his intellectual guardian, providing him not only with room and board, but also with the freedom of his library. Among its books was Théophile de Bordeu's *Recherches sur le tissu muqueux* of 1787. Exposed to the rigors of his surgical mentor's practical-*cum*-theoretical instruction, and surrounded by the medical texts of Montpellier and the new Paris school, Bichat set about assembling his own synthetic view of life under the altered circumstances of disease.

He quickly became Desault's favored student. Within a year he found himself asked frequently to substitute, when the master's presence was required elsewhere, as principal lecturer in Desault's amphitheater. Though anxious to leave the capital for the military front, he applied himself in his efforts at the Hôtel-Dieu (then bearing its revolutionary era name of Grand Hospice de l'Humanité) and into the study of surgical subjects that seemed conducive to his projected military role. Notable among those subjects were the anatomy, physiology, and pathology of the bones and joints, interests of Desault's as well. It was natural for Bichat to observe and publish upon the long line of orthopedic injuries that he saw flowing through Desault's clinic, which, judging from his later writings, included numerous fractures, subluxations of the long bones, and both rheumatic and septic affections of the joint cavities. At one point in 1795, in Desault's *Journal de Chirurgie* Bichat published an account of a patient whose "luxated" humerus had been reduced with the sudden occurrence of local subcutaneous emphysema. This short work afforded just a glimpse of the pivotal articles on synovial and other membranes that were to emerge during his *annus mirabilis* of 1799–1800.

When Desault died unexpectedly in early June of 1795 Bichat became his de facto literary executor. Largely in their late teacher's honor, Bichat and J. L. M. Alibert founded the Société Medicale d'Emulation, publishing the first volume of its *Mémoires* in 1797.

The task fell to Bichat to write the "Preliminary Discourse," which he made the platform from which to pay tribute to what he felt to be the new spirit of inquiry:

Since the changes wrought by the Revolution the march of Method, philosophical and reasoned, has been substituted for the heedless and irregular march of irreflection. One no longer flits from flower to flower like the butterfly; but, like the bee, one drains the nectar of one plant before flying off to new ones. . . .[42]

Bichat lauded the new approach to securing medical knowledge that "gives men to science who are made to push back its bounds." Here he was no doubt speaking at least in part of Desault. And when he spoke of "science" he was no doubt thinking of Desault's influential and epoch-making teaching methods, stressing bedside teaching and the importance of experience over rote learning. By now, however, in late 1797 and early 1798, Bichat was probably already concerned with elaborating a broader anatomical science as well. For now, having observed the common practice of renting dissection space and giving *cours privés,* private instruction in normal and pathological anatomy, Bichat saw an end to the perennial problem of the scarcity of bodies for anatomical dissection. That end illustrates again the conjunction of intellectual programs, professional goals, and bureaucratic initiatives that characterize the critical period of Bichat's last few years.[43]

Recognizing the needs of the new Ecoles and of the military surgeons at the front, the Directory promulgated the new law of *Vendemiaire an VII* (September 1798) regulating the *salles de dissection* and permitting the legal and inexpensive flow of cadavers into the anatomists' hands. Bichat quickly expanded his laboratory and hence his teaching activities. Henceforth he could legally remove bodies from the Saint-Catherine cemetery, from which his own remains would be ceremoniously removed a half-century later and later reinter them at Clamart. So for Bichat, the years 1797–98 were as pivotal for anatomy as the years 1793–94 had been for medical education as a whole.

In 1799, at the beginning of what proved to be his *annus mirabilis,* Bichat published a pair of memoirs on bone and joint pathology in his Society's journal. They bore striking portents. In the second "Memoir on the synovial membranes of the joints" he displayed clearly for the first time a spark of new insight into the pathophysiology of membranes. "No part of the physiology of bone is richer in hypothesis and poorer in discoveries than the account of the synovial system," he began. He then enumerated his three objectives:

> 1. To demonstrate how little foundation there is for the theories adopted up until now to explain how the synovia is transported onto articular surfaces.
> 2. To prove that it is furnished by an exhalation similar to that which takes place in serous cavities, of which the immediate organ is a membrane analogous to that of the same cavities.
> 3. To indicate the general disposition of this membrane, and its manner in particular of existence in each type of mobile articulation.[44]

Here was Bichat at a watershed in his professional and intellectual life. His early surgical concerns were here perceptibly grading over into a new physiology, and into a new system of pathological anatomy of solids and fluids mediated by membranous surfaces. The key to his new pathophysiology of the joint spaces was the relationship between the synovial membrane where the morbid appearances were localized, and the synovial fluids and effusions, or "synovia" (*synovie*), that were secreted, transuded, or "exhaled" into the joint space.[45]

Four sorts of analogies could be drawn, maintained Bichat, between the fluids constituting synovia and the membranes that produced them. An "analogy of nature" reflected the similar reactivities of the serous fluids to various chemicals, their coagulability when exposed to alcohol, acids, or heat, and their common albumin content. An "analogy of functions" denoted the lubricating function of the fluids. An "analogy of affections" obtained, such that inflammation affected like membranes in like manner – inducing adhesions, for example, leading to ankylosis in the joints, or hydropsy in the joints and other serous cavities. Finally, an "analogy of absorption" provided a means for the return of the fluids to the circulation via the lymphatic system, "after having sojourned sufficiently on their respective surfaces."

The "most striking analogy of all," though, he noted, "is that which may be observed between the synovia and the fluid that lubricates the walls of all the serous membranes, such as the pleura, the pericardium, the peritoneum, and so on." All these tissues were identifiable by their tendency to form reflections or sacs lining cavities, by their thin, polished textures, and by the capacity of their walls to form lubricating exhalations.[46]

It was a classic case of intellectual convergence. Not only was Bichat aware of the medical importance of the body humors and membranes from his readings of Bordeu and Pinel, whose magisterial *Nosographie philosophique* had just been published, but he was also well aware of Desault's surgical concerns with diseases of similar parts. As his surgical teacher's literary executor and at the widow's behest, he had just collected Desault's ephemera and brief *Journal de chirurgie* memoirs into a two-volume collection of *Oeuvres*. While most of the case discussions dealt with orthopedic problems, the collected works contained one long section on diseases of the chest. The first set of observations concerned hydropsical changes in the pericardium. It was evident that the signs and symptoms of *hydropisie du péricarde,* or pericardial effusion, often complicated by tamponade, were already understood by surgeons as well as physicians. But Bichat and Desault admitted that, hidden from the examining eye and largely from the palpating finger by the bony thorax, the disorder was hard to diagnose with certainty in a patient who was complaining mainly of the typical but nonspecific symptoms of syncope and dyspnea. Indeed, both cases in question had been misdiagnosed, one as a *pleural* effusion when the pericardial sac had been affected, and one with the circumstances reversed.

The significance of these cases for Bichat, and for the historian today, is that their implications went far beyond the mere elaboration of a physiology of absorptive surfaces. Much more than an abstracted Hallerian rubric of irritability and sensibility was involved. The clinical problem outlined here was a critical one for the hospital surgeon or physician. These patients died, and were expected to die. But if paracentesis – the placing of a needle or bistoury, such as that here attempted in the sixth left intercostal space, and the draining off of accumulated serosity or synovia – could be tried, the clinician might make a real difference in the patient's downhill course. Such an intervention, at the intersection of medical and surgical concerns, was admittedly risky. But it was potentially lifesaving.[47]

The convergence of local and global, solidist and fluidist, surgical and medical concerns that had prepared him for the *annus mirabilis* was made explicit by Bichat as he concluded his 1799 *Mémoire* on the synovia. "I may be permitted to observe," he declared,

that this method of reasoning about the organization of the parts from a consideration of their affections merits greater importance than has been commonly attributed to it. In effect, is it not evident that if an organ . . . constantly displays a diathesis attained by the entirety of a known class of organs, it must therefore be ranged within this class; and that reciprocally it is foreign to that class if it never experiences this diathesis? . . . . From which it follows that the uniformity of the affections of the living parts indicates in general a uniformity of their organization, and on the contrary the difference in one denotes diversity in the other.[48]

Working now in 1799 at a furious pitch, Bichat followed this article with another entitled "*Dissertation sur les membranes et sur leur rapports généraux d'organisation,*" postulating a tripartite classification of the membranes and promising "a quite extensive dissertation" to follow "of which this essay should be regarded as the précis."[49] As promised, the *Treatise on Membranes* appeared at the end of the year. It drew a largely, if not entirely, enthusiastic response from the Paris medical world.[50]

Despite this chiefly favorable response to his *Treatise,* Bichat found himself unable to break into the tight little circle of official and academically secure members of the *École de médecine.* Continuing at the same frantic pace, he finished the *Recherches physiologiques sur la vie et la mort* in five months, producing a work that was to do for physiology what the *Traité* had done, and what the later *Anatomie générale* would amplify, in pathological anatomy. In the final months of 1800 he continued to jockey for the assured position and income of an academic post. Two positions became vacant in early 1801, a clinical post in January, and the chair of anatomy in February. Applying for both, he was awarded only the post of *médecin expectant* at the Hôtel-Dieu. It was the only official post he was ever to hold. Undaunted, he kept up his fever pitch research and by August had completed the four densely packed volumes of the monumental *Anatomie générale.*

Bichat projected at least two further works, an *Anatomie descriptive* oriented toward regional anatomy, and an *Anatomie pathologique.* The former was completed by his disciples. The latter was not, but was projected to follow the plan of a course that he opened in September 1801 and completed on 13 May 1802. It was the last fully executed statement of the membrane model of disease.[51] His own death came just two and one-half months later.

Throughout the last lectures and writings Bichat can be seen developing his notion of histopathologic change, carefully fleshing it out, teasing out its implications, working out a full-blown membrane theory of disease and its localization.[52] Ultimately he elaborated an anatomical schema that involved the seating of disease in any one of fully twenty-one subtypes of tissue. From the *Traité,* the *Anatomie générale,* and the surviving lecture notes of his anatomy courses, a picture emerges of how Bichat viewed disease. He believed the solid tissues to be paramount in mediating disease since they were most "primitively affected by," hence "the seat of disease."[53] But the significance of the fluids – blood, lymph, and (especially) the various sorts of synovia or serosity – was never omitted in his assessment. Each of the membranes produced, he thought, a characteristic species of fluid that was disposed of in a characteristic manner by each tissue type and that accumulated excessively in various morbid affections. The fluid produced, for example, by the mucous membranes, such as those lining the oral and digestive cavities, served a protective function against foreign matter.

The membranes and the fluids they produced were in exquisite balance. Any insult in the equilibrium of organism and environment could precipitate the pathological response that characterized the tissue system affected. The mucous system would develop catarrh, polyps, or a morbid augmentation of secretion. The category of serous membranes, which came to subsume the synovium that had first attracted him and continued to fascinate above all others, produced a lymphatic dew [*rosée*]. This dewy fluid or irrigant, unlike the fluids produced by mucous membranes, was reabsorbed rather than excreted. Normally such a fluid subserved a lubricant or "humectant" function that preserved the mobility of neighboring organs, enabling them to slide past one another and isolating their resident vital principles from those of their neighbors. Mucous fluids, in short, served as physical buffers between individual organs and the external environment. Serous fluids served as buffers between neighboring structures.[54]

SENSIBILITY, IRRITABILITY, AND INFLAMMATION

Since the nineteenth century, historians have paid a great deal of attention to the physiological reasoning that Bichat developed in parallel with his pathological system. Much of that attention was focused on two related central concerns, Bichat's notion of vital properties and that of sensibility and irritability.[55] Theoretically, it would seem reasonable to suppose that his pathology, the study of dysfunction and its anatomical seats, was an extension of his physiology, the study of function. But operationally, the reverse, if anything, was true. Or, perhaps more properly stated, the two cognitive frameworks that Bichat was developing together were each related to the other in a complex and reflexive manner. I can document this contention simply enough, by focussing for a moment on the point where the two systems intersected: the problem of sensibility.

Whereas irritability usually implied contractility, the ability of a tissue to mount some sort of a motor response to a stimulus, sensibility implied an organism's ability to "feel" external stimuli, or at least to demonstrate a response of some sort (mediated in higher animals by a developed nervous system) to an irritant stimulus. The two characteristics, irritability and sensibility, were linchpins of Bichat's physiology. But why did he come to incorporate these notions with such conviction and emphasis? Did he learn of irritability simply from his reading of Haller and other, allied, eighteenth-century physiological theorists? Most likely enlightenment struck him sharply and directly, as he pursued physiological observations himself, in his observations of nature's own experiments – diseases affecting the mucous and serous membranes. Those experiments in turn were replicable in the laboratory through the artificial induction of inflammation by irritant stimuli. Here Bichat the pathologist met Bichat the physiologist.

Within a given class, Bichat averred, membranes could be expected to respond in certain characteristic ways to an irritant or inflammatory stimulus. When mucous membranes, for example, were subjected to excessive heat, he noted, "the sensibility of the mucous surface receives a remarkable heightening of energy." The capacity of a stimulus to elicit such a response depended on force of habit (*habitude*): the sound in the bladder, or the bolus of tobacco in the mouth would, after a while, be diminished by this effect. Aging had the same result: "Everything is an excitant for the infant; everything is blunted with the old man."[56] The serous membranes commanded even closer scrutiny. When their exhalant-absorbent system of lymph flow was subjected to an irritant insult, he noted, hydropsy would supervene. The normal serous fluid lubricant would become superabundant and form an effusion. One could trigger the process experimentally by insufflating air or macerating the tissue. But disease provided ample natural proof. The serous membranes observed in patients clearly had a vestigial "organic

sensibility," a sort of potentiality for position sense (*impression gén-*
érale de tact) that "transmitted not at all, or very confusedly." But,
challenged by the proper stimulus, this "first degree" of sensibility
was soon exalted to a "sensibility of relation" that brought to bear
the most exquisite tenderness known to sufferers of pleuritis, pericarditis, or peritonitis.

Departing from his surgical teacher's resolute localism, Bichat
now extended his histopathological system to a commodious and
global doctrine of sympathies. A sympathy of sensibility existed,
for example, when inflammatory irritation of one part led to pain
in another, instanced by the pain in the contralateral side of the
chest wall of a patient with pleuritis. He explained that by postmortem examination he could often rule out any actual inflammation of the painful opposite side. The sympathy of irritability
consisted of a form of action at a distance between an inflamed
organ, such as the peritoneum, and a more or less distant contractile
structure – hence the muscular rigidity and guarding characteristic
of peritoneal irritation. Sympathies of tonicity, finally, were characterized best by the spread of irritation from a point on a membrane, such as the peritoneum, to the totality of the membrane.[57]

In his never-published course of pathological anatomy Bichat
extended these ideas. Exploring specific disease settings and the
natural history of specific syndromes, he refined his system further.
He now differentiated the fluids of the organism into those produced by secretion and those produced by exhalation. The latter
included fluids exhaled in inflammation, which would today be
termed exudates, and those exhaled in hydropic maladies, today's
transudates: the milky, yellowish serosity of tuberculous pleuritis
versus the excessive but normal-appearing fluid of dropsy or heart
failure. In inflammatory affections, the serous membranes displayed a hierarchy of susceptibilities, thought Bichat. The pleura,
so often found studded with tubercle, was the most susceptible to
inflammation, followed by the peritoneum, the pericardium, the
tunica vaginalis, and the arachnoid membranes.

Affections of the membranes were similar, however, in their
symptoms, progressing from vague pressure sensations, through
extreme intensity of pain to fever and probable death. Suppuration
was more common as a terminal anatomical feature (*terminaison*)
than gangrene in these structures. It was a dire finding: "When
the ill perish this has taken place." Once such affections progressed

to the chronic stage, one noted the morbid appearances, on opening the cadaver, to have advanced still further: a liquid of variable color, consistency, and amount might be found. Albuminous flakes (*flocons*) were evident on occasion, as were adhesions between loops of bowel, miliary eruptions, and erythema of the intestinal canal.[58]

BICHAT IN 1799–1801

By the turn of the century Bichat had achieved novel syntheses both in physiology and in pathological anatomy. In just two years he had assembled a complex and suggestive skein of biological ideas, destined to become the theoretical framework for a generation of physicians. Indeed, by seizing the localizationist impulse of the surgeon and extending it through the medical doctrines of sensibility and sympathy, he sought to create something like a Newtonian synthesis in the biological sciences.[59] His views on pathology in particular were already fixed and, as I have already summarized them, expressed *in extenso* in the *Treatise on Membranes,* the unpublished course on pathological anatomy, and in the *General Anatomy*. In his private courses, propounding these views, he had already begun to influence a youthful coterie of physicians and surgeons, nineteenth-century medical men whose educational and professional experience went back no further than the reign of Napoleon.

Yet during these last few years of his brief existence Bichat succeeded in securing only one official post, that at the Hôtel-Dieu. His efforts to obtain teaching positions in the Faculty of Medicine, detailed more fully in the chapter that follows, were unavailing. Why did his influence paradoxically so belie his place in the professional world of medical Paris? It is not enough to suppose that Bonaparte and his bureaucrats did not, in essence, really mean to exclude Bichat.[60] Nor is it sufficient to wave away the Paris Faculty as an institution that enjoyed no more than secondary importance at the time. From its inception, and never more than in Napoleonic Paris, the Faculty, in fact, was of critical importance as arbiter of medical knowledge, more important than the private courses or even the hospital instruction, though both helped keep body and soul together for heads like Bichat.

The explanation of the lag in Bichat's reputation lies in the structure and function of the Paris Faculty itself, dictating a surprising corollary: the paradox dissolves away once the historical veils are removed from his career. The Faculty, along with its wholly controlled *Ecole pratique de dissection,* occupied a critical role in the processing of medical knowledge, but not in its creation. For the same reasons that Bichat's intellectual productions were vital to this most central of French medical institutions, and indeed were earnestly fostered by it, the man himself was forced to develop his career outside its doors.

2

Pathology and the Paris faculty

Had Xavier Bichat been chosen, in the early summer of 1799, for the official teaching position in what was now designated the *Ecole de médecine,* he would have been suddenly thrust into a pivotal position in the school's new program. The death of Honore Fragonard (1732–99) had vacated the post of *chef des travaux anatomiques* in the faculty's recently annexed *Ecole pratique.*[1] The physicians of the School had welcomed the subsidiary institution "into their bosom" in 1795, when the new, more ecumenical, academic regime began in earnest: Physicians and surgeons now toiled under a single institutional roof.

Since that first year Fragonard had been *chef,* directing a staff of *prosecteurs* that included André Duméril (1774–1860) and Guillaume Dupuytren (1777–1835). Both were capable young surgeons and accomplished anatomists. Later in the Napoleonic period, Dupuytren would become known as a dominant figure in his own right (Chapter 3). Though anxious to gain entry to the inner sanctum of the Ecole staff, Bichat no doubt recognized the likelihood that one of the two prosectors already in place, even though they were both considerably his juniors, would ultimately be named to succeed Fragonard, competitive *concours* or not. At the end of June, Bichat dropped out of the running. Shortly thereafter Duméril was named to the post.[2]

When Bichat withdrew his candidacy, the *Ecole pratique* was, almost to the day, a year short of its semicentennial mark. It had been founded in 1750 for the benefit of the surgeons by the leaders of that community of practitioners. It had then continued until the Revolution in a sort of ill-bounded syncytial arrangement with two other surgical institutions, the *Académie royale de chirurgie* and the *Collège de chirurgie*.[3] Arguably it was one of the two scientific and medical institutions – the other being the *Collège de France* – that survived the revolutionary attack on all vestiges of institutionalized privilege. Though legally effaced for a brief time by the suppression of the faculties and corporations, including the College of Surgery, the *Ecole pratique* had continued its instructional activities. As a result it was ripe for the picking, as a physical space and as a pedagogical idea, in 1794–95 when the new law mandated the reorganization of education. Naturally enough it was subsumed by the new *Ecole* as a constituent part of that ambitious new institutional experiment.[4]

What the *Ecole pratique* provided, especially after the new anatomical ordinance of September 1798 eased the procurement of cadavers, was concentrated experience in the manipulative and practical aspects of medicine. Paramount among these was the experience of dissection, which in turn was central to the emerging tradition of pathological anatomy. Other subjects such as practical chemistry were included as well. Perhaps the physician-dominated faculty – the *Ecole de santé* was a faculty in everything but name, and soon regained that appellation as well – was still not quite ready to cede full professorial status to those who taught the manipulative subjects. In any event, experience in the *Ecole pratique* soon brought with it as much or more cachet as matriculation in the parent faculty. The best medical students gained entrance by special concours. An educational tour of its laboratories and workspaces, whether as student, prosector, or as teaching aide, was a true *tour de main,* binding together hand, eye, and mind. This manner of aligning all the senses in learning pathology – literally absorbing anatomy through the fingertips – is what ultimately made Bichat's synthesis possible.

As I have indicated, Bichat's reformulation of pathological anatomy, in itself provided him with an important legacy quite apart from his parallel syntheses in physiology and other fields of inquiry. In the three decades following his death in 1802, Bichat's tissue theory was assimilated in the pathological works of Gabriel Andral, A. N. Gendrin, Théophile Laennec, Jean Cruveilhier, P. A. Piorry, Alexis Boyer, P.-J. Roux, probably François Broussais, and, perhaps most prominently, Gaspard Laurent Bayle (1774–1816).[5]

Again, at first it may seem curious that despite his hospital posts Bichat should have remained so marginal to the efforts of the official academic mandarinate. Yet this state of affairs aids in understanding how the Medical School – restored after 1808 to the status and title of *Faculté* – came to function between 1797 and 1822, its most vital quarter of a century. Such an analysis requires, in turn, a discussion of the structure and function of the Paris School in the years surrounding the turn of the century.

THE WORK OF THE *ECOLE DE SANTÉ*

I have alluded to the roles of some of the central figures in the rise of the Paris School: Antoine Fourcroy (1755–1809), François Chaussier (1746–1828), and Michel Thouret (1748–1810), the first dean.[6] Fourcroy was most important in the inception of the new institution, Thouret in its maintenance and stabilization over a succession of political regimes, and Chaussier in its outreach.[7] In the following section I will concern myself primarily with the work of Fourcroy and Thouret. I will discuss the role of Chaussier in Chapter 4.

When *ancien régime* structures identifiable as bastions of privilege were swept away in 1793 by the revolution, the path lay clear for ambitious men to create new ones. The groundwork for the establishment of medical teaching structures was laid in late November of 1794. On November 27 Antoine Fourcroy – nonpracticing physician, chemist, teacher, and prototypic French educational administrator – issued his penetrating and timely *Rapport et projet de décret* on the establishment of a central *Ecole de santé* in Paris. His analysis of what was needed, practical training combined with a syllabus newly meshing medicine and surgery, was a particularly deft stroke. By design it was congruent with the aspirations and sentiments of the Convention, of which Fourcroy was himself a member, and it succeeded admirably.

Disastrous epidemics, argued Fourcroy, combined with the depredations of its spreading military adventures, had placed France in a precarious position with respect to its supply of health practitioners. Such exigencies offered the Convention the "happy occasion" to create an educational regime from rudiments that had never been more than truncated and incomplete. Proper training, moreover, had been available only at great expense for those students with fortitude enough to mold multiple private courses together into something resembling a curriculum. The old academy of surgery, with its spacious amphitheater, could provide the premises for a fresh start on this project. Practical training and bedside observation would be afforded by the incorporation of three hospices or hospital *cliniques,* the *Humanité* (the old Hôtel-Dieu) for surgical diseases (*maladies externes*), the *Unité* (formerly the *Charité*) for internal medicine (*maladies internes*), and the *Perfectionnement* at the School itself for unusual and complicated cases.[8]

Fourcroy suggested twelve professorial chairs in the new school. Those chosen to hold them, should, he declared, be made sufficiently unencumbered financially that they might devote themselves to "research in the sciences that they were charged with teaching," a consummation that he devoutly wished for but never saw come to pass. His other major idea for innovation in the school, however, would be more successful:

In founding a central health school, the legislators will no doubt wish to eradicate that ancient separation between two estates that has caused so much trouble. Medicine and surgery are two branches of the same science: to study them separately is to abandon theory to the delirium of imagination and practice to blind routine. To unite and mingle them is to mutually enlighten them.[9]

In his initial report Fourcroy found no reason to spell out in detail the several steps that would be necessary to implement the plan. At the end of January, however, with the two key chairs now expeditiously and felicitously filled – Pierre Desault in surgery and Jean Corvisart in medicine – the organizers put flesh on the skeleton. Tableaux of the School's financial organization and a published *Plan générale* of the School's curriculum soon followed.[10] The elaborate *Plan générale* promulgated by Fourcroy and his committee at the end of January 1795 furnished an elaborate blueprint for the organization of instruction at the new institution. Twelve courses with corresponding professorial chairs were envisioned, including the anatomy and physiology course (initially to be taught by Chaussier), separate medical and surgical pathology courses (*pathologie interne* and *externe*), and Desault's and Corvisart's surgical and medical clinics.[11] Ongoing or "permanent" courses comprised the hospital courses at the three official School-affiliated hospices. "Nonpermanent" *cours de semestres* were to be taught didactically over contiguous six-month periods of the republican calendar, beginning with "Anatomy/Physiology," medical chemistry, and surgery (*médecine opératoire*), followed by botany and materia medica, hygiene, distinct courses in external and internal pathology, a course in medical history and jurisprudence, and the obstetrics (*accouchement*) course.

Initially the Convention set the compensation of the twelve professors at 500 *livres* per month, 6,000 per year. Though technically lacking professorial status, Michel Thouret, appointed *Directeur,* received the same salary. So, too, did the librarian, Pierre Süe (1739–1816), and the conservateur, J. B. J. Thillaye (1752–1822). Physicians and surgeons with adjunct appointments (*adjoints*) were to receive salaries of 5,000 *livres* yearly, as were the *artistes* like Fragonard in the *Ecole pratique*.[12] In late September of 1795 the Finance Committee of the National Convention issued an *arrête* raising directorial and professorial salaries to 10,000 *livres,* while those of *adjoints* and the *chef des travaux anatomiques* went to 9,000. Salaries of other *chefs* (such as *chefs* in the chemical laboratory of the *Ecole pratique*), *prosecteurs,* and *sous-chefs,* were raised about 50 percent, and standard, across-the-board student stipends, a hallmark of the early school's egalitarianism, were more than doubled from 1,200 to 2,500 *livres*.[13] It is particularly noteworthy that the posts of *directeur* and *chef des travaux anatomiques* were remunerated consistently at the same level, respectively, as full and adjunct professors.

ASPECTS OF THE NEW CURRICULUM

When the young Xavier Bichat was in Paris a scant six months François Chopart (1743–1795) and Pierre François Percy (1754–1825) began to assemble the surgical pathology course, while François Doublet (1751–1795) and Joseph-François Bourdier planned the medical pathology course. Bichat's major effort to unify the two fields intellectually (if not yet institutionally) was 5 years away. The two courses developed by the new pathology professors were mosaics of prevailing ideas, evolved over the eighteenth century, to describe and explain the diseased human frame.[14] Surgical pathology was to be divided into four sections: first, general surgical pathology, including the most important categories of lesions, emphasizing orthopedic problems, and according particular attention to the relations of the solids and fluids in their connections with disorders of the soft and hard parts of the body; second, diseases of the soft parts, such as ulcers, fistulas, and tumors; third, diseases of the hard parts, such as fractures, exostoses, and luxations; and fourth, the regional pathology of the major body cavities and extremities.[15]

In the initial plan, medical pathology was to be divided into two parts. In the first, the principles of pathology were to be explicated and developed through an historical overview. This was to be followed by considerations of the abstract notions of health and disease; the elements, including the passions of the soul, of the human organism capable of promoting health or disease; the essential natural historical typology of disease, including idiopathic, sympathetic, periodic, epidemic, and intermittent illnesses; and the standard notions of resolution or "termination" (*terminaison*) of disease. In the second part of this course the most important internal diseases would be presented according to the natural historical schema devised in the previous section.[16]

Certain features stand out prominently in this, the School's initial approach to the education of the medical student in anatomy and pathology. With the exception of the surgical pathology of the body surface and the bony skeleton, pathological *anatomy,* at least as the observer would come to think of it after Bichat, was most conspicuous by its absence. The most pervasive ills of the body, infectious and otherwise, were described mainly in the canon of eighteenth-century natural history: an essentially clinical, descriptive, and Hippocratic form of pathological discourse. Thus the problem of integrating the teaching of pathology, as well as clinical courses, could be addressed only after the devising of an intellectual *lingua franca* that could bind together the medical and surgical points of view.[17] But this latter imperative was still unmet. So for teaching purposes the divisions in pathology and the clinic were maintained. For the moment, it was enough that surgery and medicine were coequal within the single institutional framework of the *Ecole de santé.*

TENSIONS OVER THE DIRECTION OF THE PARIS SCHOOL

From the beginning those responsible for the day-to-day oversight of the School found themselves faced with a wide array of potentially divisive forces. Its central figures shared a sense of institutional mission, enlivened by their commitments to medical ecumenicism and national service through national education. But three sets of forces exerted their pull and threatened to take their toll on this sense of mission. For the administrators of the School, the first of these new sources of tension, a lobby that would have effected *de novo* the disunion of medicine and surgery, was perhaps the most important. I will discuss this particular set of centrifugal tendencies, as well as how Chaussier and others attempted to manage them by adopting Bichatian pathological anatomy, in Chapter 4.

Another source of tension, keenly felt by the *Directeur,* Thouret, and his associates, stemmed from the sheer size and rapid growth of the School. The original student body of three hundred students "destined for the armies" had mushroomed within four years to quadruple that number. The library had grown from 1,600 to 15,000 volumes. The Paris hospital system still had its unparalleled aspect as a reservoir of the diseased and dying. The *Ecole pratique* now allowed on the order of three hundred students, sprawled across fourteen dissecting pavilions, to study between three and four hundred cadavers each winter. But there were nonetheless critics of the institution's disproportion of scale when compared with the much smaller sister institutions in Montpellier and Strasbourg.[18]

The institution's critics, including no doubt certain key legislators, were clearly on the Director's mind in 1798 when the School produced a retrospect, almost certainly composed by Thouret himself, of the Paris School's first few years. There were, he acknowledged, individuals who proposed to collapse or "pluralize" (*cumuler*) the teaching functions of groups of two or three faculty members into single professorships. To do so as a means of cutting the School's operational cost to the nation, or to eliminate the paid status of the adjunct professors would, he declared, risk a serious loss of quality. As it was, he noted, the School already made do with less faculty than the two bodies the new School had replaced, the old Faculty of Medicine and College of Surgery. Available faculty was, moreover, already sorely overtaxed by the necessity to give entrance examinations to the hundreds of applicants who presented themselves each year. Merely let a few legislators come for themselves, he charged: They will see the packed amphitheater, the corridors and stairways so overflowing that the professor, cleaving his way through, might finally lecture to *la foule* as it stood, elbows shoving, pressed up against doorways, bodies sitting on the floor.[19]

Thouret saw a more insidious, and for pathology perhaps even more important, source of tension emerging within the School in the late 1790s: the question of the proper function, or balance of functions, to be reflected within the institution. Certainly the teaching mission of the School was abundantly clear. So too, no doubt, was its service function. But what of research: *"perfectionnement de l'art"*? Thouret's view was clear: The law of 14 *Frimaire* had charged the faculty with preserving this role. A series of new *Mémoires* to follow those formerly published by the *Société de médecine* and the *Académie de chirurgie* were being newly undertaken, he announced, beginning with an exhaustive description of the anatomical museum of the *Ecole pratique*. Here, too, was a function for the faculty that warranted an expansion rather than contraction of its numbers.

In his 1798 report Thouret advocated expansion, in part, no doubt, to avoid constriction. Beyond this rhetorical stance, however, lay the profound problem of projecting a research mission in an institutional vacuum. Anyone interested in the role of the central medical faculty, and seeking a meaningful research role for it, was forced to lower his expectations in time. At the turn of the century, however, there remained a tension between organizing the faculty's two functions: its esoteric function, involving the production of new knowledge; and its exoteric function, involving the processing and accreditation of knowledge produced elsewhere. In the documentary evidence one senses a pervasive tug back and forth between the two different sorts of function. This tension remained unresolved until at least the middle of the following decade. In the remainder of the present chapter I will locate this conflict against the backdrop of the organization and development of professional education in medicine from Convention to mid-Empire. I will also attempt to depict the changing link between pathological anatomy and this larger context.

COMPETING MISSIONS: RESEARCH VERSUS REGULATION

The uneasy relationship in the medical faculty between the two functions, between production of knowledge and production of certificates of competency, was always somewhat unbalanced, weighted in the direction of education and service and away from research. The unease had its roots in an equally uneasy ambivalence within the political body that established it. The Convention had never made its intentions about the structure and purpose of higher education entirely clear. One constituency, dominated by most of the *Girondins* and some of the *Montagnards,* favored a philosophy, after Condorcet, of the *véritable Université des temps nouveaux,* broadly emphasizing a philosophy embodying an *esprit scientifique et critique.* Another group, fearing the elitism they felt to be inherent in such a posture, favored a narrower vision of vocational education.[20] Outside the professional faculties of medicine and law, in fact, this state of affairs developed within a decade or so to the point where cadres of faculties of science and letters were recruited as little more than state functionaries oriented almost exclusively toward vocationalism.[21]

From the looks of things the medical school was to be spared this administrative fate. Between 1797 and 1800 the faculty itself pressed hard for the broadest possible construction of their role. In July, 1797 the professorial assembly met and authorized an official appeal to the central bureau of the interior ministry, requesting the name change to the "school of medicine," on the grounds that the new appellation would more accurately convey the faculty's scope.[22]

The shift officially symbolized the faculty's retreat from the simple, ardent ideal of hygiene and health promotion, and a return to the pursuit of all aspects of the art of healing. In their private thoughts some may have seen the name change more simply as a return to a more truthful rendition of the mission followed *de facto* all along. In the following year, pressing their advantage, the professors successfully promulgated a *projet de loi* that stipulated faculty responsibility for "the advancement of the art and the perfection of all those sciences needed to hasten its progress." The document called as well for the creation, in the Paris school and the two others, of one or more societies devoted to the teaching of science.[23]

The project bore a form of fruit in the summer of 1800. As the vestiges of revolutionary sentiment continued to ebb, the government and medical faculty formed a successor to those *ancien régime* medical organizations that had boasted the royal warrant. The new *Société de l'ecole de médecine* was primarily charged with research in medical topography and climatology. But it was nonetheless firmly planted within the medical faculty, and was envisioned as that body's arm for the pursuit of original research. The society was chartered with a membership that included the school's faculty members, fifteen key outsiders (including both Cuvier and Bichat), and the *chef des travaux anatomiques*. Two and one-half years later, in late 1803, Dupuytren would found another society, the *Société anatomique,* that included more members of the *Ecole pratique,* and promoted research in normal anatomy as a prelude to the study of pathological anatomy.[24]

But if the faculty's desires to expand the limits of medical inquiry had borne fruit briefly, and perhaps more in form than in substance, at that, it was soon to wither. If some of the members of the faculty envisioned a research role for it, that hope was soon decimated by competing demands on their energies. Without question there was a real desire to see the faculty become a source of fresh inquiry about human pathology, but during the medical faculty's second 5 years, and indeed well into the Napoleonic period, its personnel – Thouret, Chaussier, and most of their colleagues – found themselves increasingly preoccupied with the administrative burdens of what was, after all, the largest producer of health practitioners in a wartime economy. Those preoccupations and the effects they had on the teaching of pathology deserve attention next.

As early as 1797 the administrators of the faculty were beginning to be buffeted by certain harsh realities imposed by government-mandate. The new realities of this expanded mission can be characterized in terms of three sets of needs for dispersing power. One such need was demographic, wherein two studentships were committed for each geographic area. Another was intellectual, since medicine and surgery were now combined in a way that added serious problems to the task of certifying *ancien régime* students drawn from one branch or the other. And a third balancing act was political, in that the administration had to offset the demands of each of two competing ministries, War and Interior. These demands for maintaining demographic, intellectual, and political balance were perhaps in theory a major source of institutional innovation. But before long they became a major source of institutional inertia.

In much of its early period the School was thus faced with the drag effect of its own peculiar (and characteristically French) nightmare web of regulation and administration. Necessarily the situation struck men like Chaussier and Thouret with the greatest force. The experience tethered the faculty to its exoteric task of processing knowledge, much as it was tied to the closely related task of processing and passing on the qualifications of prospective students and expectant graduates. The two tasks, processing men and ideas, were complementary. Each was related organically and dynamically to the other. Withal, the preservation of the status of "old hands" and the maintenance of institutional homeostasis became an important and salutary end in itself, taking precedence over the sort of risks posed by swelling the ranks with pedagogically and administratively unproven research talent.

Three examples, variations on this theme, must suffice. Michel Thouret, the first *directeur* or dean, was perhaps the prototype of, if not the first of the French medical bureaucrats. While not unmindful of the need for scientific inquiry in the seeking of new knowledge about human disease, Thouret made his mark and reputation through service as liaison between his professional constituency in the faculty and the state patrons at the interior ministry. Napoleon's ministers expected to hold the faculty, through Thouret, on a short tether in exchange for their largesse. Quarterly detailed reports were necessary. What was more, Thouret was forced almost singlehandedly to cope with an endless line of applicants for exception to the course requirements for admission to doctoral examinations; many students took advantage of various ministerial decrees that seemed to work in their favor by taking courses in the school without formally registering. In these and similar instances, it fell to the indefatigable Thouret to adjudicate and, what was probably much worse, to prepare the endless stream of documents supporting his decisions.[25]

François Chaussier (1746–1828), by contrast, probably had a greater interest in scientific investigation. A leading anatomist and chemist from Dijon, Chaussier had collaborated with Antoine Fourcroy in mid-1794 on the educational reform project that had led to the reunification of medicine and surgery. While he remained in the chair of anatomy and physiology at the faculty until 1822, and authored well-respected works on muscle anatomy and physiology, Chaussier was of the generation born before 1750: he largely preferred the role of caretaker of knowledge, one who might sift and disseminate information as it emerged, without himself plunging headlong into research. Or perhaps, rather than saying he chose the role, one might instead note that the role chose him. For while he dabbled in physiological investigation, Chaussier also was preoccupied, much like Thouret, with the workaday questions of assessing young professionals – particularly, in his case, in the matter of staffing and intellectually charging the medical juries responsible for certifying ancillary practitioners such as *officiers de santé,* midwives (*sages-femmes*), and pharmacists.[26]

Of the faculty academicians whom I cite because of the tug each felt away from research, Guillaume Dupuytren (1777–1835) was probably the one who began with the most investigation-minded outlook. A half-dozen years younger even than Bichat, Dupuytren showed early promise as a surgeon and anatomist, becoming *Chef des travaux anatomiques* in 1801, moving up rapidly as a surgical lecturer and academician, and early on in his career conducting physiological experiments on animals at the Alfort veterinary school. But by his early thirties Dupuytren was already moving quickly away from investigation, consumed and propelled by three interlocking demands: his surgical teaching, his practice, and a paralyzing mistrust of colleagues like René Laennec, which in its ferocity approached paranoia. Yet Dupuytren enjoyed a greater degree of success both in the Paris faculty and at the flagship hospital, the Hôtel-Dieu, than either of the innovators, Bichat or Laennec.[27]

But the caution, or mere distractedness, of men like these by no means failed to promote the dissemination of new knowledge. Quite the reverse, in fact, proved to be the case. As it flowed into the Faculty, research in pathological anatomy, much of it based on the theoretical superstructure of Bichat's ideas, became bound up with the necessity of certifying lower-order practitioners. I will focus attention on that development in Chapter 3.

CRISES ARISE IN 1797–1798

The last few years of the eighteenth century brought a shift in French political winds, against which the largest central medical institution was not proof. The government in Paris had discovered that the ideological fervor of headier days required vast changes in day-to-day administration, and in 1797–1798 began to undertake such changes. Financially, the leaders in the chambers of the legislature also had their hands full. So strapped were they, in fact, that the economic supply lines to some of the more far flung military theaters were disrupted, providing opportunity for politically ambitious military leaders in the field to engage in adventures of their own devising. One such general was Napoleon Bonaparte.

Napoleon had his own agenda and his own power base. But he shared one sentiment with the republicans still in power: he anathematized the idea that royalists might regain power in the March 1797 election. Nonetheless, the election produced a majority of new monarchical-leaning members on the two ruling councils. The summer of 1797 was therefore rife with political uncertainty. It ended precipitously with a *coup d'état* on 4 September. The results are well known. The election results were vacated, the military gained greatly in power, peace negotiations with England and other enemies of the state were halted, and royalists were purged.

In this charged atmosphere the faculty of the *École de médecine* set out to conduct the fall 1798 term. Then, just three weeks after the *coup d'état,* a disturbing incident occurred in François Chaussier's anatomy course. The staunchly republican Chaussier addressed his students on "the salutary influence of liberty on the sciences in general, and particularly on medicine." What followed must have surprised him. A group of auditors or (depending on the account one believes) official students voiced their objections by hissing and scoffing at Chaussier's notions.[28] When the public got wind of the disturbance, Michel Thouret, also an avid republican but ever the conciliator, stepped in to contain any damage done to the image of the institution.[29] Writing to the Interior Minister the *Directeur* assured the government that the "murmurs" heard at Chaussier's lecture had not come from the cadre of state supported students. Responsible instead, he declared, were some of the *élèves libres,* paying students, who filled the back of the amphitheater in numbers up to a thousand strong.

Thouret promised to investigate and root out the trouble.[30] But a good deal of harm had been done already. The school's administration, committed to republican reforms both in the content of medical education and in citizens' access to it, wanted to avoid the merest hint that they were losing control. The republican journal, "*L'ami des lois,*" meanwhile wrote indignantly: "Who would believe that in Paris . . . citizen Chaussier, professor at the School of Medicine, should have been hissed and booed by students for having spoken enthusiastically of the French republic[?]" Scornfully the journal noted that only forty *officiers de santé* and one lone medical student had protested the royalist insult. "Citizen ministers," it cried, "make fewer memoranda and more purges; speak less and act more."[31]

There is little documentary evidence to suggest directly that at this early stage the school's critics, though political traditionalists, were specifically attacking the school's still controversial curriculum with respect to its merger of medicine and surgery. Veiled references in the correspondence abound, disparaging "the new mode of organization" of the school. One may still safely infer, I believe, that this most important reform stuck in many a craw. Republican reforms were impugned by association. Bold new experiment or not, came the carping from both left and right, see what a mess they are making of it. What is entirely clear is that Thouret continued to feel his institution increasingly isolated and misunderstood in the course of the fall and winter terms of 1797–1798.

In mid-March Thouret wrote the Minister a series of letters imploring him to help make the public more aware of the government's zeal for the progress of the arts and sciences as they had been advanced by the school. The Minister replied quickly, assuring the dean that the government retained full confidence in the institution's mode of organization, and that, as a result, "the school of medicine of Paris may count on the government's good will." Less than two weeks later an internal ministerial document reaffirmed the Minister's desire to support Thouret against the school's detractors. It affirmed the importance of making a published report available detailing the school's contributions. Thus the publication of the document *De l'état actuel* was in part a response to ministerial pressure.[32]

Mending fences outside the institution, Thouret recognized, was not enough. In the politically and intellectually volatile year following the *Fructidor coup d'état,* Thouret undertook a series of internal reforms as well. It was as though he recognized that internal divisions now had to be made proof against external ones. He began to stress even more firmly the importance of pathological anatomy and the other ancillary sciences in the intellectual economy of the faculty. To that end in late October of 1797 Thouret presented to the Minister the school's "plan for the extension and perfection of the *École pratique* already existing in her bosom." His notion was both to extend the availability of practical subjects to more students as enrollments swelled rapidly, and to expand the range of actual courses offered in the *École pratique*. Since pathological dissection was the linchpin of the activities of the *École pratique,* its importance would grow as the result of both measures.[33]

"THERE IS BUT ONE PATHOLOGY"

Doubtless Thouret recognized that expanding the facilities and audience of the *École pratique* would be an unexceptionable and probably popular step. Reviewing and reassessing the entire medical curriculum must have seemed a far more controversial and daunting task. But in the political climate that had now gathered around the faculty and its administration, the task had to be attempted. A *General Plan,* published in the first half of 1798, seemed a propitious point of departure. Thouret asked four men to form a committee to review the document and to recommend reforms as necessary. The members were Bernard Peyrilhe (1735–1804), Pierre Lassus (1741–1807), P.A.O. Mahon (1752–1801), and Philippe Pinel (1745–1826). The balance of the committee was significant: The first two were respected surgeons, the latter two, eminent physicians.

It is difficult to overemphasize the importance of Pinel's presence on Thouret's curricular review committee. Though already well into his sixth decade, Pinel had only recently begun to achieve the status that is now associated with his name. A few years earlier, in 1793, he had undertaken twin assignments that underscored his political and intellectual position. Irony attaches to both. The first, his appointment as Physician of the Infirmaries at the warehouse-like Hospice de Bicêtre, had led to an acquaintance with its lay keeper of the insane, Jean Baptiste Pussin (1746–1811), and two years later his transfer to the Salpetrière, the Bicêtre's female counterpart and an even larger institution.

As Dora Weiner has shown, it was the administrative genius of the layman, Pussin, and his wife, that allowed the shackles of the madmen in the two institutions to be cast off, beginning with the Bicêtre in 1797, part of what came to be known as the "moral method" of humane treatment. Pinel so depended upon the Pussins that he secured their transfer to the Salpetrière as soon as he could manage it, in 1802, and all the while gave them ample credit for the psychological benefits that immediately grew from their methods. But the physician, Pinel, nonetheless garnered most of the acclaim, in the late 1790s and in the eyes of most later historians.[34]

In contrast, Pinel received virtually no acclaim for his other 1793 effort, a *Memoir* submitted for an essay prize to which Weiner has recently redirected historical attention. This essay, entitled "Memoir on that question proposed as subject of a prize by the Society of Medicine: *Determine what is the best method of teaching practical medicine in a hospital,*" failed to win the prize and was only identified as Pinel's handiwork in 1935. But it indicates a prescience, humanitarianism, and scientific spirit that can only have greatly impressed one of its readers, Michel Thouret. It was a blueprint detailing the execution of the idealized vision for a new form of medical school, the plan that was actually proposed by Fourcroy, with Thouret looking on, late in the following year. Hence when Thouret became the medical school's first dean and director, he saw to it that Pinel was on hand to inaugurate one of the new faculty Chairs, that of Hygiene and Medical Physics.[35]

In 1798 it was natural for Thouret to turn to Pinel and his three colleagues, the quartet balanced evenly between surgery and medicine, for direction and intellectual reinforcement. On the 15th of September the commission reported its findings to the general faculty. The four members began with some preliminary observations on the desirability of revising the system of distributing the 300 "national students" among courses, particularly in the *Ecole pratique,* and on the desirability of relieving the director of responsibilities for teaching certain marginal subjects. They next supplied commentary on the most logical approaches to the curriculum, proceeding course by course. They devoted the greatest care and longest commentary to internal and external pathology. Significantly, they treated the two subjects as one ideally unified field. Of it they had this to say:

It has seemed to us that the school should not allow the opportunity to escape it to announce its works [and] to insist on this truth: that the art of healing is one and indivisible, and that as a consequence *there is only one pathology,* and that if one teaches it in two courses that is only due to the abundance of materials for this part of the curriculum[.] [I]n consequence the members of the commission had invited the professors of pathology to set forth in a few lines this regenerative idea and to apply it in their program the way a trunk is followed by its branches. They will work together to put the two parts as close as possible together in a unified whole.[36]

It was perhaps predictable that a commission selected by Thouret, and comprising Pinel and his colleagues, would produce a report that in the main endorsed and validated the school's existing structure and curriculum. Though documents of this sort, countenancing the sponsors' programs, must be read cautiously and not over-weighted, the 1798 report of Pinel *et al.* did represent at least a significant nucleus of academically-minded physicians and surgeons pleading clearly for the utility of a unified tradition of pathological anatomy. If the center was to hold, they declared, it must be placed on a solid and unitary basis. The metaphor was of their own choosing, and chosen judiciously: A "trunk" must be found to support the profession in its several branches, all nourished by the same intellectual roots.

THE TRUNK GROWS

1799

Pinel and his three colleagues had called for a new, synthetic view of pathology as the intellectual trunk from which medical education and medical practice could grow and flourish. In the months following their report to the faculty, it should be recalled from Chapter 1, three events were to have a critical impact on the emergence of pathology as this common intellectual basis. The first was the law of September 1798, greatly liberalizing the availability of material for pathological dissection, and enhancing the role of the *École pratique*. The second was the shift in emphasis in Xavier Bichat's career from surgery to medicine, reflected in the evolution from his memoirs on arthrology into the fully realized *Treatise on Membranes*. The third development was the imminent shuffle in *Ecole pratique* personnel discussed at the beginning of this chapter. That prospect was anticipated with great concern by Thouret in view of the expected demise of Honoré Fragonard, the ailing *chef des travaux anatomiques*. The first two events have already been discussed. The third occurrence, the jockeying for position as *chef* at the *Ecole pratique,* demonstrated the ambivalent relationship between the young Bichat and the faculty, and next warrants closer examination.

While various new practical medical subjects had been added to the offerings of the *Ecole pratique* by early spring of 1799, pathological and anatomical dissection remained the mainstay. Thouret was aware of this, and was further aware that he had an impending personnel problem on his hands. Ministerial documents from the month of *Germinal* show the faculty's concerns over two individuals in particular. One was the artist, Fragonard, a superb *cireur*, or wax modeller, and currently *chef des travaux anatomiques*. The other was the *prosecteur*, a sort of *sous-chef* and dissecting instructor at the *Ecole pratique*, Guillaume Dupuytren. Dupuytren was much younger and subject at any moment to conscription. He would have already been called up, had he not himself been taken ill with bloody coughing fits. But he was in the middle of preparing some irreplaceable angiological models: Could the interior minister see to it that an exception be made to the conscription law in this case?[37]

On the fourth of April the Minister of the Interior wrote, "*cher collègue*," to his counterpart in the War Ministry. "Menaced with the loss of citizen Fragonard [who is] charged with the anatomical works of the establishment, already advanced in age and in a hopeless state [*un état désespéré*], the School would be most interested in keeping nearby, for this same work, citizen Dupuytren, one of the prosectors, who combines in rare measure teaching ability, much intelligence, and an ardent love of this work." The argument, then, was straightforward: Because Dupuytren was talented and could easily step into Fragonard's shoes, he was irreplaceable.[38]

At the end of March, while these maneuvers were under way, Fragonard died. It was a milestone for the School. The artist had been *chef* since its inception. The faculty had never had to replace such a key figure in the *Ecole pratique* since that division for practical training, increasingly seen as the capstone of the entire institution, had been brought into it by the visionaries of the revolutionary period. The faculty immediately set up an administrative committee, at first, it was suggested, to include at least Fourcroy and Peyrilhe, to devise an appropriate plan for identifying and evaluating candidates.[39]

By early June the minister had formed a commission that included Fourcroy, Thouret, Lassus, Noel Hallé (1754–1822), and

Philippe Pelletan (1747–1829).[40] The commission proposed a four-step concours, relayed to the minister through the usual bureau-cratic channels. Each candidate should first compose a written memoir on some aspect of anatomical research of his own choos-ing. A second memoir would be written on an anatomical subject drawn by lot. The candidate would next be required to perform three supervised operations: a simple dissection, a vascular injec-tion, and a lymphatic injection. Fourth and last, each candidate would have to submit a previously prepared anatomical specimen.[41]

Seven candidates presented themselves. By July the commission had reduced the number to two, Dupuytren and Duméril, both "attached to the School," according to Thouret in the Faculty minutes, "in the capacity of prosectors known advantageously to all of us."[42] The two candidates were required to discourse on chemical methods necessary to the anatomist, to inject the cardiac nerves, to inject portions of the lymphatic and arterial systems, and to read memoirs on the means of best achieving the general advancement of anatomical research. On the last day of July the faculty met to hear the commission's report. A week later the fol-lowing report was issued: "Citizen Duméril, having received the majority of votes at the Professorial Assembly . . . is presented to the Minister in the capacity of *chef des travaux anatomiques* in the School of Medicine of Paris."[43]

There are two sorts of reasons for examining the details of this first, critical concours for an official post in the Paris School.[44] And two sorts of inference may be drawn. One has to do with the nature of the selection process itself. Bichat was never seriously in the running, any more than at least three others who fell by the wayside in early summer of 1799. His *Treatise on Membranes* had only just appeared, too early to have been assimilated by the med-ical leadership. The nomination of two prosectors, however, cre-ated a genuine contest, one that seems to have been conducted fairly. Though the early correspondence suggested that Dupuytren would have an edge, the faculty chose Duméril for his performance in the *concours*.

A second reason for examining this affair is that it points up the sort of knowledge expected of the candidates for positions in the teaching of anatomy. Those expectations were still most congruent with the surgical anatomy of the eighteenth century, coupled with a nod to medical doctrine as far as it was reflected in practical chemical methods of anatomical preservation. Less than a year earlier Pinel had pleaded for a single science of pathology that could undergird the ideological foundations of the new School. The tissue pathology of Bichat was ultimately to provide that new science, but it was too early for this new constellation of ideas to have begun to seep into the anatomical tradition. The latter tradition was now, if anything, growing stronger in the *Ecole pratique*. Bichat himself was still teaching it in his own private courses in anatomy.

1801

The situation a year and a half later, when the next major anatomical post became vacant, was a good deal more ambiguous and complicated. Paul Mahon died in the early winter of 1801. With Pinel and the others, Mahon had been a member of the commission responsible for the quiet manifesto urging development of a new pathology. His death now left vacant the position of adjunct professor of anatomy and physiology. In the middle of February Thouret recorded in the faculty minutes the progress that had been made toward replacing Mahon. The names of ten candidates had been suggested by various members of the faculty, including, notably, Duméril, Dupuytren, Bichat, and Anthelme Richerand (1779–1840), the rising young physician, physiologist, *idéologue*, and sometime antagonist of Bichat.

They were all youthful. Indeed, Bichat was the eldest of these four candidates. He was also now a name to be reckoned with: He had been Desault's protégé, he had successfully navigated the transition from chiefly surgical to medical interests, and he had produced an impressive stream of books and memoirs including the influential *Recherches physiologiques sur la vie et la mort*. What followed is, therefore, hardly surprising: When the faculty assembled, Bichat polled as many votes as anyone, in a tie for the highest vote count.

There was much talk of *mutation,* or internal reshuffling, the process by which Mahon had moved from the marginal professorship of historical and legal medicine into the one now left vacant.[45] The faculty met in mid-February and, by a complex rating procedure in which a lowest score denoted the highest assessment, the nineteen members in attendance narrowed the list to three candidates: Duméril and Bichat, who scored 14 points each, and Dupuytren, who scored 16 points. These were the three finalists. Beyond this the faculty assembly refused to go, leaving final selection in ministerial hands.

The matter left the ministry and its bureau of instruction with a nice dilemma. Dupuytren and Duméril were already part of the faculty system. But Dupuytren had been ranked last by the faculty. Were the faculty's assessment followed slavishly, Duméril and Bichat would have been appointed. But Bichat, a disciple of both Desault and Pinel, was still an outsider, though by now, as a member of the new *Société de l'ecole,* certainly a "near-outsider." And, while Bichat was in the process of inventing a new medicosurgical tradition, that of pathological anatomy, Duméril, who also taught at the *Muséum d'histoire naturelle,* represented an older anatomical tradition with close links to comparative anatomy, natural history, and zoology.

Intervention on Duméril's behalf came from just those quarters. Less than a week after the faculty's deliberations, Georges Cuvier (1769–1832) addressed the minister with a spirited plea for the *chef des travaux anatomiques.* Napoleon's exact contemporary, Cuvier was already a trusted colleague. They had entered the Academy of Sciences at virtually the same moment in 1795. Sixteen months later Bonaparte was to appoint Cuvier Commissioner of Public Instruction and, in 1808, to the Council of the Napoleonic Université de France. Under the Empire he would move on to a further series of influential posts including membership in the *Conseil d'état* in 1813.[46]

Though not yet ensconced in these positions, Cuvier was nonetheless, by 1801, already an influential "gatekeeper" in the scientific community. Since his youthful training in management in the 1780s at the Caroline Academy in Stuttgart, he had honed his skills in the art of administrative persuasion. "I hope you will pardon," he now wrote with practiced phrases, "the interest that the science of anatomy, and my particular attachment to Citizen Duméril, inspire in me [to take] the liberty of reminding you of his entitlements to the place of adjunct professor of anatomy and physiology. . . ." Cuvier admitted that Duméril had published nothing, but noted that in comparative anatomy "I owe him the justice of saying that a large part of my own comparative anatomy comes from him, absolutely from him. . . ."[47]

Cuvier went on to note that in the other two candidates' work there was no doubt much that was estimable. Perhaps, he declared,

Dupuytren and Bichat could even be credited with contributions that were indeed superior to Duméril's. But the object of their work was "more philosophical and medical than anatomical," while Duméril was a superb anatomist in the traditional mold: His dissecting skills and knowledge of comparative anatomy – the stamp of the natural historian – were unsurpassed. Cuvier pointed out that the new job would hardly be more lucrative, since that of *chef* had provided free lodging; this perquisite could perhaps be split off and used to help one of the other candidates. He reminded the minister that Bichat and Dupuytren, as practitioners, had more options open to them than Duméril, who lacked clinical experience. And finally, Duméril had rendered assiduous service to the School and now deserved recompense by advancement to a professorial post.[48]

Under the new Bonapartist political regime, decisions regarding appointments of this sort had often come to flow directly from the highest echelons of the bureaucracy. It was, indeed, over the First Consul's signature that Duméril's appointment came down a month later, along with that of Dupuytren to fill the slot of *chef* thus created by Duméril's promotion.[49] The upshot was that two staunch members of the School's staff had moved, through the classic system of *permutation,* to new positions that each considered a form of advancement, while Bichat remained a part of the periphery, albeit the near periphery. It seems clear in retrospect that Cuvier's intervention on Duméril's behalf was a critical if not a necessary or sole condition in preserving the latter's standing within the faculty. What is less clear is why the ministry selected Dupuytren over Bichat for the post Duméril vacated.

But there is a logic of sorts to be found in this sequence of events. There was little question even then about the importance of Bichat's innovations in tissue pathology. And there is little question now, if there was any question in 1801, about the fact that he was in the middle of creating the new medical tradition of pathological anatomy. But in the event there were two sets of inertial forces arrayed against him. One was simply the inertia of the institution itself, maintaining its integrity and internal equilibrium as the political winds outside its doors continued to shift. To retain both Duméril and Dupuytren offered a positive advantage in this regard; both had put in time and were well-known figures to others among the institution's "regulars."

Second, in a real sense, Cuvier had been right about the three candidates' relative qualifications. To bring Bichat into a position seen by many to center on traditional anatomy raised a thorny problem of institutional "fit." Pathological anatomy did not yet, after all, officially exist. That Bichat was investing it with new meaning, through a tissue pathology that could integrate surgical and medical concepts, did not immediately confer advantage when it came to perpetuating the standard regime of instruction in the medical school. Thus its proponents had to contend not only with institutional inertia but also with a sort of disciplinary inertia, of which Cuvier's patronage of Duméril was emblematic.

A still broader point may be made with respect to the manner in which Duméril and Dupuytren remained in the institution, by a form of *permutation,* while Bichat remained out. It relates to what one might call the norm of polymathy. Just weeks before the concours that I have been discussing, the *Société de l'école de médecine* had been formed to promote investigation: to foster the stretching of the bounds of knowledge by those in the School's employ, and to bring them into contact with near-outsiders, such as Bichat. But the overwhelming function of the Faculty remained, as I have said, an exoteric one: it remained a central clearing house for knowledge in other quarters. Pathological anatomy was part of that knowledge, yet officially it was not to exist in the Faculty, in fact, for decades to come.

Such a state of affairs could exist because medical knowledge had few fixed internal borders. When a concours was held it was for a faculty post in an area related in some measure to clinical knowledge, and not for a departmental or specialty position. As the 1801 concours demonstrated, there was no real "lobby" for specialized knowledge as a factor conferring added value in considering new faculty personnel. Most holders of chairs were clinicians with knowledge in a variety of areas, the best of them true polymaths. This was still the case, indeed, in 1811 when a range of candidates, most of them already active within the institution as *aides d'anatomie,* declared themselves for three vacant professorships. The candidates included important younger figures like François Magendie (1783–1855) and P. A. Béclard (1785–1825), Bichat's disciple. The victors again achieved appointment to the various posts by a process of *permutation,* still an accepted routine for selecting faculty. Indeed, the ability to range widely was still regarded at least as highly as the ability to produce breathtaking new medical theories.

What is odd is that Bichat had both abilities. But he died in 1802, having completed a remarkable corpus of work ranging over normal anatomy, normal physiology, and pathological anatomy. His work in the last of these subjects, though it never gained him a position in the faculty or even its *Ecole pratique,* nonetheless soon did become a vital part of the school's intellectual life. The scaffolding of the new pathological anatomy, erected on his several works and on his teaching, already bid fair to be that basis for a unified medicine, the common trunk Pinel had eloquently called for a few short years before.

The necessity for such a new pathological anatomy was already becoming apparent to many by the time of Bichat's death. But the importance of the new tradition was amplified a year later. In 1803 a new law was passed concerning the regulation of practice by the subclass of practitioners known as *officiers de santé.* At that point the question of what medical personnel should know became even more vexing, as I shall demonstrate in Chapter 3. And the role of the Faculty of Medicine, as it would soon once again be known, became even more that of a clearing house. Less than ever could it play the esoteric role envisioned by the founders of the *Société de l'école de médecine.*

As for Georges Cuvier and Xavier Bichat, a final, ironic counterpoint marks the curious story of men and reputations. Though two years older than Bichat, Cuvier long survived him. After Bichat's death, the famed biologist, having stepped in the path of the pathologist's career at a critical early stage, had done little or nothing to foster the tradition begun by the younger man. Three decades after Bichat's death, the biologist came to his own life's end in 1832. Bichat's body was to remain at the Saint-Catherine cemetery for another dozen years. Perhaps someone had already been told of the disappearance, or nonappearance, of Bichat's head. Whether by his own direction, or that of his heirs, no such fate was allowed to befall Cuvier's body. He was buried with an iron cage over his head.[50]

3

Pathology in the middle

Bichat's death in 1802 did not go unnoticed. While not yet a totem for the pride and aspirations of the community, he was still lamented by many in the medical community who felt a claim on his memory. But what sort of claim was it? Had Bichat's ideas, the tissue pathology and the extended canon of pathology that crystallized around his teachings, as yet become insinuated into the marrow and sinew of Paris medical thought? It is not an easy question: Pathological anatomy, ironically, had no formal institutional structure, no official vehicle, until the mid-1830s, when my story in this volume stops. Because institutional changes evolved over such a long time, conventional institutional history cannot account for many of the subtle intellectual shifts that occurred. Such approaches fail adequately to track the infiltrative process through which the internal structure and external audience of the Bichatian system grew.

Yet when people, historians or the historical actors themselves, choose their heroes, they seldom do so randomly. In surveying the growth and assimilation of Bichat's ideas, I will therefore offer not only description of that infiltrative process, but I will also tender some tentative contextual explanations *why* those ideas were appropriated in certain ways by particular groups and individuals. In this chapter and Chapter 4 I will offer such an analysis for Bichat's intellectual heirs in Napoleonic Paris. In subsequent chapters I will attempt to do the same thing for the British medical men who began to stream into France after 1814.

★ ★ ★ ★ ★

Even though Bichat's ideas on the anatomical seats of disease were already beginning to circulate in the Paris medical community, their institutional inroads are difficult to track. They worked insidiously, in the teachings, more often than not outside the Paris Faculty's official confines, of men like Gaspard Laurent Bayle (1774–1816), Pierre Béclard (1785–1825), and Théophile Laennec (1781–1826). As I noted before, formal institutional structures changed at a glacial pace. The generation in power during the Napoleonic era, and even the one that followed, saw few changes in formal curricula. Where discernible at all, those shifts in the "official" teaching of pathology were of little consequence. In those years external and internal pathology, the abstract theory of the physicians and the arch-localism of the surgeons, continued to be taught separately.

But if the intellectual inroads traced by Bichat's tissue pathology remained shallow in the early days of the Paris School, by slow degrees its features did begin to appear. How did the tradition of pathological anatomy, introduced by a man consigned at least early on to the outsider role, begin thus to deepen and reach its full amplitude? In the medical culture of Napoleonic France what allowed the new pathological anatomy to etch a permanent pattern on the map of medical thought?[1]

It seems clear that the answer lies in two aspects of the intellectual map of the Paris medical scene in the early years of the nineteenth century. First, not for many decades would pathological anatomy evolve into a separate laboratory science of the sort that physiology, for example, was about to become. Instead, pathology remained an integral part, indeed in France it was the cornerstone of clinical medicine. Hence it becomes possible to understand the observation that Laennec's *Mediate Auscultation* was most profoundly a work of pathological anatomy. I will show, in fact, that that epochal publication grew out of Laennec's pathological labors in every bit as meaningful a sense as it did out of his much briefer, roughly three-year, series of physical diagnosis experiments using the *cylindre* or stethoscope.

A second feature of the cognitive map available to guide any young, anatomically oriented French medical student during the reign of Napoleon was the choice (depending on his clinical inclinations) of what were essentially two pathologies. The first was an official, or "headquarters" pathology dominated by such surgeons as Guillaume Dupuytren (1777–1835) and his disciple Jean Cruveilhier (1791–1874), and harking back to such late eighteenth-century luminaries as Giovanni Morgagni (1682–1771) in Italy or Matthew Baillie (1761–1823) in England. This official pathology continued to dominate the Paris faculty; it was essentially that taught in its courses in "external pathology" as well as in the all-important pathological components of instruction in the *Ecole Pratique*.[2]

The new pathology of Bichat, Gaspard Bayle (1774–1816), and Théophile Laennec (1781–1826) did not, on the other hand, represent the old, theoretical and natural historical "internal" pathology still taught in somewhat creaky fashion by various lights (including Philippe Pinel) of the Paris faculty.[3] It grew up, rather, in the interstices of the system: in the several private courses in pathological anatomy taught by Laennec and others, in the memoirs presented to the equally diverse newly formed medical societies, and in the contributions found in the pages of journals such as Jean Corvisart's (1755–1821) and Alexis Boyer's (1757–1831) authoritative *Journal de médecine, chirurgie, pharmacie etc.* That said, it is probably better to look upon the official, surgically oriented pathology as one pole of a spectrum that found its opposite pole in the new pathology adumbrated by Xavier Bichat in 1799.

No doubt one reason for the lugubrious pace at which Bichatian pathology was incorporated was the fact that, while it partook of some of the localism of official, surgically oriented "external" pathology, it was as almost nonvisual as the old, general "internal" pathology of the physicians. Indeed, the visual and pictorial characteristics of the pathologists' labors as they evolved along this spectrum supply useful clues to understanding the morbid appearances as they appeared to those learning and teaching pathological anatomy. For that field became an ever more visual one in ensuing decades; there is a certain irony to explaining this (with normal anatomy) most graphic and depictive of the medical sciences in purely verbal terms.

One might begin to foster such a visual understanding of this scale of possible pathologies by comparing styles of illustrations. Bichat and Cruveilhier represent the antipodes of the available approaches. For artistic depiction of the pathological changes so laboriously described in both works, Bichat observed the principle of parsimony. His art budget was admirably low. He omitted illustrations. In Cruveilhier's *Pathological Anatomy of the Human Body* (Fig. 3.1), by contrast, the picture told (and was designed to tell) much of the tale. It would have served well as an atlas, not merely of pathological anatomy, but also of normal anatomy and indeed of surgical anatomy, stopping just short of serving the operative surgeon as well.

★   ★   ★   ★   ★

I purposely choose styles of illustration, from Bichat to Cruveilhier, that span precisely the chronological period with which my discussion is concerned. It would be an easy assumption to seize on the *cognitive* scale subtended by these two ways of seeing pathological anatomy, and to translate it into a *developmental* scale: to infer a genetic principle whereby the nonvisual evolved into the visual. That is a tempting, classic error. For when all is said and done it will not be Cruveilhier, the grand pictorialist of disease, but Théophile Laennec, more modestly depictive, who brings the narrative to a close. Cruveilhier's *Anatomy* may be seen as the limiting case, and probably the perfection, of an official pathology that, while it never entirely faded from a central institutional po-

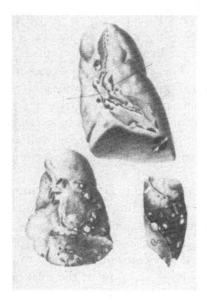

Figure 3.1. See text

sition, eventually did so intellectually. It would prove to be Laennec's *Mediate Auscultation,* as a work of pathological anatomy, that provided the synthesis and hence the culmination of the process by which the new, Bichatian pathology was slowly integrated into the older, organ-based model.

In the following sections I will show how it became possible for a variety of ecumenically minded medical men to combine and recombine various elements of the official pathology and the new pathology. I will suggest that it was both professionally and intellectually decisive that they had the option to amalgamate the surgical and medical approaches at the actual level of *explaining disease processes.* I contend it became increasingly expedient, for physicians in particular, to demonstrate the utility of a localizationalist approach in the practice of internal medicine. Finally, I show how the new pathology remained, even in the hands of Laennec himself, and despite its growing acceptance, an "exoteric" body of knowledge: innovation that continued to be generated at the periphery and imported as needed into the central "knowledge-processing" institutions.

THE DYNAMICS OF CHANGE

From the earliest days of the new Paris Faculty to Michel Thouret's death in 1810, and arguably for another decade yet to come, the inner dynamic of Paris medicine was determined by three crosscutting sets of forces. The first, already sketched briefly earlier, involved the stabilization of expectations and resources within the Faculty itself. These pressures were largely economic, centering on the distribution of state resources between the education sector and others (notably the military), as well as within each educational subsector such as medicine, law, engineering, and science.

For Thouret and the members of his faculty, this meant constantly exercising vigilance, the minding of fences, and demonstrating the ever-felt need for expansion. Garnering the several academic coins of the realm, salaries, key "gatekeeper" positions, bricks and mortar, also served as a constant source of motivation to expand the circle of knowledge and power, the relationship of one to the other understood intuitively. The new system of centrally supported medical education was one of the first cases in which the state made demands, impersonal and essentially devoid of cognitive content, that were passed through to a faculty body which, as though by some strange alchemy, might then transmute them into a coherent system of shared ideas and favored beliefs about the body's ills.

In the two decades after the Revolution, then, there were forces that fostered conservative, dogged tendencies among the Paris medical elite and especially among its knowledge brokers in the Faculty. Another, second set of forces, however, affecting the evolution of Paris medicine, grew out of just the opposite pressures to create innovation in the intellectual content of medicine. Medical theory, I will contend, was not merely a sort of *jeu* for the well-placed elite of French medicine, who had the luxury and time to speculate on the arcane reaches of pathology. It was also, and most significantly, a cognitive product with direct implications both for practice and for the structure of the profession.

What I want to emphasize, however, concerning these pressures to innovate is not just the new pathology in and of itself, but also the location of its production and, most important, the directions in which innovation flowed. Under Napoleon a vigorous countercurrent of thought developed in support of the notion that the Paris faculty might appropriately function as a key vehicle for research progress: what was commonly called *perfectionnement de l'art*. Such sentiments could be heard being voiced most passionately in the precincts of the medical faculty, at the meetings of the *Société de l'ecole de médecine* and the *Société d'anatomie*.

The two societies deserve close scrutiny. Had their organizers fully realized their aspirations, the Paris medical faculty would have become the very epicenter of the center, since the city of Paris had within a decade achieved recognition as the capital of progress in the practical sciences. But this current of ideas, suggesting that ideas should be created in the center and flow centrifugally outward toward the periphery, remained generally a narrowly held one, confined to a few organizers within the faculty. Poised against it was a broad array of centripetal streams of entrepreneurial effort, exemplified by those who, like Bichat before them, innovated for the preparation of their *cours libres* and then filled their monographs with the ideas they wished to disseminate. These men provided the ideas and techniques that "perfected the art" and, if adopted by the Faculty, brought their authors notoriety, perhaps even an eventual Faculty appointment.

A third set of forces was unleashed when the timeworn issue of surgery, medicine, and the proper relations between them, pitted medicosurgical ecumenicists against separatists. Since the reforms envisioned by Pinel and Fourcroy, and then sparked by the Revolution itself, there had been no dearth of detractors. Now, in the new age, those opponents of medicosurgical integration found themselves in the rear guard. They were no less vociferous for it; their brief hinged in part on the argument that the amount of overlap between the two professions was not significant enough to maintain integrated curricula. Thouret, Fourcroy, and their allies depended upon making the countervailing argument: that undergirding medicine and surgery was a common foundation of ideas about disease. For surgeon and physician alike, they felt, such pathological ideas would have to be so close to coextensive that to sunder them risked doing irrevocable violence to the medical man's proper understanding of the true order of nature.

THE GODFATHER

Medical historians take as a virtual given the role of Jean Corvisart in stimulating the practice of physical diagnosis. Through his 1808 translation of Leopold Auenbrugger's (1722–1809) *Inventum Novum,* and through his reintroduction of Auenbrugger's method of percussion in his own *Essay on Diseases of the Heart* (1806, 1818, 1839), Corvisart has been recognized as a major source of impetus for the integration of pathological anatomy and physical diagnosis. The active ferreting out of antemortem findings and careful description of morbid appearances postmortem: these are well and properly identified as among Corvisart's influential early extensions of the Bichatian method into the semiology of the living patient, into the search for signs of disease.[4]

Corvisart also deserves to be known, however, for his role as a benign ecumenical presence, the vigorous yet conservative champion of the new medicine, linking the Napoleonic bureaucracy and patronage system with both the mandarins and the footsoldiers of the Paris medical community. In 1799, when the *coup d'état* of Brumaire catapulted Napoleon into power through the establishment of the Consulate, Corvisart was already in his mid-forties and (since 1797) holder of two key chairs: the centrally important physician's chair of *clinique interne* at the recently renamed *Ecole de médecine,* and the medical chair at the *Collège de France.*[5] Now, with Pierre Barthez (1734–1806), he was named both government physician and chief physician to the First Consul.[6]

Two years later, in 1801, his power assured, Corvisart took further steps that would position him perfectly to play the role of godfather. The two measures, separated by no more than a few months, were his assumption of both the sponsorship of a new medical organization, the *Société d'instruction médicale,* and the editorship (with Boyer) of the crucially important *Journal de médecine.* The *Société d'instruction* was one of several new societies arising to satisfy an array of newly identified (or redefined) needs.[7] Though not necessarily more influential than some of the others, the *Société d'instruction* nonetheless added to Corvisart's lengthening list of platforms from which to oversee the progress of the new medicine, and a money prize, the *prix d'encouragement,* was furnished by the state for the production of innovative medical ideas and methods.

Corvisart was a member of all the organizations, and with his second major new activity of 1801, the journal editorship, he secured his near-Olympian status as adjudicator and publisher, with Boyer and shortly thereafter, with Thouret's successor J. J. Leroux as a third editor, of technical innovations, manifestos for educational change, sundry disputes, reviews, and news of the profession.[8] In its first number, Corvisart and his colleagues set forth their conception of the function of a medical journal:

A journal of medicine is a type of *public bureau,* where each company of men, cultivating medicine and the accessory sciences of this art, where each author . . . can fix a date [of priority] for his work. . . . It should offer the means of remaining up-to-date. [In footnote] We declare once and for all, that we give the name of Medicine to any man having demonstrated a degree of knowledge and possessing a legal title, whatever part of the healing art he practices.[9]

As if to underscore the ecumenicism announced in their journal's title, the editors went on to admonish themselves publicly about the risks of confining the data they intended to publish to one hospital, the *Charité,* or as it was then known in the temporary rhetoric of revolution, the *Unité,* and to two professional groups. But the journal should serve as a depository, they declared, for others' work from a wide range of institutions, augmenting that work "to lead to a single goal: *the interest of medicine,* and, by necessary extension, *the interest of the sick.*"[10] But the interest of medicine, it soon developed, did not always imply absolute unanimity of opinion. Rather, Corvisart and Boyer wished to offer clinicians and pathological anatomists, be they physicians or surgeons, a sphere of neutral territory in which to articulate their views.

If those views differed, as would soon be the case between Laennec and Dupuytren (I will return momentarily to their dispute), the editors would remain impartial, allowing the open expression of opposing, if not indeed hostile, views. It was through his carefully nurtured position above the fray, even more than his equally carefully modulated support of the new pathology (or any other single innovation), that Corvisart created a critically important forum. It was a locus for hammering out territorial issues, thorny questions of how expertise ought to be distributed, without the combatants demanding total submission or, perhaps worse, simply seceding from the intellectual game.

To Corvisart and his small circle of protégés and colleagues the winter and early spring of 1801 were critical. The winter term of that academic year, a period always devoted to feverish anatomical activities in anticipation of the putrid deadhouse summers, was part of Bichat's last full year in Paris. The young pathological anatomist was giving, for what seems like the last time, his private winter *cours particulier* in normal and pathological anatomy. At about the same time, Théophile Laennec arrived in the capital. Within a month, in early May, the young Breton had registered at the *Ecole de médecine,* started to follow Corvisart's *clinique interne* at the *Charité,* and, on the side, begun following the private anatomy course organized by Guillaume Dupuytren. Dupuytren, it will be recalled, had also just been named *chef des travaux anatomiques* at the *Ecole pratique,* after the revealing *concours,* discussed in the last chapter, in which the faculty selected him over Bichat.

The stage was set. The key actors were in place. Corvisart, secure in his several roles, presided benignly over the process by which a fractious medical community squabbled but ordinarily sought consensus where possible. Bichat was approaching the point of his own final illness. Gaspard Laurent Bayle, in Paris since 1798, joined Dupuytren and Laennec in the *tour de main,* the round of dissections and anatomy courses that formed the unstructured but essential basis for the several possible configurations of pathological anatomy. In another two years new alliances would begin to form, shift, and re-form. Dupuytren would, in 1803, add the duties of assistant surgeon at the Hôtel-Dieu to those of *chef*, and would take on Bayle as his *aide d'anatomie* at the *Ecole pratique*. Laennec would take his medical doctorate, win both first prizes offered by the Institute of France in clinical medicine, for internal medicine and for surgery, and would then, at year's end, begin his own course in pathological anatomy.[11]

Those inclined toward the study of internal medicine, exemplified by Laennec, and those favoring the study of surgery, exemplified by Dupuytren, saw the body in different ways. The discrepancies in their daily rounds and the cases they saw insured such discordant perceptions. Yet they had found, in pathological anatomy, a common language. Within that language it soon became clear there was room for dialectical variation and tension. Part of the purpose of the remainder of this chapter is to describe and explain that variation in terms of the factions that continued over the next generation to propagate their own, parochial interests within the larger medical community. But an equally important purpose is to discover how this *lingua franca* cohered and, in so doing, served to buoy the larger community by binding physicians and surgeons into an integrated professional body.

THE FORMATION OF NEW SOCIETIES

The abolition of the academies and corporations in the early 1790s had left an organizational void that many acknowledged would have to be filled through one means or another. In the decade between the establishment of the *Ecoles de santé* and Bonaparte's 1804 coronation as Emperor, a spate of new societies were created. They replaced and reinforced some of the important internal elements of the medical community's badly eroded old superstructure. Coalescing around each of the potential interests of the community, several student groups came together around 1800, and so, too, did several faculty organizations.[12] In the former group figured the *Société d'instruction médicale*, formed around students in the clinics; the *Société médicale d'émulation*, particularly imbued with Bichatian lore and soon in turn emulated by the faculty and students of Edinburgh; the *Cercle médicale*, a shadowy group that is difficult to trace in detail, and the *Société d'anatomie*, a particularly intriguing group composed of students of the *Ecole pratique*.[13]

Of the new faculty-dominated societies the most important was already mentioned in connection with Corvisart, the *Société de l'ecole de médecine de Paris*. Formed, as one observer noted, in order "to console *la science* for the loss of the former Royal Society [of Medicine], and of the Academy of Surgery," this Society was pulled together at the behest of the Interior Minister, Napoleon's brother Lucien Bonaparte.[14] The internal arrangements of the *Société de l'ecole de médecine de Paris* were carefully laid out so that political balances would be struck between both medicine and surgery, and between the faculty and outside medical savants. It comprised forty associate members: the twenty-four professors of the *Ecole de médecine;* its librarian; the *chef des travaux anatomiques;* several *docteurs–régents* of the old, *ancien régime* faculty; members of the former academy and college of surgery and of the Royal Society of Medicine; as well as selected "*savans*" [sic] of the "accessory sciences to the healing arts."[15] In addition sixteen adjunct members were planned to be chosen from the coterie of rising young physicians and surgeons practicing in the Paris community.[16]

Though its makeup was carefully designed to be ecumenical, the Society's first charge from Lucien Bonaparte echoed the old Royal Society's mission. This was made explicit when, on June 15, 1800, the Interior Minister wrote to a group of interested physicians,

I invite you to occupy yourselves without interruption to carefully collect and compile the topographical descriptions that had begun with the Society of Medicine. . . . [T]he observations that you will gather will have as their principal object that which relates to the salubriousness of the air, dietetic regime, the nature of nutriments, physical education, and so on. . . . If the means at your command are insufficient . . . I will with pleasure procure for you all those available to me. . . . The Society will undertake a correspondence with the doctors and physicians of the Departements.[17]

By October the faculty had filled out ranks of the Society in such a way as to bring its total membership to forty-three and to insure the presence of the requisite expertise in climatological medicine. This expertise was of the classic, Hippocratic sort, based on a natural historical model of describing and classifying disease, and was about as far from the new pathology as one could get.

French governments both before and since the Revolution could predictably be expected, however, to require medical experts drawn particularly from the physicians' ranks, much as the battlefield practice could be expected to draw from the surgeons', to limn the "medical constitutions of Paris" or of other French locales and regions. This longstanding patronage was again now given formal structure through the channels of the new Society. The net effect was to create small informal networks of observers who could be relied on by the Society, and by Corvisart, publishing their findings in his journal, to provide the detailed medical reports and natural historical findings regularly expected by the government.

The initial collaborators in the project were J. J. Leroux, Gaspard Laurent Bayle, Louis-Aimé Fizeau (1775–1864), and Théophile Laennec.[18] Hence the outwardly (and probably also in many respects inwardly) ecumenical Society of the Paris School of Medicine served as the nexus for individuals with two interlocking sets of interests. The first was *"perfectionnement de l'art,"* the euphemism for what later came to be known as research, and a sure boost for an academic career. The second interest lay in locating research that reflected physicians', rather than surgeons', habits of thought. It was no more of an accident and no more incongruous that the most important champions of Bichatian pathology grew out of this concertedly *medical* milieu than it was that Laennec published his first major piece of theoretical medical writing on the doctrine of Hippocrates.

For physicians jealous of old prerogatives, dimly remembered from the *ancien régime,* the *Société de l'ecole de médecine* was a link with the past. Equally important, it was a careful and measured attempt to hold on for the day when the Paris medical elite would return to function as a cadre of expert investigators. Both the membership and the immediate activities of the *Société de l'ecole* reflected such a role. The *Société d'anatomie* complemented the role perfectly. Less information is available with which to trace the details of this organization's history between 1803, when it was founded by Dupuytren and others, and 1809, when it ceased to exist. But the broad outlines of its program are nonetheless available in the manuscript notes for the welcoming address delivered, probably by Théophile Laennec, at the beginning of academic year 1808–1809.[19]

At this first meeting of the new term in 1808, the member-initiates of the *Société d'anatomie* heard Laennec tell something of their organization's history and a summary of its mission. The purpose of the society, he declared, was to review anatomical cases

in detail and at length. In most cases these cases would be expected
to illustrate well-known lesions and anomalies. Repetition would
and should not be penalized. It should be understood, Laennec
noted, that this was not a *société savante*. Its membership, therefore,
need not be confined to some tiny, investigative elite, but, to the
extent that students' fitful interest allowed, open to all anatomically
inclined young physicians and medical students interested in self-
instruction in this growing field. To such an end, newly registered
students in the *Ecole pratique* and hospital *internes* were invited to
join, with former years' members carried as "resident members"
and the newly fledged as "associate members"; the former made
the rules.[20]

A major purpose of the *Société d'anatomie,* then, was to reach
out to rank and file students in the *Ecole pratique,* and to inculcate
the basic tenets of both normal anatomy and the nascent science
of pathological anatomy. But exactly what sort of anatomy did
the leaders of the *Société d'anatomie* want to foster? At pains to
orient the new members to the style and outlook of their predecessors, Laennec created a window through which the future historian might recover the meaning of anatomy outside the rigid
central curriculum. As befit the circle of individuals centered at
the *Ecole pratique,* the vision of anatomy Laennec now described
was far broader than that offered at the central school, its ancient
name of faculty of medicine now restored.[21]

With a nod to the organization's founder and erstwhile opponent
Dupuytren, Laennec noted first that the society could be expected
from time to time to occupy itself with comparative anatomy,
though the emphasis must remain human anatomy. Still, "no one,"
he emphasized, "can ignore the light shed on human anatomy [by]
the dissection of animals and the comparative examination of the
organs of one and another [of them]." He went on to discuss briefly
what he called "practical anatomy and physiology," which he ad-
vised his new colleagues to study "in all their extent" as "sciences
worthy of full attention and meditation of the physician who is
truly worthy of that name." This approach, one may infer with
reasonable certainty, was the standard, dissection-oriented anatomy
of the *Ecole pratique,* as taught by the various aides, prosectors,
and the *chef* himself.[22]

Laennec laid out the proper path to be taken. The "objects of
study" mentioned thus far, he insisted, were not the only preoccupations of the *Société d'anatomie.* "A vista [*carrière*] more vast,

more fecund, and richer, especially, in facts immediately applicable to clinical medicine opens up beyond them. I mean to speak of pathological anatomy[,] of this science without which diagnosis [is] always either impossible or prone to uncertainty." Opening up cadavers and communicating one's findings to like-minded colleagues, these were the only means of refining the advance intelligence available from the few extant texts and of bringing precision to clinical medicine. The diagnostic certainty gained would astonish those finding it more convenient to heap scorn on anatomical studies than to engage in them. The foundation of the society's activities was bedside observation followed by postmortem examination.[23]

What is most striking in Laennec's presentation of anatomy is the manner in which it extended Bichat's model of pathology to link pathological anatomy with the clinic. Not just professionally but also conceptually, they were, he felt, a seamless whole, inseparable in practice and in theory. At the same time it must be said that, while Laennec was pushing pathology in the direction of bedside internal medicine, the same claim could be made for surgery. Dupuytren's move in 1812 to the surgery chair vacated by Raphael Sabatier (1732–1811), for example, was analogous in important respects. But there was a major difference in style between the pathological anatomy identified with Dupuytren and that identified with Bayle and Laennec. The former spread his version far and wide through his domination of teaching at the Paris Faculty and the Hôtel-Dieu, consistently emphasizing applications to the surgeon's craft. He wrote little or nothing on pathological anatomy, though he had projected a *Traité d'anatomie pathologique* as early as 1803.[24] For their part, Bayle and Laennec disseminated their version, as had Bichat, through extensive publication as well as through the private courses in which the new pathology was tested and expanded.

DUPUYTREN VERSUS BAYLE AND LAENNEC

The tensions between medical and surgical cultures persisted from the *ancien régime* into the Napoleonic period. It is probably not putting too fine an edge on it to see those tensions mirrored in the differing interpretations given pathology by Dupuytren, on the one hand, and Bayle and Laennec on the other. If the sense of polar opposition between the two camps seems forced, it is no doubt partly due to the dearth of text on the one side and the plethora of it on the other. Yet there are ways of smoothing out this seeming asymmetry between surgical pathologists who practiced without writing and pathological anatomists who wrote prolifically. All of them made programmatic statements at one time or another about the nature of pathological anatomy. In such statements one finds important clues, even among the laconic surgeons, to the manner in which each group chose to "read" the morbid appearances of the human body.

In late 1801 or early 1802 Dupuytren, recently appointed *chef des travaux anatomiques,* reported to the assembled members of the *Ecole de Médecine* on pathological anatomy as he saw the field developing. Exemplar of what was to become the school's official pathology, Dupuytren defined the field clearly and simply as what the *Ecole pratique* actually did on a day-to-day basis: dissect myriad cadavers, and then identify the morbid appearances in the organs of the deceased. Pathological anatomy sustained an important, but purely operational and subsidiary role in the institutional economy. Dupuytren employed certain graphic *tableaux* as *aides-mémoires* to direct the pathological anatomist's work, summarized as follows:

1. Indicate the respective number of lesions in involved organs and apparatus, to further the work of the physiologist (who seeks causes of disease) and the clinician (who seeks means of preventing or curing disease).
2. Determine the nature of affections in each organ and compare them with those found in other organs.
3. Establish the simultaneous presence of lesions in different organ systems –for example, fatty liver in association with pulmonary phthisis – to furnish physiologist and clinician glimpses of the reciprocal influences between those organs.
4. Arrange the morbid appearances in a nosological order [so as to] render the classification of disease more exact; peripneumonia, for example, should be defined in patients with typically indurated lung parenchyma, even in those cases lacking the classic symptoms.
5. Avoid attempting to assign the proximate cause of death; the causes of certain lesions of organs may be expected to be different from the primary disease process.
6. Correlate lesions observed in large numbers of patients postmortems with the seasons in which they died; these "anatomical constitutions" should be coextensive with the "medical constitutions" observed by physicians.
7. Correlate the lesions of patients with their age and sex; particularities of organization may be found to obtain in the fetus, the child, and so on.[25]

It is readily apparent that Dupuytren's last three desiderata for the pathological anatomist were equally as applicable to the physician's work as they were to the surgeon's, if not more so. Indeed, a physician in the amphitheater listening to Dupuytren would have found little if anything objectionable, especially when the latter elaborated on the subject of pathological anatomy in the service of nosology. But in Dupuytren's lexicon there was no overarching theory of pathological anatomy, no intrinsic notion of the body economy, that could serve to redirect the physiologist's or clinician's conception of disease. For the surgical pathologist the lesion, the local morbid appearances, dictated the nature of the disease as well as the intervention most likely to be beneficial.

In 1802, though, Dupuytren saw pathological anatomy not as a field with its own separate existence, but as an auxiliary of the clinic, no doubt most especially the surgical clinic that he would soon undertake at the Hôtel-Dieu. Even his staunchest supporters recognized this. His disciple and main beneficiary in the new chair of pathological anatomy, Jean Cruveilhier, would later write that the chief reproach to Dupuytren was in acting as though *"la chirurgie, c'est moi."*[26] And, again, there was that final irony: It was ultimately Dupuytren whose financial legacy would, some three decades later, establish the new science of morbid appearances, "so long an accessory to the pathology and clinic courses," as a separate discipline within the Paris faculty.[27]

At the same time that Dupuytren, from his vantage point of *chef,* was holding forth on pathological anatomy, Théophile Laennec, four years younger and still a student in the *clinique interne,* was investigating a critical pathological issue: inflammation of the peritoneal membrane enveloping the abdominal cavity. In an age in which tuberculous and suppurative diseases dominated, his interest was especially appropriate. "Under the eyes of Professors Corvisart and Leroux," Laennec detailed several cases of young males, ranging in age from seven to forty, suffering from *douleur de ventre,* abdominal pain. Vivid descriptions of these patients' agonies, "uttering horrible cries and the whole body trembling," were followed by the ritual *ouvertures de cadavres.* In these Laennec demonstrated the inflammation of the serous membranes, their relations to the mucous membranes, and the presence of the "false," adventitious, or "accidental" membranes (the shaggy, organized pseudomembranes), that so often appeared in such cases.[28]

In the next volume of Corvisart's journal, taking pains to address his remarks directly to Dupuytren, Laennec expanded these observations to the affections of membranous sheaths of other viscera as well, discussing, for example, the state of "carnification" of the pleura in certain peripneumonias. Haller and Bordeu, he declared, had been too vague on these subjects, as had all other authors;

"that is why I decided to describe them and to offer this description to you."[29]

Dupuytren's immediate reaction can only be guessed. What followed in 1803 and 1804, however, when Laennec established his own private course in pathological anatomy, can be traced in detail. Corvisart, scrupulously maintaining neutrality, published blow and counterblow in his journal. That Laennec's incursions into anatomical science rankled Dupuytren deeply now became plain to see. Late in December of 1804 Laennec stood before the *Société de l'ecole de médecine* and presented a broad, programmatic statement on pathological anatomy. By now he was a *docteur–médecin,* recent laureate of the both medical and surgical first prizes, with his private course now well on the way to a second cycle of dissection lessons. In his lecture to the society recognized as the elite most devoted to "the perfection of the art," research, Laennec laid out a classification of disease that was both eclectic and venturesome (Fig. 3.2). It was a framework for not merely describing but attempting to understand the morbid appearances seen at autopsy. The essentials of this framework were to remain fixed in his and others' minds for the rest of his career.[30]

What Laennec said to the *Société de l'ecole de médecine* was this. Morgagni's successors, in France and abroad, had refined and extended his knowledge of pathological anatomy without really "coordinating its materials through systematic linkages." Bichat had sensed this deficit and attempted to rectify it, providing the initial basis in the *Treatise on Membranes* (none of this had ever been mentioned by Dupuytren), and extending it in the *General Anatomy.* "Each mode of lesion," for Bichat, "always offers the same observations in all organs belonging to the same system." Bichat had thereby himself fallen heir to certain errors because he had imputed to each system a large number of unique affections, and, further, had reduced the number of general or common affections to two, inflammation and scirrhus (*squirrhe*).[31]

Repeated pathological dissection, however, now disclosed to Laennec a more complicated system. The four possible sorts of pathological "alterations" included those of nutrition, form or position, foreign bodies (be they inanimate or, a favorite of Laennec's, invading insects and worms), and, lastly, alterations of texture. The term "texture," used particularly in English-language treatments of tissues, was synonymous with the array of tissues and membranes emphasized in the new pathology. And it was precisely

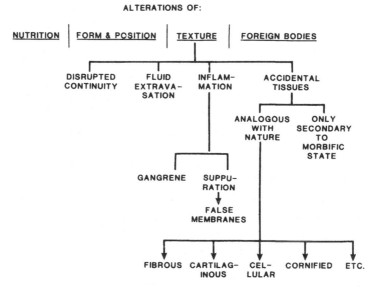

Figure 3.2. Partial schematic of Laennec's system of classifying tissues and disease states, emphasizing specific disorders of "textures" (tissues). Note Laennec's attention to membranes exhibiting property of analogy between normal and morbid states, and those not occurring in nature.

this category of pathological alterations that Laennec now proceeded to develop, in the 1804 presentation and thereafter. He divided tissue changes into four subgroups, with the "accidental" tissue, such as tubercle, looming as the most important. "It is mainly in this last order of lesions," he wrote, "that one encounters the most pervasive, the most deadly, and the most difficult to distinguish of them all."[32]

Angered at what he perceived to be usurpation, Dupuytren felt compelled to counterattack. He had always harbored esteem and admiration toward Laennec, he declared. But now it was necessary to claim priority for the ideas Laennec had enunciated, precisely and only because Laennec had pointedly proclaimed himself the first to have presented this classification in his first private course. Six years before, he, Dupuytren, had projected the reorganization of pathological anatomy. He had done so after having been stimulated by reading Morgagni and hearing the lessons of Corvisart, "who, one of the first, had inspired the taste for pathological anatomy, and who joined to this first merit the merit of having created several parts of this fair science."[33]

What was more, according to Dupuytren, Laennec must have known of this project, both from Dupuytren's course that year and from his well-publicized announcement in late September, 1803, of his intention to produce the definitive *Elementary Treatise of Pathological Anatomy*. In the fall of 1804, furthermore, he, Dupuytren, had presented an overview of his principles to the *Société de l'ecole de médecine*. Laennec had written him a letter thanking him for the 1802 course taken under him, and had then proceeded to begin his own course two years later, bringing with him the precepts learned during many conferences and consultations. Many reliable sources had reported that Laennec's course included only those precepts. As for Bichat, "whose name is repeated in [Laennec's] note with an affectation whose motive everyone concedes, in my forthcoming *Treatise of Pathological Anatomy* I will render homage to [one] to whom I intended to offer it before death struck down his brilliant career; but I will praise only those things he truly accomplished." But, he hastened to add, he wished to do justice to Laennec's contributions, and would have adopted the latter's modifications of his ideas had they not been couched in such vicious terms.[34]

Later that year Laennec responded and, once more, Dupuytren countered. The charges and countercharges became even more shrill in this last published exchange, also aired in Corvisart's *Journal*. Laennec found Dupuytren and his work "estimable," but the latter's "rather strange assertions" attacking Laennec's personal character did not establish his priority. The published record must tell the tale, Laennec pointed out, though he also took some pains to exonerate his role in the activities behind the scenes, in the earlier courses and dissection rooms. "I declare in advance," concluded Laennec, "that I will respond no further" to additional charges.[35] Dupuytren responded with claims to priority on all counts, including publication, and with charges of treason: Laennec had come into the inner sanctum, promised to collaborate, in a subordinate role, on a textbook, and had further promised to supply a series of observations on the affections of serous membranes, important observations, no doubt, but observations never delivered as promised.[36]

In tracing this steamy little dispute, I have no desire to establish "anteriority" as claimed by either party. The point is how such a priority dispute illuminates the distinctions between habits of thought and styles of investigation exemplified in individuals who came to count as archetypes of different parts of the medical community. Throughout the dispute the opponents were talking past one another. Laennec's views were more theoretical in content, and he underscored this fact by locating himself consciously in the wake of the newly emerging tradition symbolized by the figure of Xavier Bichat. He spoke, in a way, like a member of a political party that was powerful but unencumbered by public office. Without having to run an *Ecole pratique,* Laennec was freer to stretch the bounds of the very meaning of pathology, rendering it more anatomical than the nosological and semiotic school of Philippe Pinel, yet more theoretical and holistic, more oriented to the "body economic," than that of Dupuytren and his fellow surgeons.

★ ★ ★ ★ ★

Laennec was as good as his word. He never did respond further in print to Dupuytren's accusations. But years later, in 1812, Laennec was asked to write a summary of pathological anatomy for the *Dictionary of Medical Sciences* of Adelon et al. Though he included the early piece, the piece that had so annoyed Dupuytren, nearly verbatim from the *Journal de Médecine,* he changed a few things. He expanded upon the most complex and ramified part of the classification, the accidental tissues, in the terms incorporated in Figure 3.1. He used language that provides a clue to the gradual development of his thinking in pathology over the years prior to his discovery, just four years later (1816), of the stethoscope.[37] And, a minor but telling point, he expunged Dupuytren from his own account: In 1803–1804 he had written of the parallel discoveries, by Xavier Bichat and Rene Dupuytren, of accidental (that is, ectopic or clearly abnormal) serous and mucous membranes in, respectively, certain cystic tumors and certain fistula tracts. Now, in 1812, Laennec credited the latter discovery to John Hunter.[38]

After 1804, despite the growing recognition of his ideas on pathology, Laennec was constrained for financial reasons to go into private practice. Hence it is no great surprise that his ideas on pathological anatomy evolved more rapidly before 1804 than afterwards, and that the similarities between the two versions of the essential text outweigh the differences. The most striking feature among their similarities is the use, evident in 1804 and even more so in 1812, of the metaphor of the "body economy." The point of pathological anatomy, he asserted, was to create a framework for understanding disease based on firm observation and fashioned for appropriate application to practical medicine. Accomplishing this goal would mean distinguishing those *genres* of tissue pathology that would likely lead to different outcomes (*terminaisons*), and distinguishing different alterations of tissues according to "their different effects on the body economy." Although it might be possible to "map" this quintessentially internal medical approach onto any number of political or socioeconomic trends of the Napoleonic period, I prefer simply to map it onto the daily exigencies of the practicing physician. The internal medicine Laennec now practiced full-time, demanded that he think of the body in an ecological and economic, as opposed to an extirpative and hence exclusively localistic manner. What the new pathology did, by distributing the several essential tissue types through the body, was allow physicians to localize disease and yet generalize its consequences.

Like Dupuytren, and unlike Bichat or Laennec, Gaspard Laurent Bayle left few textual clues to his interpretation of the anatomicoclinical method espoused by the several stalwarts of the new pathology. As Ackerknecht has noted, Bayle produced only one monograph, the influential but highly focused *Researches on Pulmonary Phthisis,* which was in turn drawn from his presentations of a large series of *Charité* hospital cases in November 1809 through January 1810. Personally and professionally Bayle found himself trapped in a delicate position between Dupuytren and Laennec. But so far as it was applicable, Bayle adhered closely to the general outlines of the emerging framework represented by the latter's pathological classification of disease.[39] In a concluding section, for example, he described a series of cases of "chronic pleurisies [*pleuritides*] that one might have mistaken for phthisis."[40]

Illustrative is one of Bayle's clinical cases, that of the unfortunate young coachman Antoine C., probably suffering from an abscessed right lung, with severe pleuritis. Four years earlier, at age twenty-eight, the patient had experienced the onset of cough and malaise, progressing slowly and inexorably downhill, becoming marasmic and edematous, and finally expiring on the nineteenth of May in his thirty-third year. At autopsy the right pleura was opaque, white, and greatly thickened, while the lung parenchyma within, its architecture all but destroyed, was covered with a white accidental membrane masking the shrunken viscus inside. The patient did not have tuberculosis, noted Bayle, but a chronic pleuritic condition mimicking its symptoms. "If we had made but a superficial examination of the chest at the time of autopsy, we would have been intimately persuaded that the malady was truly a phthisis that had completely destroyed one of the lungs."[41]

In a companion piece to one written by Laennec in Adelon's *Dictionary,* Bayle further expanded on the utility of the new pathology for clinicians. What Bichat had done in systematizing the tissues of the body economy, and what Laennec had done for the classification of diseases based on Bichat's system, Bayle now did for the categories of clinical reasoning about the framework of pathological anatomy. He first distinguished between two sorts of lesions. Vital lesions derived from perversions of vital properties and were not ascertainable at death. That left only organic or physical lesions as the province of pathological anatomy. Clinical observation allowed the physician to infer certain vital lesions, while both clinical observation and the opening of cadavers allowed him to infer physical lesions. Somehow one had next to link symptoms with the organic lesions that could cause them.[42]

From this point of view, Bayle noted, there were three sets of conditions under which pathological anatomy should become instrumental for clinical reasoning. First, in instances similar to those described in the example drawn from the phthisis monograph, symptomatology often misled the physician when similar symptoms accompany clinical presentations with discordant causes: Symptoms alone were insufficient to distinguish such specific conditions. Second and conversely, differing symptoms may proceed among different patients from similar underlying diseases and similar specific lesions. Finally, in a sense synthesizing these points, Bayle provided a rule of thumb for denominating specific diseases: A condition observed in two different patients could be counted the same if the presence of both the same symptoms and the same underlying lesions could be determined.[43] A process of mutual or "reciprocal rectification" (the term is Bayle's) allowed the clinician, who was also the pathological anatomist, to move usefully back and forth between antemortem findings (Bayle's "physical symptoms") and the postmortem examination.[44]

Bayle added some additional diagnostic caveats to his classification of anatomoclinical reasoning. Two in particular stand out. The anatomical lesion, he noted, establishes the class and possibly the specific type of a disease entity, but not its origin. Final causes must remain obscure. So, too, in many instances, must *immediate* causes. It is often impossible to state the nature of the terminal event; only the organic lesions that (presumably) preexisted are discernible, and it is assumed they become causes of death only through some sort of mediating mechanism. Only rarely are the organic and inciting (that is, inciting to death) lesions one and the same, as, for example, in cases of ruptured aneurysm or acute cerebral hemorrhage.[45]

For Bayle, then, pathological anatomy was the touchstone of diagnosis, though he agreed with Laennec that there were many remaining areas of uncertainty and gaps left unfilled. Bayle and Laennec embodied pathological anatomy at the point to which it had developed in the late years of the Empire, just as Bichat was the avatar of medical change in the early Napoleonic years. By degrees, the tissue pathology adumbrated by Bichat was being integrated into the clinical world view of the internist. All the while the pathological anatomy of the faculty's *pathologie externe* course and, most particularly, the *Ecole pratique,* continued to hew closer to the surgical vision of what I have called official pathology. The former was useful in the diagnostic efforts in which it was pressed into service. The latter was equally useful and adaptive in two interrelated efforts with which *it* was allied. The first of these efforts was the anatomical pedagogy based in the *Ecole pratique* and designed for future surgeons. The second was the actual practice of extirpative surgery requiring, above all, an intimate knowledge of *local* anatomical relationships as the operator sought to avoid impinging on vulnerable neighboring structures.

There were thus two pathologies or, at least, two opposing tendencies in pathology that developed during the Napoleonic period. Indeed, pathological theory and practice could have become a divisive force in the Paris school of physicians and surgeons. Yet they did not. The two pathological traditions did not whirl apart but instead became part of a sort of dialectic of the human body, in which the leaders of the school continued to seek common ground. Efforts to mesh medicine and surgery were paralleled by efforts to braid together the two strands of pathology. In Chapter 4 I detail some of the efforts by which these two sets of steps, one professional and one cognitive, were aligned.

4

The center holds

On arriving in Paris in 1822 with my condisciple A. Robert,
I gave myself entirely to the studies for the career that was
imposed on me . . . . Robert, having apprised me one morning
that he had bought a *subject* (a cadaver), took me for the first
time to the dissection amphitheater at the *hospice de la Pitié*.
The sight of that horrid human charnel-house, those scattered
limbs, those grimacing heads, those half-cracked skulls, the
bloody cesspool in which we walked, the revolting odor
pouring out, the swarms of birds fighting over scraps of lung,
the rats in their corner gnawing on bloody vertebra, filled me
with such dread that, jumping from the amphitheater window,
I took flight and ran home all out of breath, as though death
and her hideous procession were at my heels.
      – Hector Berlioz (1803–1869), *Mémoires*.

ATTEMPTS TO DISARTICULATE MEDICINE AND SURGERY

Throughout the Napoleonic period Michel Thouret, the Paris faculty's director and later dean, would have to struggle, alongside
his patron Antoine Fourcroy and his lieutenant François Chaussier,
to keep the institution they had crafted on course. Avid republicans
all, these men formed its core, provided its ballast. They fought,
as did Thouret's successor J. J. Leroux after the first director –
dean's 1810 death, to preserve their creation against a series of
revanchists. In coming together in 1794, the medical and surgical
communities had each had to give up something. Each yielded
part of their autonomy, if not in the daily practice of their art,
then in the process by which their educational leaders answered a
crucial question: What does the product of our pedagogy need to
know? That medicine and surgery were now taught in tandem,
with a root of anatomical, chemical, and physiological knowledge
commonly held by new students, did not by any stretch of the

imagination mean that the foes of such ecumenicism would now abandon their opposition.

After the fall of Paris at the end of March 1814, the debate over the resegregation of the faculty grew and redoubled in ferocity. Closely tied to Napoleon, Corvisart retired to the country, there to endure a decline that lasted until his death in 1821. Chaussier lost some of his subsidiary positions, notably those of physician and chemistry professor at the *Ecole polytechnique*. He was already on the path to the final loss of his faculty post, with the suppression of the faculty in 1822, and with it his health in a debilitating stroke.[1] What followed within the year 1814 was a flurry of broadsides both *pro* and *con* on the by now entrenched 1794 system of teaching. The latter, its detractors, now a generation removed from their dominance of medical education, seem to have been the most vociferous. One advocate of separation wrote that the "penury" of "physician savants" and "distinguished practitioners" owed directly to the well-known "corruption of teaching" that had occurred in the twenty-five years since medicine and surgery were reunited.[2]

Another formerly disenfranchised physician, emboldened by newfound royal patronage, decried the indecisiveness of direction, the diffuseness of lessons, and the profligacy of expenditures in the faculty. If one could not be both physician and surgeon, then the educational reunion of the two was *ridicule*. The only visible reason for retaining the present ecumenical arrangements, indeed, was "that they want to conserve the administration of the schools, the cumulation of [professorial] positions, their independence, their salaries, and this absolute empire which they have exercised for twenty years in both branches of the healing art."[3] Against such threatened incursions the faculty could only reinforce and rely upon the barricades already in place: the basic inertia of the place, and the proclaimed intellectual necessity of following a common root and trunk before branching out into a clinical field. Faculty apologists were willing to offer certain modifications with which to "perfect" the art of healing and the educational system without dismantling it, primarily by dividing the two professional streams somewhat earlier than before.[4]

To trace this debate in any detail would lie outside my main purpose.[5] Here I seek only to sketch the canvas against which men like Leroux, Chaussier, and Laennec (though the latter was, next to the others, more of an outsider vis-à-vis the faculty) were striving to make the center hold. Two points bear making on this struggle that reawakened under the Restoration. First, the efforts of the central faculty elite were, in the end, proof against the threats of professional and educational revanchism. The center *did* hold, for reasons both political and intellectual. Second, listening to all these noises about medicine and surgery, one begins to filter out the grinding of a related but different axe. The faculty, many felt, had over the years simply accumulated too much power. It was undoubtedly this sense of an excessive accretion of authority, especially over clinical instruction, that stimulated many to the pitch of invective reached in the late 1810s. Again, the best defense the faculty had with which to protect itself was its own entrenchment – and the single, powerful intellectual contention that the healing arts had but one rootstock.[6]

Is it possible to specify the steps by which this accretion of power took place? Can one identify the new pathological anatomy as a key component of the rootstock of ideas developed by the faculty as proof against divisionists? And were the two processes of accretion, political – institutional in the first place and technical – intellectual in the second, related in some organic and verifiable manner? To the first two questions the answer seems clearly positive, to the last, perhaps a bit more qualifiedly so. For the years bracketing the first *Société d'anatomie,* 1803–1809, also marked a pair of critical developments in the role of the Paris faculty as "knowledge processor." In the two following sections I wish now to return to those changes and to glance at how the faculty's administrative burdens also became its ballast against the storm.

A FACULTY ROLE IN CERTIFYING DISTANT KNOWLEDGE

For most categories of subphysician health practitioners in Napoleonic France, the famous or – depending on the ox being gored – infamous law of 19 *Ventôse an XI* (11 March 1803) set new standards for the provision of credentials. The most controversial role among the lower orders of practitioners was that of the *officier de santé,* or health officer. Having previously straddled an unregulated morass of potential duties and roles, the health officer now submitted to a rigid set of requirements that stipulated where, when, and how he could practice.[7] By 1803 the problem of lack of regulation was exacerbated with ever greater severity by the sheer numbers of practitioners at the level of physician and surgeon, but even more so at the level of auxiliary providers. The scale of the problem had been magnified in the main by the needs of the military and by the sheer overflow effect as practitioners with uncertain or no credentials poured out of military service and back into civilian life.[8]

Since my aim is primarily to comment on the faculty's role in processing the *officiers,* and thereby processing their basis of knowledge, the briefest account of their collective vicissitudes must suffice. Before 1803 the situation in French medical or surgical practice was not unlike that soon to develop in Jacksonian America: Second-class practitioners went nearly unregulated, particularly in the rural areas outside Paris. Conversely, there were unregistered and uncredentialed physicians and surgeons who had obtained much of their expertise during years of military practice, and who did possess skills equivalent to those of products of the three major schools. This group had no clear-cut channels for proving their competency, nor did they possess clear access to appropriate credentials.

The law of *ventôse* dramatically changed this state of affairs. Previously there had been disquiet in some quarters over the lack of regulation, and already in some quarters opposition formed to the unification of medicine and surgery. These tensions did not disappear after 1803, but now an identifiable group of auxiliary practitioners emerged to draw the opposition of physicians and surgeons alike. Throughout the nineteenth century the corps of *officiers de santé* would continue to be a thorn in the side of a unified profession pulling together to confront the interlopers' threat. Even when the relative numbers of *officiers* were reduced by well over twofold, as the century wore on, the increasingly overpopulated ranks of regulars in successive generations redoubled their attacks. In 1892, nearly a century later, they succeeded and the *officiers de santé* were abolished.

The greater part of the 1803 law was penned by Antoine Fourcroy. It assigned a ponderous series of duties to certain members of faculties in the existing schools of medicine. *Jurys médicaux,* examining boards set up in the *départements,* were established under the supervision of such key figures as François Chaussier. The juries were carefully balanced panels of physicians and surgeons whose duty it was to determine which practitioners, usually already practicing as provincial surgeons, could be registered as duly certified *médecins de deuxième classe.*[9] To preserve the faculty's medicosurgical balance in the field, the juries were designed to reflect the ecumenicism observed at home. "Each jury," wrote one planner (probably Fourcroy or Thouret), "will be composed of five members, three physicians and two surgeons for the medical examinations, three surgeons and two physicians for those in surgery," with analogous arrangements for pharmacy and other fields.[10]

For Thouret, Leroux, and others, the new duties connected with regulation of practice were two-edged swords. They were sources of enormous power, since they bestowed on those who organized and implemented the medical juries across the country both the authority to define and adjudge the range and level of expertise for each type of practitioner, and the remuneration (Fig. 4.1) that went with it. This exercise in the politics of expertise was as important at the "micro" level – the details of what a physician, surgeon, or *officier* was expected to know – as it was at the "macro" level, which mainly defined the hierarchy of professional relations. Of course the sword had another edge as well. Particularly for those sitting in the dean's offices, simply having to sift through applications of practitioners for diploma equivalencies, and to respond to each such application on an individual basis, performed iteratively scores and indeed hundreds of times over, became an extraordinarily onerous task.

★   ★   ★   ★   ★

Beginning a few years after the creation of the *Ecoles de santé,* Thouret had become inundated by appeals from students and military corpsmen seeking exemption from or leapfrogging within parts of the new educational regime.[11] In a report published by Thouret simultaneously with the promulgation of the new law in 1803, the dean had voiced his strong support of the new regulation, decrying the presence of "hordes of empirics" and the "horrid anarchy during the long silence of the law." Thouret affirmed the notion of a centralized system for the standardization of expertise. The linchpin of the system would be a coterie of commissioners.

Jury members were often drawn from the central faculties. Deployed in the service of each of the juries, commissioners' char-

RÉSUMÉ des Travaux du Jury de médecine, présidé en   par M.
        Professeur de l'École de médecine de
        et des Réceptions, dans le Département d

ÉTATS	SOMMES	MONTANT DES SOMMES versées OU RECEVEUR de l'hospice.	
des Officiers de santé, des Pharmaciens, des Sages-femmes et des Herboristes reçus ou examinés dans le département d et des sommes qui sont provenues de ces examens et réceptions.	payées au Président et aux Examinateurs, pour les droits qui leur sont accordés par l'article 4 de l'arrêté du Ministre de l'intérieur sur la convocation des Jury.		(Dans cette colonne, le placement indiquera les jours d'entrée et de clôture du session du jury. Il fera connaître si une somme ne se rapporte pas au chef-lieu du département, et à quelle distance du lieu des dépenses principales elle a été faite. Il chargera des personnes qui ont une profession sans examen, et quel est, dans ce dernier cas, le droit de ....)
Nota. Exprimer en chiffres le nombre d'examens et réceptions.			
Réception d'officiers de santé, à 200 fr. chacune, ont produit.	fr.		
Réception en vertu de l'article 21 et de la loi du 19 ventôse, à 66 fr. 66 cent. chacune, ont produit	Payé au président, pour droit de présence aux examens et réception d'officiers de santé, la somme de	fr.	
Examen de premier degré, avec ajournement, pour le reste, à la prochaine session du jury, à 60 fr. chaque, ont produit	Au même, pour droit de présence aux examens et réception de pharmaciens, la somme de		
Examen de deuxième degré, avec ajournement, pour le reste, à la prochaine session du jury, à 70 fr. chaque, ont produit	Au même, pour droit de présence aux examens et réception d'herboristes, la somme de		
Examen de troisième degré, avec ajournement à la prochaine session du jury, pour la délivrance du titre de réception, à 70 fr. chaque, ont produit	TOTAL	fr.	
Réception de sages-femmes	Payé aux examinateurs, pour droit de présence aux examens et réceptions d'officiers de santé, la somme de		
Réception d'herboristes, à 30 fr. chacune, ont produit.	Aux mêmes, pour droit de présence sur les examens et réception de pharmaciens, la somme de		
Examen Probatoire, non ajournement, il a produit, à 30 fr. chaque, ont produit.	Aux mêmes, pour droit de présence sur les examens et réception d'herboristes, la somme de		
Réception de pharmacien, à 100 fr. chacune, ont produit.	TOTAL		
Examen de premier degré, avec ajournement, sous le			

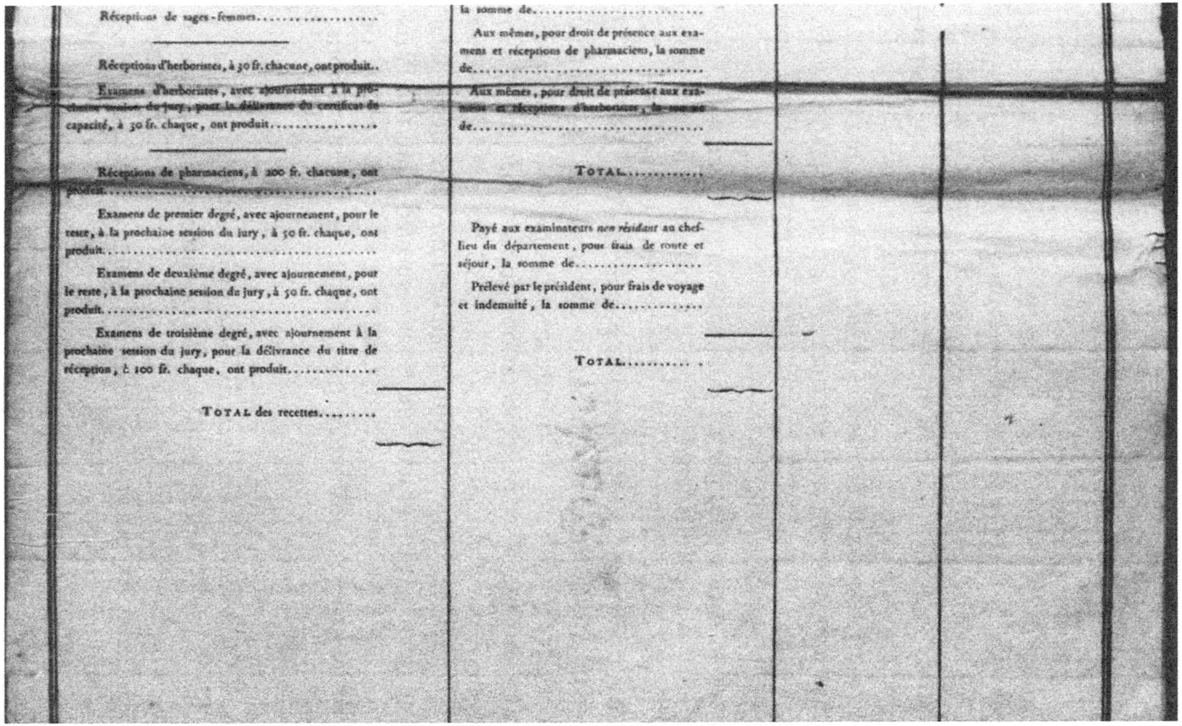

Réceptions de sage-femmes..............

Réceptions d'herboristes, à 30 fr. chacune, ont produit.

Examen d'herboristes, avec ajournement à la prochaine session de jury, pour le déplacement du candidat, à 30 fr. chaque, ont produit.

Réceptions de pharmaciens, à 200 fr. chacune, ont produit.

Examen de premier degré, avec ajournement, pour le cas, à la prochaine session du jury, à 30 fr. chaque, ont produit.

Examen de deuxième degré, avec ajournement, pour le reste, à la prochaine session du jury, à 30 fr. chaque, ont produit.

Examen de troisième degré, avec ajournement à la prochaine session du jury, pour la délivrance du titre de réception, à 100 fr. chaque, ont produit.

TOTAL des recettes..........

la somme de..............

Aux mêmes, pour droit de présence aux examens et réceptions de pharmaciens, la somme de..............

Aux mêmes, pour droit de présent aux examens et réceptions d'herboristes, la somme de..............

TOTAL..............

Payé aux examinateurs non résidant au chef-lieu du département, pour frais de route et séjour, la somme de..............

Prélevé par le président, pour frais de voyage et indemnité, la somme de..............

TOTAL..............

Figure 4.1. Format of medical juries' résumé for reporting examinations.

acteristics were also balanced, to the extent possible, by the appointment of a physician and a surgeon in tandem for each *département*.[12] For the *département* of the Seine, around Paris (the same held true for Hérault, around Montpellier), three commissioners instead of two were appointed: Michel Thouret, R. B. Sabatier (1732–1811), and C. B. Leclerc (1762–1808), all collaborators in the reorganization of anatomical teaching.[13] And lastly, a small, select group of supercommissioners were assembled to act as peripatetic presiding officers over the jury deliberations. The jurisdiction (*arrondissement*) of the Paris *Ecole de medecine* contained two divisions, comprising ten and fourteen *départements* respectively. The first was given to Pierre Lassus (1741–1807), the latter and larger to François Chaussier.[14]

The medical juries provide an uncommon glimpse into how medical theory was manipulated and how information flowed from one place to the other. The faculty imported knowledge from the private laboratories and studies of elite physicians like Bichat and Laennec, while the juries exported it to the masses of provincial practitioners. If they did not distribute knowledge wholesale, they at least disseminated a set of expectations about what the *officier* candidates and others might need to know to get past the juries (Fig. 4.2). These expectations would then be a measure of medical theory as understood by practitioners far removed from the Paris elite. In this light the critical desiderata are the *procès-verbaux* or minutes of the juries' examination proceedings and deliberations.

★ ★ ★ ★ ★

Although the archives do not exactly belch forth holdings on the subject, what exists is choice. In Isère, for example, in late October of 1805, the jury held its third séance of the day to scrutinize three surgical candidates for the *officier* certificate. One was asked to discuss tooth-pulling: how to correlate the choice of teeth to pull with the presence or absence of pus in the maxillary sinuses. A second was asked about simple fractures: no elaboration. The third was asked, quite simply, "What is paracentesis? How does one accomplish this operation?" Buried in this telegraphic recording of the questioning is a critical piece of information: for the operation of paracentesis was the most important intervention of an invasive sort, at times diagnostic and at times therapeutic, that was available to clinicians. In a sense, with respect to clinical intervention, it was the closest thing to the purely technical analogue of the new theory of pathological anatomy.

The operation of paracentesis regularly and frequently illustrated, always tacitly and sometimes explicitly, the interdependence, the organic integration, of medicine and surgery. For the practitioner, proper understanding of the efficacy of this procedure for penetrating the belly or chest by insertion of a hollow trochar, depended upon the localism of the surgeon as well as the tissue theory of the physician. Presently I will show how Laennec used it in his *Mediate Auscultation.* Here, between fifteen and twenty years earlier, when a provincial second-class surgeon was being asked about paracentesis, there was a clear indication of the jury members seeking the common ground between their own areas of expertise.[15] Similarly, though with less specificity of detail, ten candidates in the Gironde were each asked about pathological anatomy in 1816 in order that the jury might assess the theoretical trunk of their practical knowledge.[16]

By the 1820s it was common practice in the juries to require knowledge about just that – *pratique commune,* the common ground where every practitioner had to tread. Observe, for example, the proceedings of the examination of six Grenoble area *officier* aspirants in 1821. On 13 October the six candidates were assembled for the third part of the examination, on "practice in common," and posed the following:

Le Sieur Fourrier: what is hydrocele, its different forms, the operative procedures for the two species of it? Le S[r] Antoine: What is peripneumonia? In what ways does it differ from pleurisy? What is its treatment? Le S[r] Dupasquier: What do we mean by hydropsy, and what are the different forms of this malady considered in relation to its anatomical seat? What are the general means we use for combatting it? Le S[r] Massot: How do we treat wounds made with sharp instruments? Le S[r] Calvat: What is inflammatory fever? and what is the appropriate treatment for it? Finally le S[r] Galvin: Enumerate the means that the art uses for the union of simple wounds made by cutting instruments.[17]

This document provides a particularly illuminating account, both for what it includes and for what it leaves out. It would not have done to ask these practitioners, for example, about the finer details of climatologic medicine or of nosology as some physicians still construed it. Nor would it have done to ask them, for example, about the intimate details of classical surgical anatomy, for the

TITRE DE RÉCEPTION
DE PHARMACIEN.

ARRONDISSEMENT
de
réfecou de médecine
d

JURY MÉDICAL
du département

Nous soussignés, composant le Jury médical du département d ... en exécution des lois des 19 ventôse an 11 [10 mars et 11 avril 1803], certifions que le Sieur ... âgé de ... après avoir suivi, conformément à l'article XV de la loi du 21 germinal précité, les deux examens de théorie; savoir, le premier sur les principes de l'art, et le second le ... sur la botanique et l'histoire naturelle des drogues simples, s'est présenté le ... à l'examen pratique, lequel a consisté en opérations chimiques et pharmaceutique qui lui ont été désignées, et qu'il a exécutées lui-même; dans lesquels actes probatoires, et qui ont eu lieu publiquement, le Sieur ... ayant donné des preuves de son savoir, nous le déclarons pourvu des connaissances exigibles par l'exercice de la pharmacie, et à cet effet lui délivrons le présent titre.

À ... ce ...

(cachet : ARCHIVES NATIONALES)

Commissaire de l'École de médecine d
Président du Jury.

Membre du Jury.

Membre du Jury.

Membre du Jury.

Membre du Jury.

Membre du Jury.

Membre du Jury.

TITRE DE RÉCEPTION
D'OFFICIER DE SANTÉ

DSSEMENT
de
m médecine

MÉDICAL

Nous soussignés, composant le Jury médical du département d ... en exécution de la loi du 19 ventôse an 11 [10 mars 1803], certifions que le Sieur ... âgé de ... après nous avoir exhibé la preuve de ... années d'études

a suivi, conformément à l'article XVII de la loi précitée, les examens ordonnés; savoir :

Le premier, le ... sur l'anatomie ;
Le second, le ... sur les élémens de la médecine ;

Le troisième, le ... sur la chirurgie et les connaissances les plus usuelles de la pharmacie : Dans lesquels examens, qui ont été soutenus publiquement, le Sieur ... ayant fait preuve de capacité, nous le déclarons pourvu des connaissances suffisantes pour exercer les fonctions d'Officier de santé; et, à cet effet, nous lui délivrons le présent titre.

À ... ce ...

(cachet : ARCHIVES NATIONALES)

Commissaire de l'École de médecine d
Président du Jury.

Membre du Jury.

Membre du Jury.

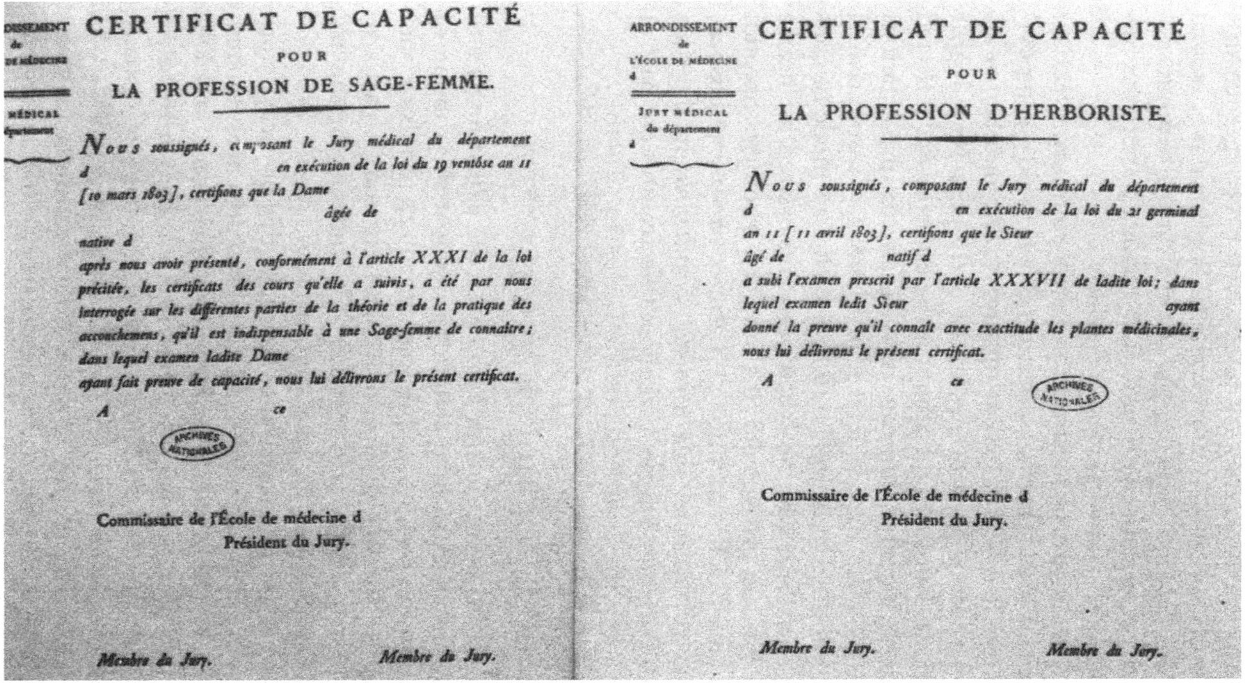

CERTIFICAT DE CAPACITÉ

POUR

LA PROFESSION DE SAGE-FEMME.

Nous soussignés, composant le Jury médical du département d en exécution de la loi du 19 ventôse an 11 [10 mars 1803], certifions que la Dame âgée de native d après nous avoir présenté, conformément à l'article XXXI de la loi précitée, les certificats des cours qu'elle a suivis, a été par nous interrogée sur les différentes parties de la théorie et de la pratique des accouchemens, qu'il est indispensable à une Sage-femme de connaître; dans lequel examen ladite Dame ayant fait preuve de capacité, nous lui délivrons le présent certificat.

A ce

ARCHIVES NATIONALES

Commissaire de l'École de médecine d
Président du Jury.

Membre du Jury. *Membre du Jury.*

ARRONDISSEMENT de L'ÉCOLE DE MÉDECINE d

JURY MÉDICAL du département d

CERTIFICAT DE CAPACITÉ

POUR

LA PROFESSION D'HERBORISTE.

Nous soussignés, composant le Jury médical du département d en exécution de la loi du 21 germinal an 11 [11 avril 1803], certifions que le Sieur âgé de natif d a subi l'examen prescrit par l'article XXXVII de ladite loi; dans lequel examen ledit Sieur ayant donné la preuve qu'il connaît avec exactitude les plantes médicinales, nous lui délivrons le présent certificat.

A ce

ARCHIVES NATIONALES

Commissaire de l'École de médecine d
Président du Jury.

Membre du Jury. *Membre du Jury.*

Figure 4.2. Specimen "certificates of capacity" for ancillary professions according to the law of 19 *Ventôse* 1803. In the entrance certificate *[titre de réception]* for *officier de santé*, particularly noteworthy is the specification that candidates be tested in each of the three fields: medicine, surgery, and anatomy.

physician membership of the jury might well have regarded that line as excessively specialized. What was left? For one thing, wound healing was emphasized: Suppuration and the care of wounds, despite the relative peace of the Restoration period, was always uppermost in medical and surgical minds alike.

One then comes to the questions on peripneumonia, pleurisy, and hydropsy. What is their significance? There is no strong evidence that there had been a recent upsurge in the number of affections of the serous membranes in the early post-Napoleonic years. Rather, it seems, the meaning of the enterprise is reflected in two features characterizing this array of clinical presentations and descriptions. First, they all represented lesions of tissues central to the economic system of the body, the Bichatian mode of conceptualizing disease that by now had been emphasized for nearly two decades by the proponents of the new pathology. Second, though his name was not mentioned, Laennec had just published, less than two years earlier, his *Mediate Auscultation*. In the final sections of this chapter I argue that these two features are part of one phenomenon: the apotheosis of the Bichatian system.

LAENNEC EXTENDS THE BICHATIAN SYSTEM

Though I have brought the story down to the adjustments and accommodations medical men sought to make at the coming of the Bourbon Restoration, it is appropriate briefly to turn back once again to Laennec's strikingly productive early period, circa 1803–1804. Towards the end of and just after his student years he had fully intended to publish his own authoritative *Treatise of Pathological Anatomy*. From the partial manuscript of this projected work it is clear that project was based firmly on his experiences teaching pathology in the circle of Corvisart and, at that point, still Dupuytren. It is equally apparent that it was firmly rooted in Bichatian pathological theory, even if Laennec took certain pains to distance himself from the earlier model in some matters of detail.[18]

What the first part of this *Treatise* shows, commencing with Laennec's survey of the recent, dramatic history of the emergence of pathological anatomy, is that Laennec was self-consciously seeking to extend the canon of this new field. In it he saw a wholly new way of mapping out the body and its morbid appearances, and of doing so in a manner clearly set apart from that employed by the traditional "descriptive anatomists." Toward this latter group Laennec clearly bore his share of scorn. Bichat had begun the task of transforming pathology, but, if anything, had not taken it far enough. Other young medical men had sought, since Bichat's death, to follow in his footsteps, in France and abroad, but with mixed results. A translation of Matthew Baillie's work, under the title *Traité d'anatomie pathologique du corps humain,* had received some degree of notice, as had the lecture notes of Samuel T. Soemmering (1755–1830) from the period 1796–1798. The latter bore certain resemblances, declared Laennec, to the ideas of Bichat on inflammation, especially in the serous membranes, but was incomplete, careless, and lacking in rigorous method or enough detail.[19] That left Bichat's *Anatomie générale* as the acknowledged leader.

Why had pathological anatomy continued to lag? Laennec offered the following hypothesis. "Until now all the authors who have written on pathological anatomy," he wrote, "have, in the exposition of the lesions of organs, followed the order in which they present at the dissection of the human body. This method borrows from descriptive anatomy [which], besides entraining a mass of repetitions, turns away from medical progress which, to the extent possible, classes diseases according to their nature rather than their seats." Bichat himself had not entirely escaped blame in this regard, confining his analysis, for example, of general affections – those that could attack whole systems rather than individual organs – to two, the scirrhous and the inflammatory. It should soon be possible to locate each type of lesion in all the systems of the body, with appropriate modifications according to tissue type.[20] For these reasons, Laennec determined, he would approach pathological anatomy without rigid adherence to traditional anatomical divisions except as they could be used as "auxiliary methods."

The alternative strategy that he chose was in essence that set forth at the *Société d'anatomie,* discussed in the previous chapter. It was a clinical strategy, and a medical one, yet more anatomical than any the old nosological school would have accommodated. But in 1803 it was a strategy already less oriented to the dissection table and more to the clinic than that of the "headquarters" school of pathological anatomy. Even had Laennec not lost the taste for producing a separate treatise in pathology as a result of his public antagonisms with Dupuytren, he was already on the path toward a synthesis of medicine and pathological anatomy. Just as Bichat had, after Desault's death, veered from surgery toward medicine, Laennec now was partly drawn, both by inclination and by necessity, away from teaching anatomy and toward the daily practice of *clinique interne*. The resulting synthesis can be seen growing year by year in his reports from the several hospitals in which he performed postmortem dissections. It was a synthesis visible in both the literary and the professional pinnacles of his career, the *Mediate Auscultation* of 1819 and the 1822–1824 pathological anatomy lectures at the Collège de France.[21]

A typical postmortem case in which Laennec recast the morbid appearances in Bichatian terms was that of the cleric, Cardinal Vincenti, whom he saw in March of 1811. The case illustrates certain points worth considering before Laennec arrived at the use of the stethoscope as a correlative tool in such efforts. First, it represents Laennec's thinking before the Restoration; second, it represents his thinking before he began his serious experiments with the *cylindre;* and third, it represents his interest and involvement in religious matters. This last tendency was with him a life-long one. It was consistent with both his Breton background and his family's innate religiopolitical conservatism. Lastly, the case reflects Laennec's already spreading reputation as a diagnostician who based his inferences about the presence of disease in bodily tissue systems on the principles of the new pathology.

The seventy-five-year-old priest Vincenti had been seized with a bout of peripneumonia on March 18. Laennec was called in four days later, just after the patient's personal attending physicians had performed phlebotomy and removed about a pound of blood. Adopting the "Hippocratic" approach to the patient that he staunchly supported, Laennec noted the old Monsignor's flushed facies and his moderately full pulse, then described the exceedingly blood-engorged liver and the twice-normal-sized left kidney. These findings he apparently discerned before the patient's death sometime in the following six days. Then, at the *ouverture* performed on March 24, the diagnostician confirmed the general state of tissue engorgement that he had predicted.

The cranial contents bore out his supposition, with the vessels in all three membrane layers surrounding the brain and spinal cord gorged with blood. The ventricles and several neighboring cysts were brimming with "liquid serosity." The abdominal cavity was full of greasy matter, the stomach and intestines forming a "voluminous mass" moderately distended by wind. One kidney, apparently the left one, showed stone formation. The heart, finally, demonstrated an adherent serosal membrane, though Laennec did not comment on whether he could adduce evidence of cardiac tamponade. The lung, on the other hand – note the compulsion to remark on the *absence* of serous membrane disease – demonstrated no pleural adhesions.[22]

From this period in Laennec's career until his death a decade and a half later, his casebooks and autopsy records bristle with cases of peritonitis, pleuritis, pericarditis, as well as other serositides and mucositides. Hardly a cadaver, and hardly a body cavity, was opened without clear or purulent serosity pouring out onto the table, not to mention the onlookers. Small wonder that many of the pathological anatomists, Bichat and Laennec included, probably succumbed to the "phthisical" condition that afflicted their patients so ubiquitously.

LAENNEC AND THE RESTORATION (1815–1819)

The beginning of the Bourbon Restoration was a momentous period for Théophile Laennec. Corvisart's departure in early 1814 to a forced rustication, and the hundred days, a year later, had set the stage for a new political context within which the Paris medical community had to learn to live. Laennec, never known for the sort of liberalism that now besmirched men of the Chaussier mold, fared well, taking over the *clinique interne* at the *Charité* in April 1815 and the physicianship at the *Necker* in September 1816. His observations in the months immediately following were probably critical in determining how he would incorporate the introduction of the stethoscope into his canon of pathological anatomy.

When he began using the "cylinder" after 1816 or so, Laennec must have soon realized that he had hit upon the perfect diagnostic tool for further elaborating the new pathology. Again, at this point an interest in pathology implied the investigation of both antemortem *and* postmortem findings; pathological anatomy was not now and (unlike the nascent science of physiology) *never would be* exclusively the domain of the laboratory worker. The stethoscope was now, rather, zealously pursued by Laennec and a few close associates – ironically, his friend Bayle had just died in May of 1816 – as a means of establishing the likely anatomical findings

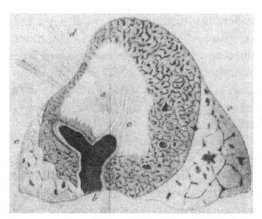

Figure 4.3. Illustration of lung from *Mediate Auscultation*.

antemortem that usually could be expected to be soon confirmed at postmortem. This correlative approach was the fundamental purpose of the *Mediate Auscultation* when it finally appeared between two and three years after Laennec began accumulating additional cases at the *Necker*.

The text of the *Mediate Auscultation* may be considered in several ways. Three approaches in particular deserve attention, for each provides fresh insights into the importance of Laennec's pathological system. A first perspective from which to look at the *Mediate Auscultation* is the pictorial view. Figure 4.3 depicts a typical illustration from Laennec's text. That the two volumes contained any sort of pictorial content at all already represents a concrete extension of the Bichatian tradition. The problem of rendering pictorially the body economy and, particularly, the relationships between normal and abnormal membranes, as opposed to the parenchymal organs that dominated the old pathology, becomes immediately apparent.

In the figure Laennec shows the reader the whole panoply of morbid alterations to which a lung in far-advanced stages of phthisis might be subject. The pleural membrane is carefully limned at point 'd,' but is a subtle appearance, overshadowed by the gross cavitary and fibrotic lesions elsewhere in the lung. That was simply a fact of scientific life for physicians like Laennec, but was not in the least inconsistent with their emphasis on the complex relations between the solid and fluid parts of the body, mediated by the diaphanous membranous that bounded the solids and exuded the fluids.

Another perspective on the *Mediate Auscultation* is found in the theoretical plane on which the text was pitched. It is probably not excessive to emphasize again that, theoretically speaking, the book was in considerable measure an effort to establish the legitimacy and the expanding boundaries of the new pathology. It is presentist to see it exclusively, or even primarily, as a work designed to popularize an instrument which, as it happened generations later, would end up dangling from virtually every medical neck. Medical historians and physicians trained in the Anglo–American tradition are at a disadvantage in this respect. Reared on John Forbes's celebrated English translation of 1821, which is an entirely different sort of book for reasons discussed in a later chapter, we see the stethoscopy magnified because the pathological anatomy and the tissue pathology supporting it have been shorn away. But the *Treatise on Mediate Auscultation* as it appeared in 1819 was a work of pathological anatomy.[23]

Lastly, from the theoretical and the general one must move to the level of particularities – that is, once again, to the case descriptions themselves as Laennec formulated them for his original edition between 1816 and 1819. One may take the case, for example, of one J.-M. Potu, a 30-year-old former soldier described by Laennec as being "of a fine constitution and a sanguine, lymphatic temperament." The young man had first come down with an intermittent, quotidian fever while imprisoned by the Russians on the Eastern front. Initially the soldier's fever had broken, immediately following a crisis during which he drained pus from his right ear. After the peace of 1814, Monsieur Potu had come to Paris to look for work as a porter.

In May of 1817 Potu came down with what was at first thought to be a *rhume* or cold, but a month later he became increasingly short of breath and a month after that experienced the onset of a hectic cough. He spent several weeks at each of the central hospitals, first the *Charité,* then the Hôtel-Dieu, and finally the *Necker,* where he came under Laennec's direct care. Laennec's first physical examination on the third of November revealed a pale, debilitated, tachycardic young man with a wretched cough. Examination with the *cylindre* showed diminished breath sounds on the right side of the chest, where Laennec also noted the transmission of whispered sounds, which he termed pectoriloquy.

For the rest of that month the patient continued to go downhill and as he did Laennec noted increasingly resonant percussion sounds in the presumably affected lung. From this he inferred the presence of a cavitation process and made the diagnosis of "tuberculous phthisis." He also suspected the presence on the right side of an effusion of fluid, and added to his diagnosis the note, "pleurisy with effusion and pneumothorax."

The patient lingered on; on the twenty-fifth of January Laennec shook Potu's trunk and heard a splash "like that produced by a half-full bottle," again localized to the right side of the chest with the stethoscope. At this point Laennec attempted to treat the effusion of fluid. Unnamed diuretics were little availing. Laennec at this pointed called in a series of consultants, including the new Dean of the Paris Faculty, Leroux, and the physiologist Récamier. As a result of these consultations he called in a surgeon, one Monsieur Baffos, to do the operation of *ponction* – in modern parlance, thoracentesis. When the surgeon's trochar reached the pleural cavity, some two pounds of purulent liquid poured out, affording Potu a measure of relief.

On the twentieth of February Laennec noted for the first time the presence of abdominal pain in this patient. Five days later he was agonal, and on the next day, the twenty-sixth, he died. On the twenty-eighth Laennec conducted the *ouverture* in the presence of several of the medical notables of the Paris community. An ounce of serous effusion fluid, or *serosité,* was discovered in the pericardial sac. The peritoneal cavity contained a pint of murky serosity, and the stomach and bowel were somewhat distended by gas. Laennec noted the presence of a false membrane, whitish and quite easy to detach, covering the right iliac fossa as well as parts of the upper aspect of the liver.[24]

The case of the unfortunate young soldier Potu illustrates important additional points about Laennec's project. This and similar cases were, among other things, exercises in medicosurgical consultation. The physician and the surgeon were participating in complementary and mutually reinforcing enterprises. The diagnostician could localize the accumulation of liquid serosity now in the antemortem state. The surgeon could now bring out his trusty trochar and perform the merciful operation of thoracentesis. And here lies the second, critical point of the project: the therapeutic dimension.

From time to time, in the era of high technology medicine, one hears the inquiry: Why did Laennec *bother* with so much effort to refine diagnosis when the patients inevitably died? To pose the question this way is to miss two key motives in the enterprise. The great preponderance of these patients, mostly afflicted with terminal tuberculosis, did indeed die. But the anatomicoclinical method (the clinicopathological correlation) offered two complementary means of making the physician and the surgeon useful nonetheless. It permitted Laennec and his colleagues, first, to establish *prognosis,* and to tell patient or family just how bad things had gotten. Equally important, it permitted them in limited degree to undertake therapeutic intervention. To perform thoracentesis, or abdominal paracentesis, or even pericardiocentesis – and each of these was a relatively frequent occurrence – to remove excessive "serosity," was to buy time by influencing the economic balance of fluids and solids in the body. The new pathology portended actual therapeutic benefits not unlike those inherent in the process by which, in the twentieth-century, cancer cytopathology would guide the choice of palliative treatment.

LAENNEC AT THE COLLÈGE DE FRANCE

Like Bichat before him, Laennec spent most of his life without the key position of a central chair in the Paris medical faculty. Confronted with this fact, one might point to his accession to two chairs in late 1822 and early 1823. But his assumption of the medical chair at the Collège de France in December 1822, and the professorship of *clinique interne* at the Paris Faculty, must be carefully considered through a reconstruction of the social and political context in which they took place.

The larger political context was that of the resurgence of strong antiliberal sentiment in the Villèle regime, especially strong among individuals who counted in the governance of academic institutions. At the medical faculty a series of disruptive events at the inaugural academic session of 1822–1823 gave the royalists the opening they needed. They closed the faculty for a short period in November and ordered its reorganization. In January Laennec accepted the clinical professorship, which, as the result of a royal ordinance the following month, became one of an enlarged number of full-time chairs: There were now twenty, and Laennec was one of ten new professors.[25]

The Grand-Master of the University and the Minister of the Interior, Corbière, were not averse to placing their hand on the scales when the death of Jean-Noel Hallé vacated the medical chair at the Collège. During the same tempestuous academic year that the Faculty found itself upended, Laennec became even more centrally involved in a political fracas. Ever since 1821, when Hallé had steered Laennec toward the celebrated Duchesse de Berry as her personal physician, the Breton had considered himself the leading candidate to replace the aging incumbent. But when the Collège's professorial assembly met in March to nominate a successor, only six of twenty votes were cast for Laennec. Chaussier had eight. Bertin, who would soon be the focus of another furor at the faculty, received four, and the young François Magendie, not yet thirty years old, received two. Laennec's name was misspelled.[26]

Between March and July various individuals and groups made their interests known. The Academy of Sciences weighed in with the recommendation that Magendie be appointed. On July 31 the Minister of the Interior seized on the Academy's recommendation to promote Laennec as a consensus candidate. "[T]his savant," he noted in his report to the King, "presented by the Grand Master of the University, has balanced M. Chaussier [against Magendie] in the deliberations of the Collège Royal. Consequently, I have the honor of proposing to Your Majesty the attached plan for an ordinance." The ordinance was immediately forthcoming and Laennec began his first and only course at the Collège that autumn. He chose as his subject an exhaustive synopsis of pathological anatomy.[27]

Before discussing Laennec's lectures at the Collège de France I wish to return momentarily to the social and political contexts of which I spoke, by way of explaining the royal intervention that netted him the position in the end. Laennec himself later explained the sudden, unexpected setback in March by placing it in context of the swirling liberal *versus* conservative politics that had made all alliances so unstable in early 1823. He felt that he had lost three critical votes from professors who sided with the liberal wing when they felt their independence threatened from above.[28] But another, less global, political, explanation, a more mundane one, is equally plausible.

Put simply, Chaussier was a more central figure within the *medical* establishment. He had paid his dues with the juries and a hundred other institutional connections. Laennec was the relative outsider, the producer of valuable esoteric knowledge. But, with his now once again appropriate religious and political leanings, he was not long to be denied. The two explanations, indeed, are hardly mutually exclusive. It is true beyond anyone's doubt that the royalists did intervene on his behalf, so that royal patronage was the deciding factor.

What is more interesting is the reason for the setback that required such an intrusion. There Chaussier's liberalism was probably no more important than his centrality in the faculty's essential role, that of "processing" the knowledge generated outside its walls. Both factors, micro- and macropolitics, may have played a role. Their relative importance remains unclear. One should probably discount neither – neither the importance of the politics of knowledge in a particular institutional array, nor the importance of more traditional forms of ideology, exemplified in Laennec's case by the politics of monarchical tendencies and economic valencies.

LAENNEC'S COURSE AT THE COLLÈGE DE FRANCE

Laennec used his lectures to develop a two year course of pathological anatomy, given in 1822–1824 and begun again in 1824–1825. It was unlike any ever given before, by him included. The notes for these lectures were scrawled hastily. They are at times difficult to read, and, more of an obstacle, they are divided between two repositories of which one is especially difficult to use.[29] They are nonetheless of considerable interest and handsomely repay the time spent examining them, and not merely because of the extraordinary international audience that they attracted. These lectures represented the full flower of the new, medical pathology that now posed an important complement and parallel to the old (and still viable) surgical pathology of Dupuytren and Cruveilhier.

Laennec approached the Collège lectures as though composing his valedictory. He recapitulated the recent history of pathological thought from Boerhaave to Bichat. He emphasized the "accidental" tissues that formed in various disease states, forming, for example, false membranes or serous cysts with tissue linings capable of exuding fluid into their cavities. These considerations dominated the first year of lectures. In the second year Laennec began to weave in the techniques of physical diagnosis as an adjunct of pathological anatomy.[30]

The discussion of the physical diagnostic sign known as *râles* is instructive. This sign, one of several "bruits foreign to [normal] respiration," was formed, he contended, by the murmur or passage of air across "liquid mucosities" – a sign, in other words, of catarrhal states. Such states were the equivalent in the mucous membrane system of the vigorous outpourings of serous fluid in the synovial and serous systems. In addition to the "sonorous" ("musical" to the mid-twentieth century physician) *râles* found in certain conditions, auscultation might also disclose "cavernous" *râles* if the stethoscope were placed over a cavitary lesion of tuberculosis, or "mucous" *râles* if the instrument were located over smaller bore airways.[31]

By the forty-first lecture Laennec had moved to the core of his concern, to the pleural membranes, the pleural cavities they delimited, and to the morbid appearances of the serous system. The problem with diagnosing the agonies of the dyspneic patient, he pointed out, was in differentiating those with hydrothorax – the *épanchement* of serosity into the pleural cavity of which he spoke repeatedly – and those with blood, thick pus, or air in the same cavity. Distinguishing between "latent pleurisy," a form of isolated inflammation of the pleura, and hydropsy (what might now be called pulmonary edema), was a common and potentially dangerous error. Such disturbances of the body economy were best understood by analyzing the subtle checks and balances between membranous systems, and between fluids and solids of the body economy, characteristic of the new pathology.[32]

It was a grandiose scheme. Laennec himself had precious little time to expand it further. In 1824–1825, preoccupied with a number of personal matters, he began a second two-year cycle of lectures, presenting the same wealth of material he had feverishly assembled two years earlier. Late 1825 found him preparing the second edition of the *Mediate Auscultation* for the printer. By April of 1826 he was ill. In that month he used his cylinder on his own chest and noted the presence of an ominous finding, a sign he had described in the book: *bruit de coeur perceptible à distance*. On April 20 he wrote his last will and testament. He died on the thirteenth of August.[33]

Even though the first chair in the subject was a decade in the future, pathological anatomy, in both its strains, that of Bichat and Laennec as well as that of Dupuytren and Cruveilhier, was by now deeply entrenched in the French medical consciousness. A new generation of clinicians applied both modes to a variety of entities, often melding and recombining them in novel and useful ways. That story, symbolized by Feyen-Perrin's illustrious depic-

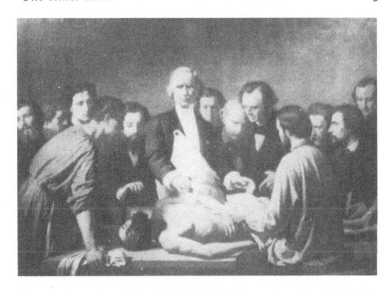

Figure 4.4. Auguste Feyen-Perrin's "The Anatomy Lesson of Dr. Velpeau," painted in the mid-nineteenth century, depicts the practices associated with the tradition discussed in this chapter.

tion of "The Anatomy Lesson of Dr. Velpeau" (Fig. 4.4), is a straightforward one. Less straightforward is the story of the fate of pathological anatomy in other national contexts, especially those in which medicosurgical rapprochement was more primitive. The single most important example of this phenomenon was the English medical community, many of whose members came to hear Laennec at the Collège de France. Liberated by peace into a state of wary mutual admiration, the two nations circled round one another. So, too, did their medical elites.

PART II

Channel crossing

5

The context of English pathology, 1800–1830

The intellectual and professional circumstances of English medicine in the late Georgian period were dramatically different from those across the Channel. That this was so does not necessarily reinforce the invidious comparisons many English observers at the time made at their own countrymen's expense. Indeed, the truth of the matter was that by the late eighteenth century English hospital planning, medical reform, and surgical anatomy teaching all had had significant impacts on their continental counterparts. Even so, the medical communities of England and Scotland, as the age of Napoleon drew to a close and its members began more broadly to engage the outside world, was in a rather fractious state. In re-engaging, English medicine produced a suite of new professional structures. Those new structures, institutions, societies, and a number of other enterprises, including a rash of new medical journals, jostled one another and their ancient predecessors, while their various patrons and designers pursued a variety of interests. Among such interests were the tasks of fostering pathological anatomy and certain other elements, notably chemistry, of an emerging nineteenth-century scientific culture.

The desire to bring pathological anatomy, French-style or otherwise, into medical education and medical practice must be understood against the backdrop of the professional changes that were sought by the new men and their organizations. Intellectual aspirations were tightly interwoven with professional aspirations, neither necessarily antecedent to the other. The rise of the surgeon–apothecaries[1] and the emergence of the new medical journals, for example, were at once vehicles that promoted the new pathology and outlets benefitting from it. More broadly stated, the new culture of science became a resource, lending authority to the professional enterprises of medical men. Their success or failure, in turn, clearly influenced science's legitimacy in the eyes of medical educators and practitioners.[2]

Bracketing all these efforts to change English medical ideas, organizations, and professional relations, was the crucial, encompassing fact, the tripartite division into surgeons, physicians, and apothecaries. Not until long after pathological anatomy began to enter the medical curriculum in the 1830s did this stratification of English medicine cease, in broad outline, to dominate. For much of the nineteenth century it would remain the formal pattern within which factions of the profession sought to rearrange the boundaries of knowledge and expertise. Each caste, and each alliance between castes, was forced to work within these straits throughout the early decades of the nineteenth century. In France the energy derived from scientific culture had been used to suppress boundaries where walls had stood before 1794. Here in Britain that same energy was expended in battering away at walls that, quite concretely, still stood fast.

This chapter begins with a look at the circumstances of English and Scottish medicine before 1815. It next sketches some of the terms of the professional debates that exercised English medicine between 1812 and 1832. It appraises the interested parties' concepts of the appropriate expertise for practitioners. It assesses in particular the role of the surgeon–apothecaries, their aspirations within the divided medical house, and the increasing complexity of English medicine after 1815 as those aspirations were partly fulfilled. This assessment leads to a consideration of medical journalism, one of the most important aspects, other than the surgeon – apothecary's or general practitioner's changing role itself, of this increased complexity.

In a subsequent chapter I therefore extend the portrait of the medical journal literature that blossomed in the period after 1815. That enterprise was an important forum for reformers of various stripes. It was a platform for debate on the ostensible decline of English medical science, and for proposals to reverse the tide. Within that larger debate, concerns over the state of pathological anatomy in England soon became a major focus. One thus comes full circle: The new journals, those who built careers on them, and their prominent role in both collecting and disseminating intelligence about continental medical science, became part of the means for diffusing knowledge and power through the English medical profession in the post-Napoleonic period.

THE ORGANIZATIONAL BACKGROUND BEFORE 1815

Efforts to achieve reform before mid-century, to the extent they met with success, relied on practitioners' abilities to form coalitions cutting across loyalty to the three regulatory and examining bodies. Since both intellectual and social coalitions served similar interests, the distinction between them was often blurred. Only recently has the importance of this sort of coalition politics been fully recognized as an important source of the mediation between knowledge and power, especially as it proceeded in the years around 1815.[3]

Hence the English medical profession began to change organizationally, usually by forging new "linkage" organizations rather than amalgamating old ones, long before the three bodies that regulated its members began to reflect those changes. So to change was a matter of adapting to new circumstances in both of the worlds of the physician: in professional society and, even more particularly, in the natural world of disease and the body. The new circumstances had been apparent by the late eighteenth century. The beginnings of adaptation by English medical culture, through the formation of new organizations, had become apparent at the same time. While the French were conceptually and administratively integrating medicine and surgery beginning in the 1790s, English medical men were forming more informal and voluntary groups like the Society for the Improvement of Medical Knowledge.[4] Founded in 1793 by John Hunter and George Fordyce, surgeon and physician, respectively, the Society was a coalition of the surgical and medical elites of London. It represented not so much a conjunction of their expertise as of their professional resources and interests.

If the Society for the Improvement of Medical Knowledge exemplified an early coalition of physicians and surgeons, its ecumenicism lacked both the intellectual breadth, and its elitism the professional depth, that would eventually foster the desire to promote pathological anatomy on English shores. An intermediate step toward this sort of catholicity of interest was the formation in 1805 of another, larger coalition, the Medical and Chirurgical Society. Founded with appropriate high moral purpose "for the purpose of conversation on professional subjects, for the reception of communications, and the formation of a library," as well as to counter "the unhappy state of [James Sims's] Medical Society of London," the new group installed Dr. William Saunders as its first President. Its charter membership reflected an exquisite balance and symmetry – hardly accidental, one must suppose – between its surgical and medical factions. The former group included Astley Cooper and William Blizard, while the latter faction numbered Saunders, Matthew Baillie, John H. Hunter (d. 1809), and William Babington among its more eminent members.[5]

The Hunter–Baillie circle, of which Saunders was a key member, dominated the Medical and Chirurgical Society. When Saunders resigned in 1808, Baillie himself succeeded to the presidency. It is not surprising, therefore, that the organization was the most receptive of its time, and continued to be so through the Napoleonic era, to the original, indigenous interest in English pathological anatomy that had long characterized this circle of surgeons. But the characterization was an eighteenth-century one: The Medical and Chirurgical Society was formed by men educated before 1800, men who were most comfortable discussing pathology in the natural historical style that extended to their pathological anatomy.[6]

So the alliances and valencies of the Medical and Chirurgical Society were transitional between those of the Society for the Improvement of Medical Knowledge and those of the new men educated after 1810. On one hand, the leaders of the Medical and Chirurgical Society locked official horns on at least one occasion with the College of Physicians, staunchly and consistently maintaining its independence from both colleges.[7] When pathology enthusiasts like Richard Bright and John Bostock came along, they were quickly drawn into the Society's membership and officership.[8] But on the other hand, the new, more theoretical pathological anatomy emanating from France was not embraced by the Society even when later, younger figures began to favor it. Indeed, in 1846, when the Pathological Society was founded, its members would move with delicate, minuet-like footwork to placate the older, more clinically oriented Society. For their trouble, the upstart so-

ciety's members found themselves fended off most unceremon-
iously.[9]

Scottish science played three different roles in this story: first *in
situ* in Edinburgh, second in its effects (mainly through the Hunters)
in London, and third in its leaders' fondness for Paris medicine.
In this section I discuss late eighteenth-century Edinburgh. In the
next section I discuss the impact on English medicine of the Scot-
tish-born John Hunter. In the chapter following this I consider the
impact of young surgeons' and physicians' direct experience with
Paris medical study, with a look at how early nineteenth-century
Edinburgh educators carefully primed young medical minds to
make that journey.

But before there was Hunter, and before there was the Paris
hospital of Bichat and Laennec, there was the unique Edinburgh
medical fraternity, and there were the Munros. Beginning with
surgeon Alexander *primus* and continuing with his physician son
and namesake, the Munros developed a remarkable concordance
of education in anatomy, physiology, and surgery in their University courses. As Christopher Lawrence has shown in his extensive recent studies, these courses were accessible (they were
taught in English) and popular. Both *primus* and *secundus* based
their lectures on pathological dissection, which in the latter's case
extended to theoretical concerns with pathophysiology.[10]

During the ascendancy of Munro *secundus,* in the final decades
of the eighteenth century, the University was joined by the increasingly important Royal Infirmary, founded in 1729 but grown
to pedagogically useful proportions only in the second half of
the century. Bedside teaching potentiated and complemented the
instruction conducted in the medical school's lecture rooms and
surgical amphitheater. And interlocking directorates insured a
continuum between the interests of hospital and school, if not
necessarily of the patients: As Guenter Risse notes, by the 1790s
a fifth of the infirmary's income came from student admission fees.
And it was simple enough for university faculty to delay discharges
or to arrange transfers to insure an appropriate and timely flow
of teaching cases.[11]

The late eighteenth-century Scottish picture was to remain largely unchanged in the early decades of the nineteenth.[12] But even though the Munros personally presented a *tour de force* in which *primus* already, in Lawrence's words, "consummated the marriage of medicine and surgery," and even though they emphasized necropsy findings in their own didactic teaching, Edinburgh offered neither a commodious milieu for the widespread development of pathological anatomy nor, for that matter, the deep interpenetration of medicine and surgery. Munro *secundus,* for example, saw to it that the surgical incorporation was excluded from university surgical instruction.[13] And postmortem dissections, when they were performed, were oftener than not rather cursory, desultory affairs. Mortality rates were relatively low and patients' families were frequently obdurate about permitting postmortem dissection of their deceased relatives. Consequently, students of physic could expect to observe firsthand no more than a handful of autopsies during their clinical course, while the surgeons fared perhaps a bit, but not a great deal, better.[14]

INTELLECTUAL AND INSTITUTIONAL ROOTS BEFORE
1815: HUNTER AND THE HUNTERIANS

I have characterized the anatomical outlook of the English medical elite before 1815, anchored by the Hunter–Baillie, circle, as essentially "natural historical." Yet the man who came to occupy the same sort of talismanic stature in Britain that Bichat came to enjoy in France, John Hunter, left a legacy of morbid anatomy that was considerably more complex than that suggested by any such catch-phrase. It is hence worth pausing to examine that legacy, from Hunter's Scottish origins through his death in 1793, and ultimately to his monumentalization by various followers for a century and more thereafter.[15]

Like another Scot, James Carmichael Smyth, Hunter was interested not only in local pathological lesions, but in their general effects on the tissues of the body, both solid and fluid. In the nineteenth century he was often compared to Harvey, even to Newton, because of the emphasis he placed on the role of the bloodstream in health and disease. That emphasis was reflected in the title of his perhaps best known work, the *Treatise on the Blood, Inflammation, and Gun-shot Wounds* published in the year of his death.

That text may serve, in fact, as a sort of map in which one may trace the subtle shifts in direction Hunter sought to impart to surgery. Such shifts, as L. S. Jacyna has recently shown, were largely responsible for the polemical reconstruction of Hunter's reputation.[16]

The *Treatise on the Blood* made much in particular of what was undoubtedly the paradigmatic pathophysiological *process* of the nineteenth century, from Hunter and Bichat to Joseph Lister, namely, inflammation. Hunter was well aware of the role of the vasculature in mediating between local inflammation and its distant effects on the rest of the body. He was concerned with the origins of suppuration and adhesion formation in inflammatory responses to injury, and performed multiple experiments on animals in an attempt to elucidate these processes. He expatiated at length, not only in the *Treatise* but also in his surgical lectures, and in his *Observations on Certain Parts of the Animal Oeconomy* on the manner in which animal heat was depleted or augmented by inflammatory or other affections, linking local morbid occurrences with overall changes in the body economy.[17]

In a long chapter, for example, on "the adhesive inflammation," Hunter described how the blood could serve as a "uniting medium" in the formation of adhesions. The blood, he noted, if "thrown out of the circulation from an inflammatory state of the vessels," mediated the formation of false membranes and adhesions, especially in the major body cavities. In his observations of the human organism afflicted with "natural" military wounds, and the experimental injury of animals he studied by analogy, it is clear that he frequently encountered phenomena such as pleural adhesions in the chest, and bowel adhesions in the peritoneum.

Hunter explicitly used the latter, peritoneal inflammation, as an example of this form of pathological change. "The following I shall give as an example," he stated, "which I have often observed on the peritoneum of those who have died in consequence of inflammation of this membrane." In such cases he observed that the intestines became "more or less united to one another," in a manner that was stronger or weaker depending on the stage and explosiveness of the inflammatory process. "In some it is so strong as to require some force to pull them asunder; the smooth peritoneal coat is, as it were, lost, having become cellular, like cellular membrane."[18]

Inflammatory disease was also characterized by differential effects on different organs, depending upon their role in the body economy. If, for example, the heart or lungs were to become inflamed, "either immediately, or affected secondarily as by sympathy," the disease would affect the constitution more violently than the same amount of inflammatory change located outside the vital parts, "or was in one with which their vital parts did not sympathize. . . ."[19]

Reasoning of this sort, repeated often in Hunter's work, makes two things clear. First, as early as the 1780s and 1790s the surgeon Hunter was not unaware of the interpenetration of the local and the general in disease phenomena – the subtle, complex interrelations between surgical wounds and constitutional illness. Second, he explicitly used the language of tissues and textures that some historians have come to identify with the French, others with Britons such as Smyth.[20] And yet on balance, when texts such as those just discussed are placed back in the context of Hunter's full body of work, he cannot be perceived (any more than can his direct spiritual heir Matthew Baillie) as an originator of modern morbid anatomy or of systematic tissue pathology. Hunter's central concerns rather remained the local treatment of abscesses and gunshot wounds, the local vasculature of aneurysmal or inflammatory lesions, the comparative anatomy of normal and diseased structures, and – most importantly, on the very basis of these several abstract interests – the clear demonstration of the scientific basis of surgery.

Here lay the key distinction between Hunter and the French. John Hunter folded enough physiological theory into his surgical system to make clear to all professional comers the elevated, esoteric status of surgical science. The Hunterian Orators who followed at the College of Surgeons in the nineteenth century seized on this program much as their counterparts at the College of Physicians had done before and since. No physiological theory could be put forward without considerable reference to Hunter's "animal oeconomy." That did not *necessarily* translate, however, into the further step, taken in France but not in Britain, by which surgical theory might methodically be integrated into medical theory.

Recent scholarship, particularly the work of Othmar Keel, Susan Lawrence, and L. S. Jacyna, has gone far toward clarifying this state of affairs. The latter's recent, deft examination of Hunter's reputation represents a more complicated and satisfactory account of the views of British surgeons. In this important article, Jacyna retrieves what he aptly calls the "polemical context" within which the afterimages of John Hunter were conjured up for various, sometimes self-serving ends. What were those ends? Jacyna's argument hinges on the way in which Hunter furnished an overlay of "scientificity" for the professional status of the elite, questing surgeon–anatomist. In some sense Hunter was for the eighteenth-century surgical professional man what William Harvey was for the physician a century and more earlier. Beginning with the authors of the Hunterian orations from the mid-1810s on, accounts of Hunter's life work evolved into a sort of comfortable, holographic image. Intellectually minded surgeons of the nineteenth century could mirror their own careers against the Hunterian hologram and come away with flattering reflections.[21]

Susan Lawrence further corroborates the notion of an English establishment of "separate but equal elites." In her discussion of the intellecutal and professional succession in the Hunters' extramural lecturing school at Great Windmill Street, Lawrence documents the short-lived nature of the amalgamation of medical and surgical lecturing from 1810 to 1812. From 1813, she shows, in a "collective desertion" of physicians, medical lecturing moved to the "Medical and Chemical School" across the way to No. 42. In this location the medical men could spread out a bit, provide their medical and chemical courses, and still bask in the patina of the prestigious, nearby anatomical theater, still warmed by a Hunterian glow.[22]

★ ★ ★ ★ ★

By the end of the eighteenth century, then, in the Edinburgh of the Munros and William Cullen, as well as in the London of their compatriots John and William Hunter, there were "perfect conditions for the potential interchange of medical and surgical ideas."[23] That sort of interchange could indeed be discerned in pronouncements of elite medical authors on whom most historians of the period focus their attention. But Lawrence's term, "potential," remained the operative one for most of the rest of the medical community, for two simple reasons. First, despite the efforts of men of high station (especially well-placed surgeons) to render surgery and medicine more scientific by melding their insights and theories, the two professional groups remained separate in training.

As long as training remained separate, so too, in most cases, did outlook.

Second, pathological anatomy, as a potential vehicle for any such merger, gained adherents in both Edinburgh and London, but still failed to attain the pride of place that it already enjoyed in turn-of-the-century Paris. In some hands, largely surgeons', the morbid appearances of the human frame were beginning to work at all three levels, theoretical, practical, and professional, to integrate the world views of physician and surgeon. As long as physicians were less likely to take part, however, and autopsies remained (for whatever reasons) an afterthought in the hands of those who did perform them, this effect was truncated. The powerful integrating tool of pathological anatomy sustained an impact that was more often potential than real.

PROFESSIONAL ROOTS BEFORE 1815: THE SURGEON–APOTHECARIES

If one wished to look elsewhere for evidence for a more pervasive impact of pathological anatomy, where might one seek it? One obvious place would be the apothecaries and, in particular, that subset of the apothecary community known as surgeon–apothecaries. The apothecaries' attempts, beginning in 1815, to achieve status more closely approximating that of the surgeons and physicians, formed fertile soil for the implantation of new ideas. I pause, therefore, to consider their program in some detail.

Most accounts of the apothecaries' efforts, viewing them in the context of the English medical profession circa 1815, look forward to the emergence of the general practitioner as an ascension from the lowest order in the medical hierarchy.[24] The apothecary, fore-runner of the general practitioner, is therefore the pivotal figure in such accounts. Some historical studies place greater emphasis on the view from this pivot point of 1815 looking toward the path beyond. Hence, the Act of Parliament enacted in July 1815 reg-ulating the certification and practice of the apothecaries, is taken to be the first all-important step toward assuring their mobility up the social, economic, and intellectual ladder. According to this view such an assurance was possible because from its Olympian height, the elite College of Physicians, having become a haven for obstructionists opposed to reform legislation, was caught napping.

The College suddenly found itself smartly sidestepped by its low-born pursuers.[25] According to this view, the Apothecaries Act was a victory for the nascent general practitioner and a spur to the formation of the reform-oriented institutions that were soon to spring up in London.[26]

More recent studies, marshalling impressive evidence, view the pivotal events of 1815 and the apothecaries' role in those events from the path below. Arriving nearer the mark in important respects, these accounts point out the apothecaries' fear of encroachment from below by those purveyors of base trade, the druggists and chemists.[27] Accused by the apothecaries of peddling unpredictably formulated or adulterated wares, the chemists antagonized and overtly opposed them, even though the two groups' expertise was by now more complementary in fact than competitive. Because the 1815 Act, in the version finally enacted, excluded the chemists and druggists from its regulations, and because it obfuscated the definition of the apothecary, revealing the conservative manipulating hand of the College of Physicians, the more recent view of the Act considers it "a reassertion of the theory of 'orders' at the very moment that this theory was crumbling in the face of the new social structure."[28] The Apothecaries Act was, in short, not a victory in this view but a blow that "tended to degrade" the apothecaries; the new institutions of the 1820s and 1830s must then be explained via broader socioeconomic arguments.[29]

Both versions of the roots and consequences of the 1815 legislation become inadequate in their analysis of the bill's principal supporters, and of how those supporters perceived its effects in terms of their own intellectual aspirations. In the struggle for and against the proposed "Act for Enlarging the Charter of the Society of Apothecaries" that described medical London in early 1815, the group that fervently backed the legislation was not the Society of Apothecaries but the three-year-old Association of Apothecaries and Surgeon–Apothecaries.[30] Just before the bill's passage one of the leading central members and chief spokesmen of the Association, Robert Masters Kerrison, who later (1820) changed his spots and became a physician, wrote that "many Apothecaries have gone through a regular course of instruction in Surgery, and combine that with their other occupation. They are, on this account, more extensively useful, particularly in thinly populated districts of the country, where there could not be possible subsistence for three persons – the physician, the mere surgeon, and the mere apothecary."[31] This argument for complementarity and upward mobility was coupled with a parallel argument for quality control: certification to separate out and suppress the chemists and druggists, tradesmen pure and simple, whose encroachment from below was feared above all else. The surgeon–apothecaries' professional goals were thus threefold: a higher ceiling, a higher and less leaky floor, and more room to walk about.

The surgeon–apothecaries' interests were far from coincident with those of either of the two licensing bodies that certified them.[32] Kerrison was at pains to emphasize both the numerical strength and the separateness of his group. "The term surgeon–apothecary," he declared, "is intended to designate those who practise as apothecaries, and are also members of the Royal College of Surgeons. They are now the most numerous part of the profession in town and country."[33] He then recalled how the Association, whose steering committee had been pressing for reform for over two years, had met with a cold shoulder from *all three* examining bodies in London, the two Royal Colleges and the Company of Apothecaries.[34]

What, then, were the surgeon–apothecaries seeking? It seems clear enough that in 1815 they had to settle, after the rough-and-tumble of Parliamentary maneuvering, for half a loaf in terms of their program of professionalization and that they had to cede the licensing and regulatory functions to the Society of Apothecaries, given legislative unwillingness to bring about a major, 1794-style *bouleversement* in the formal structure of the profession. It seems equally clear that the 1815 Act was not so much a giant stride as a consolidation of slow, creeping gains won de facto in the previous quarter-century by the apothecaries, essentially through the failure of juridical authorities to prosecute them as they inched their way onto physicians' and surgeons' territory.

As I have already noted, however, earlier interpretations of 1815 are predicated on the notion of the apothecary-to-general practitioner evolutionary sequence. If one sets such a notion aside to ask instead about the surgeon–apothecaries' interests at the time, as measured by certain intellectual pursuits and forged in the consensus politics of the surgeons' and apothecaries' mutual concerns, a different picture begins to emerge.

What was this mutuality of concern? Again, the surgeon–apothecaries' aspirations were recognized as so sufficiently foreign to the Society of Apothecaries that the latter body resisted their program. (It should no longer be surprising that "the apothecaries were militant but their controlling body slumbered,"[35] since the "mere" apothecaries were not the dominant lobbying force to begin with.) But the cognitive substance of that program is yet to be elucidated. To answer the question more fully one need only take the surgeon–apothecaries and their spokesman Kerrison seriously and survey the world as it appeared to them. As Kerrison knew, his Association had not been the first organization seeking to loosen the Colleges' viselike grip on the apothecaries' practice. Both in the 1790s a General Pharmaceutical Association and again in the first decade of the new century an "Associated Faculty" had come together briefly, purporting to raise and regulate professional entry standards. By 1811, however, all such efforts had foundered.

The surgeon–apothecaries were different. It may be that the "torch was taken over" by them, but they were, like the Medical and Chirurgical Society of London a decade earlier, brought together as a self-conscious *coalition* of individuals and groups of individuals who perceived their interests to be complementary and convergent.[36] Professionally, they all sought opportunity. Intellectually, they sought integration of the physicians' humoral lexicon with the surgeons' localistic, anatomical lexicon. As an alliance between partly competing but partly cooperating interests, the surgeon–apothecaries wished to avoid any act that would "interfere with any of the rights . . . vested in [the existing examining bodies]."[37] That the majority of the participants belonged to both groups assured such circumspection.[38]

The surgeon–apothecaries' circumspection was not evident in their early meetings, stretching at frequent intervals from midsummer 1812 to midsummer of 1813. They had convened initially in July 1812 at the Crown and Anchor, a tavern in the Strand where the apothecaries had met since the eighteenth century. The concerns voiced here quickly transcended mundane but troublesome matters such as the price of glass, and the focus of the Crown and Anchor discussions soon turned to the problems associated with finding "the best mode of placing the profession under a proper superintendence."[39] Those present and those otherwise represented (over 1,000 paid-up members drawn from over the nation, comprising apothecaries, man–midwives and surgeon–apothecaries), had developed skills and knowledge no longer matched by the three examining bodies. All three bodies were nevertheless approached on repeated occasions. After a year and more of hearing their entreaties go unanswered, however, the surgeon–apothecaries' circumspection began to erode.

As a result, at some point late in 1813 the surgeon–apothecaries' steering "London Committee" actually toyed with, and publicly proposed, the notion of a fourth examining body. The new body was to consist of a decentralized panel of Boards of Medical Practitioners.[40] Each such Board would be empowered to examine candidates in the categories of practitioner whose expertise no longer corresponded to any one of the three existing bodies. "It should be understood," they noted, "that no fourth legal body was contemplated until the present Colleges had refused to join in the application to Parliament for a Bill."[41] At this point there were two strategies for getting a Bill passed. The more radical was the fourth-body strategy, linking the surgeon–apothecaries tightly with ideal institutional forms that would match their current expertise and bend existing power relationships to conform. The more conservative strategy was to appease the power structures, accept regulation by one of them, and bend their cognitive and instrumental concerns to conform. In the face of a stone wall the surgeon–apothecaries resolved, on November 19, to fall back on the latter strategy.[42] At this point their die was cast and events set in train toward the legislation enacted some twenty months later. For all the reasons given above, the resulting Act was conceded at the time to be a compromise, the fruit of an "arduous and most unsatisfactory struggle," but its "first object, . . . in some degree, gained."[43] It was half a loaf, in short, but nutriment of a sort for the further development of their plans.

THE SURGEON–APOTHECARIES' PROGRAM

Under the continued hegemony of the three examining bodies, the surgeon–apothecaries' program unfolded in uneven fashion. It is important to distinguish, therefore, between those aspects of their program that, properly sanctioned, became law and immediately had an impact on medical education and practice, and those aspects that remained keenly held but unfulfilled intellectual aspirations. It is equally important to recognize that both aspects, aspirations realized and aspirations carefully held in abeyance, reflected the self-perceptions of the new men. Outlines of the new self-image thus emerge both from events and pronouncements regarding the surgeon–apothecary's career after 1815.

It would be too simple to suggest that the Apothecaries Act, given the surgeon–apothecaries' desire to dissect, sent young Englishmen packing off to France with the blessing of the English accrediting bodies. That they did in fact hie themselves off to Paris is discussed at length in Chapter 6. But to suggest a causal connection entails the *post hoc ergo propter hoc* fallacy: The suggestion is too simplistic because the College of Physicians was much too threatened by the new pathological anatomy to allow a windfall for the supporters of this increasingly foreign tradition.

In theory, this sort of windfall might have been possible for anyone with the audacity to set up shop in the French manner right at home, on English shores. Would not the students and young surgeon–apothecaries come running? But the paucity of dissection material would have limited such an enterprise at home even if the surgeon–apothecaries were suddenly required to dissect there.[44] Legislation reshuffling the requirements could, however, have a major impact: This was demonstrated in the Company of Apothecaries' interpretation of the 1815 Act's requirements for study in an entirely separate area, a field more congenial to the English medical temperament: botany.[45]

Physicians' native interest in natural history and pharmacognosy, and the imperative for standardization of the apothecary's knowledge, together mitigated for a much greater emphasis on formal botanical instruction immediately after 1815. William Salisbury, author of an 1816 *Botanist's Companion* and himself proprietor of an "herbarizing school," described the 1815 Act as "having made [botany] indispensable to all the younger branches of the medical profession."[46] The result was an explosion of field classes in botany, supplying instruction to hordes of medical students from all over Britain, seeking tutelage in English plant lore. According to an extensive recent study of the British natural history school, this explosion was of an order of magnitude sufficient to reshape British field botany. It was the critical factor in the future growth of that field, both for the botany instructors in their newly created posts, and for the many new students attracted to the field by their studies under those instructors.[47]

But no such explosion occurred in morbid anatomy. Asked in May of 1828 why the Court of Examiners of the Apothecaries still required no dissection, its Secretary, John Watson, responded that they were "desirous not to throw any obstruction in the way of persons about to be examined . . . because, by the law of the land, as it at present stands, dissections cannot legally take place."[48] He added that he was certain that the requirements would be tightened as soon as the legal impediments were removed. Enabling legislation removing those barriers would only be passed finally in 1832.

Instruction in pathological (or even normal) anatomy with dissection was not to be actually required before the mid-1830s, on the eve of the era of microscopic histopathology.[49] Even then the matter was hardly one of routine. As late as the mid-1834 deliberations of the Parliamentary Select Committee on Medical Education, one of the Apothecaries' examiners, John Ridout, could testify that anatomy examinations required no "demonstrative," i.e., dissecting, skills even though it appeared by now that "students pay very great attention to anatomy, quite as much as their opportunities for dissection will afford to them."[50] Hence the market for knowledge of botany was significantly different than that for pathological anatomy. In the former case the demand was created artificially, in some measure at least, by the apothecaries' 1816 requirements, with a rapidly inflated supply of instruction that may have even pulled the market along further. In pathological anatomy, by contrast, the demand grew from two sources: from the official requirements of the College of Surgeons, and from within the ranks of students, for reasons quite apart from the officially sanctioned canons of knowledge.[51] This demand far outstripped the abilities, intellectual and material, of the "suppliers in the hospitals and private schools of London."[52]

Remaining as they did under the thumb of the powerful preexisting examining bodies, the surgeon–apothecaries thus advanced a program that was neither professionally nor intellectually as aggressive as would have been the case had they been able to sustain their short-lived fourth body strategy. But from their pronouncements over the years 1814–1823 nonetheless emerge the outlines of a new self-image, defined not merely by events but also by aspirations.

As Justice Sir James Park would later point out, in 1815 there were legally and administratively only "four degrees in the medical profession, physicians, surgeons, and chymists and druggists."[53]

But the self-perception inherent in the surgeon–apothecaries' view of those four orders prompts some analytical remarks that reveal the picture to be more complicated than Park allowed. First, as Robert Masters Kerrison was at pains to note in his 1814 *Inquiry*, the surgeon–apothecaries wished to distance themselves from *all four* orders, the upper three with their respective courts and examiners, and the unregulated tradesmen at the bottom. Kerrison provided each of the four in turn with assurances of unthreatening fealty from the new men. Among the recipients of the surgeon–apothecaries' assurances was the "*Regular* Apothecary, who has an honourable solicitude for the welfare of his patients."[54] Second, there is a clear indication of the surgeon–apothecaries' displeasure with the elitism of the "Hospital, or consulting Surgeon[s]" who controlled the Court of Assistants of the Royal College of Surgeons. That the elite cadres of hospital surgery, dominated by the Astley Coopers and Benjamin Brodies, were virtually as aloof and refractory toward reform as their medical counterparts was therefore a further stimulus for cohesion within the coalition of surgeon–apothecaries.

THE SURGEON–APOTHECARY AND THEORETICAL INNOVATION

Coalitions become most cohesive, arguably, when, in synergistic fashion, their self-perceptions combine intellectual and professional–political expectations. It is not surprising, therefore, that the surgeon–apothecaries, far from giving up the ghost after 1815, continued to elaborate an intellectual program of increasingly rich detail, and that they presented it *in extenso* in the "Introductory Essay" to the new journal that they sponsored beginning in 1822–23. The question posed in that essay, probably penned by Kerrison, and a related one by Thomas Alcock (1784–1833) was essentially this: What should a general practitioner uniquely *know*?[55] But

the Association no longer expects to gain their object by a direct application to Parliament at present. They see that the time is not come for such a proceeding, and they believe that by steadily following their present plan, and by affording proofs of the evils to be remedied to the public on the one hand, and exciting their compeers to a further improvement in the knowledge of the healing art on the other, they are not only adopting the one most likely to be ultimately effectual, but are laying open a field well worthy of being cultivated by men even of the highest attainments.[56]

Thomas Alcock echoed many of the same views in his own "Essay on the Education and Duties of the General Practitioner in Medicine and Surgery":

The division of diseases into the provinces of medicine and surgery is purely artificial and not founded in nature; in nature the mutual influence of local and constitutional derangements upon each other admits of infinite gradation and variety. Hence it will be ascertained, whenever the physician or the surgeon is really qualified to secure to any sufferer the full measure of benefit which the science of medicine is capable of affording, that he effects it by no narrow or partial views, but by concentrating, as it were, the resources which are artificially assigned to separate departments of the profession.[57]

Alcock (1784–1833) shared a number of important characteristics with many of the surgeon–apothecaries who came of age in the 1820s. Like James Clark (1788–1870), James Johnson (1777–1845), John Farre (1775–1862), Charles Thomas Haden (1786–1824), and like his collaborator Kerrison (1775/6–1847), Alcock was part of a generation of provincials seeking professional advantage in the thriving, postwar metropolis. Most in this generation of surgeon–apothecaries had seen service as military and naval surgeons, posts in which they had enjoyed a great deal of independent responsibility for general patient care. Almost all of them had traveled extensively on the Continent during or just after the hostilities, and some of them, such as Clark and Haden, had studied or lived there for extended periods. Mustered out and arrived in London, they suddenly confronted a closed system. The College of Physicians granted a number of them the lesser certifications of licentiate or extralicentiate,[58] but remained a tiny, increasingly otiose group presided over by the ultra-Tory Henry Halford (1766–1844). A stiff and pompous aristocrat, Halford could be relied on to resist not only physical diagnosis and pathological anatomy, but virtually any innovation of any description. Almost as resistant to change was the governing elite of the College of Surgeons, whose Court of Assistants followed the whims of the powerful chief hospital consulting surgeons. The power of this latter group was as enviable and invidious as its patronage was seductive within a system still mired in nepotism.

When they were faced with the straitened prospects imposed by this system, a system that reigned *de jure* long past 1815, it was natural for the new men to question the viability of old theories, old therapies, and old career patterns. The physicians' traditional antiphlogistic treatment regimens and drug therapy seemed, if possible, even less adequate than the hospital surgeons' more anatomical, localistic, and extirpative approaches. In any case, the surgeon–apothecary usually found the avenues of approach to both medical and surgical posts studded with hurdles.[59]

THE WORD

[T]his is a reading age . . . . It would almost seem that the chimerical project of equalizing ranks, rights, and riches, had now changed to the equally chimerical project of placing all classes of society on a level, in respect to knowledge. Thus we see some engines at work to debase the faculty in the eyes of the populace, while others are endeavoring to elevate the populace, (in their own eyes at least) to rank with the faculty in medical lore! . . .[This] will be attended with one *good effect* at least – that of forcing all classes of medical society to an increased cultivation of the science they profess. Thus, while blunders may probably become more numerous among the people themselves, it is likely that error will diminish among their medical attendants.[60]

In the England of the 1810s and 1820s, the broad front along which medical knowledge and society were changing extended to an increasingly important facet of professional culture: the printed word. It is impossible to understand either the context or the content of English pathology without a grasp of the rise of new literary forms during this period. There was a crucial relationship between pathology as an evolving body of knowledge and the evolving medical journal, and the relationship was a reflexive one. Each needed the other. An expanding market for practical information in a readily and cheaply available format entailed in its wake an enlarging space for theoretical medicine as well. Some of the new medical theory would come from the pens of domestic writers. Much of it would come, particularly after 1816, in a new review literature drawn from continental sources rendered into English.

In all of the new journals, those turned toward foreign developments and those turned inward, pathology, especially pathological
anatomy, was in turn one of the new fields whose importance
served as the rationale for the growth of the medical publishing
industry.

This growth had dimensions that far exceeded mere gestures of
intellectual experimentation among medical elites. More was involved than a generation of medical moderns burning to spread
the new wisdom. Printing technology had entered a new phase.
After 1810 steam-driven printing presses were introduced into the
publishing industry. As this new technology was developed and
put into routine production of the printed word, costs declined
dramatically. The effect on publishing was slow but dramatic.
Obstacles remained, only to be withdrawn piecemeal. The economic dislocations imposed by the war with France was one such
obstacle in the period 1810–1816. The printing machines themselves were improved in slow stages, with a twentyfold increase
between 1810 and 1830 in the rate at which they could produce
printed text. High taxes on paper production and on the periodical
press remained a fact of life, abominated by utilitarian reformers
and many others, throughout the 1820s, before the Reform Parliament of 1832 finally matched its political energies to the economic ones of a resurgent publishing industry.[61]

The process of resurgence was well under way, however, by
1816, with signs of it in view even by 1810. A major expansion
of publishing in general was a nearly inevitable consequence of
technological advances pushing it, coupled with new markets
pulling it. The professional middle class was no small factor in
establishing such markets before 1832. A flood tide of books,
magazines and journals, from bird-watching to the study of geological formations, responded to an audience of those with the
affluence to buy them and the interest, be it amateur or professional, to support them. The number of medical journal "starts"
grew steadily throughout the period, reflecting the recognition of
a potential market for medical information, under a new set of
economic circumstances in the publishing world.

Medical publishing expanded rapidly as well. Publishers bent
on moving into the medical market, while foregoing to some extent the opportunity for sudden and rapid capital appreciation, were
able to reduce their financial risk in a business riddled with un-

certainty.[62] Medical editors, after 1815 almost always youthful reformers trained in the postwar period, saw their new posts as viable means of forging and reinforcing their medical careers.[63] They also saw the editorships as platforms from which to popularize scientific innovation. The readership, in turn, gained access to new techniques and ideas in a format and manner that not only sped the information to the physician's desk, but also amplified its impact because the volume of literature was growing so fast.

One might conveniently divide the spectrum of early nineteenth-century medical periodicals into four genres, each with a role in disseminating pathological anatomy. The first type to emerge was the Baconian repertory of observation and fact, often as the record of some formal or informal association. Generally published annually or less frequently still, this type dominated medical periodical publishing in the eighteenth century, declining in the early decades of the nineteenth. The importance of any particular title was in proportion to that of the association for which it served as a vehicle; perhaps the most enduring was the *Medical Essays and Observations* (1733), which evolved into the *Edinburgh Medical and Surgical Journal* (1805).

The second genre, and the first to emerge in the nineteenth century, the publication of the proceedings and transactions of medical coalition organizations, antedated the post-1810 (i.e., post-steam engine) growth spurt of the periodical literature. It was typified in the first instance by the *Medico-Chirurgical Transactions* begun in 1809 by the syndics of the Medical and Chirurgical Society of London. It grew fitfully in parallel with the small group of medical organizations that it reflected. When the formation of those organizations was a function of coalition politics, which was the case with the Medico-Chirurgical Society in a socially narrow-gauged fashion and the Surgeon–Apothecaries in a broad-gauged manner, their journals' editorial contents tended to reflect the consensus of the organizations' component interests.

Pathological anatomy was often the convenient theoretical equivalent of the coalition product. Only after 1815, however, did the field begin to take on the more cosmopolitan cast of continental theoretical pathology. The third genre of medical periodical, the abstracting and reviewing journal, coincided with and may have fostered this development. This species of journal, typified by the *Medical Intelligencer* and the *Quarterly Journal of Foreign Medicine and*

Surgery, provided more direct and straightforward access to foreign material, and eliminated the mediating agency of medical societies and their elite leadership. Pathological anatomy now arrived with but the single coat of varnish provided by the editors' own sensibilities.

A fourth genre of medical periodical was the journal dominated by the reformist impulse embodied in *The Lancet,* founded in 1823. Approximated by no other journal for sheer pluck and spleen, *The Lancet* quickly became notorious for publishing the introductory lectures of English medical academic poo-bahs without the authors' approval, hence presenting their ideas and techniques unvarnished, and without recompense. But *The Lancet's* founder – editor, Thomas Wakley (1795–1862), was less interested in importing new knowledge than he was in showing that he could disseminate the old wisdom without effective trammels from the London hospital elite: a snub of its monopolistic practices. Wakley was, with occasionally constructive results, a curmudgeonly fellow who took aim whenever possible at the "hospital bats . . . in their dreary recesses."[64] The running feud between the chagrined, frequently litigious hospital consultants and the eccentric, often churlish Wakley provided neither party with much incentive for probing the new medical science.[65] Thus, the major source of pathological anatomy, both as career and as cognitive style, were left primarily to the medical journals and the moderate reformers who staffed them.

THE "VORACIOUS BATS" AND WHAT THEY
THOUGHT: THE BEGINNINGS OF THE
MEDICO-CHIRURGICAL TRANSACTIONS

The first number of the *Medico-Chirurgical Transactions* displayed prominently, in front of its prefatory material, a list of the members of the Medical and Chirurgical Society of London from its formation to March 1809. In addition to the hospital squirearchy of London – figures like William Babington, Alexander Marcet, and Astley Cooper of Guy's, William Blizard and John Yelloly of the London, and Henry Cline of St. Thomas's – the list included stalwarts of the Edinburgh school such as James Gregory, Thomas Charles Hope, and Andrew Duncan. It included as well the essential core of the Hunter–Baillie circle (notably Matthew Baillie and Everard Home), and useful local nonmedical worthies like Humphry Davy and Sir Joseph Banks.[66] The first volume of the *Transactions* contained a carefully balanced array of medical and surgical contributions, ranging from John Bostock on blood chemistry to Astley Cooper on carotid artery aneurysm.[67] Edward Jenner contributed two pieces on rabies and smallpox.

The "Case of a Foetus Found in the Abdomen of a Boy" presented by George William Young (d. 1850), reflected as well as any the sort of cognitive product that was possible in the coalition of elite physicians and surgeons. Speaking to the hospital elite in March of 1808, Young went beyond the anecdotal sort of case description that would have sufficed in the not-too-distant eighteenth-century past. Young told of the hapless infant John Hare, born a healthy and apparently normal infant on the eighteenth of May in the previous year. When the boy had begun vomiting and over the summer a protrusion in his abdomen gradually had become increasingly prominent, his mother finally sought Young's advice in early September. The surgeon discovered a tense, movable, fluctuant mass in the left epigastrium, extending down toward the umbilicus. Young considered the boy most likely to have a congenital mesenteric cyst, distended by the fluid contained in its cavity. He foresaw no cure, and counseled expectant therapy, observation without specific surgical treatment, in an era when the peritoneal cavity of the living human was never broached by the reputable surgeon.

Young lost track of the boy and his mother until January of 1808, when the child was brought back to him in a shocking state. He was now a "mere skeleton clothed in skin with a face of age and anguish."[68] His mother explained that during the autumn his abdomen had increased in size until its girth, swollen by tumor, reached a yard around. The distension was tensest opposite the projecting mass. But suddenly, on December 23rd, the mother discovered that the projection was diminished, the child's flanks were bulging, and the boy was suddenly able to void large quantities of urine, which continued over a week's time. Then the process reversed itself once again and the child's belly again began to swell. Young felt that he could palpate another cystic cavity filled with fluid and containing a hard tumor floating within it.

Through the next month-and-a-half the situation gradually worsened until finally, on February 25, the emaciated child succumbed. Assisted by the Mechanics' Institutions and London University founder, George Birkbeck (1776–1841), Young conducted a postmortem inspection twelve hours later. They noted a cystic cavity whose wall was in places thin and transparent, and elsewhere "thick, dense, and perfectly opaque."[69] After describing its location and attachments in fine-grained anatomical detail, Young punctured the cyst, withdrawing 78 ounces of a "limpid fluid having the colour of an infusion of green tea."[70] He then declared that "it may be easily conceived that we were greatly surprised on finding that this substance had unequivocally the shape and characters of a human foetus."[71]

The dissection of the fetal monster discovered by Young was described in considerable detail in his case report. Though these morphological details are inherently interesting, more significant yet is Young's pathophysiological view of the morbid events during the infant Hare's illness. In January, on first observing the child's deteriorating condition, Young had surmised the following sequence of events to explain its clinical course: The tumor had "consisted principally of a fluid contained within a distinct cyst; that this cyst was ruptured on the 23rd of December; that its fluid contents escaped into the cavity of the peritoneum, and that the absorbents of this extensive membrane rapidly removed them."[72] Weeks later, when the postmortem examination had made it clear that the neoplasm was far more than a simple cyst, Young could sharpen his clinicopathologic correlation. He could verify by observation that the cyst wall had torn, leaked, and resealed. He could note the membranous quality of its internal serosal coat, capable of exuding the serous fluid that bathed the foetus; and he could liken the cyst to a structure that "answered the purpose of a placenta."[73]

The class of pathological phenomena typified by this case was as common in England during the Napoleonic period as it was in France, and indeed remained as universal long since: body cavities, cysts, and potential spaces filled with fluid; solid, tissue parts and humoral, fluid parts of the body interacting to create normal sites of lubrication, or abnormal sites of inflammatory exudation, painful distension, or tamponade. In 1809, addressing an audience of both physicians and surgeons, and attempting to explain the events in a diseased body's tissues and fluids, the surgeon Young sought to do so in terms that would be congenial to the widest segment of his audience. The resulting notion that fluid could undergo exhalation and then absorption by way of the surface of a membranous tissue was hardly novel in Young's account or in Britain in 1809; in part it harked back to the late seventeenth-century physiology of lacteals and intestinal absorption, and was hardly more dependent on foreign ideas than was the basic notion of the appropriateness of doing clinicopathological correlation.[74]

What was lacking from Young's Lexicon, however, and from that of his many medical and surgical colleagues who presented cases and investigations to the Medico-Chirurgical Society, was the sort of *systematic* tissue pathology that was then emerging within the Paris school. The approach remained rather that of the natural historian. A serous membrane was functionally linked not with other, analogous tissues susceptible to pathologic transudation or exudation, but to the placenta, an organ functioning at an entirely different level of complexity. At some inchoate level, a *lingua franca* between physicians and surgeons, a way of seeing pathological events was perhaps being formulated. But the formulation linking tissues and body fluids was as yet neither generalized nor, in the form seen here, easily generalizable.

6

Channel crossing

Anatomie Vivante; or, Skeleton Importation Company
   These are the days of speculation: one of the most profitable,
has been that of the Skeleton Importation Company. It appears
that some of our half-pay captains, whose former duty it was,
to "eat Frenchmen alive," have lately changed their occupation,
(in conformity with these piping times of peace,) to that of
picking the bones of a French skeleton; and good picking they
have! Between three and four hundred of the hydra-headed but
little-witted multitude of John Bulls – or rather John Gulls,
have run daily to Pall Mall to get their half-crown share or
sight of the living skeleton! In short, no Frenchman ever before
excited such curiosity on these shores – except Napoleon
himself. The living skeleton may therefore, in this respect, be
considered as a second *Bony*-parte.
               – Medico–Chirurgical Review (1825), **3** (n.s.): 600

THE EXODUS

By the 1820s the British medical world was becoming aware of
an exodus of many of its brightest students to France. A migration
of this magnitude was repeated and surpassed only a half-century
later when a larger number of American, Japanese, and other student groups began trekking to Germany to observe the new laboratory medicine. The earlier migration of a large segment of
young medical professional men to France in the decades after Waterloo is still of considerable interest. It touches on the nature of
"influence," not merely as the dry transfer of ideas, but as a whole
array of interactions between national cultures, practitioner communities, and medical traditions.

   Pathology in the post-Napoleonic period is difficult to discuss
in the disciplinary terms that seem comfortable for scientific medicine after the midcentury mark. Neither the French school of

Xavier Bichat and Théophile Laennec, nor the English work of Robert Carswell and Thomas Hodgkin resembled a modern scientific discipline or specialty, though pathology was later to evolve in both those directions. Nor was pathology by 1820 a coherent body of written knowledge susceptible to the tools of comparative literary history. Yet the juxtaposition of texts has been the principal tool of comparativists concerned with the reception of ideas generated in one culture and assimilated into another.[1] If this method is no longer sufficient, what tools are suitable?

One point of departure may at first glance seem too diffuse and obvious, but soon gains in explanatory power: whether conceived as the theory of disease, as the practice of anatomical pathology, or as clinicopathological correlation, pathology was part of clinical medicine before becoming enshrined in a separate discipline. It was to remain so until the advent of microscopy. At that point, new institutions were to form, first in Germany, around a range of new techniques, whereupon the circumstances of the field changed dramatically.[2]

In the Napoleonic period, however, and for a long time thereafter, pathology was part of the everyday armamentarium of practitioners. Physicians who made their daily rounds and attended patients at the bedside were the same as those who tested the boundaries of knowledge about pathological anatomy. It was understood that pathology texts were the result of clinicians' investigations. In the medical mind of the 1810s and 1820s, pathology was linked inextricably with a series of central problems of clinical medicine. After 1820 it came increasingly to be linked as well with the new techniques of physical diagnosis developed in the wake of Théophile Laennec's and others' work. Hence it is not surprising to find John Forbes's compendium of cases, drawn from his own experience with the stethoscope and percussion as well as from the findings of Laennec, Auenbrugger, Corvisart, and Collin, described in at least one prominent journal under the rubric of "pathology." *On the Diagnosis of Disease by Means of the Stethoscope,* by Forbes, was thus recommended to British readers "as containing a magazine of most accurate and useful pathology."[3]

When French clinicians wrote important pathology texts, they were in most cases translated quickly into other tongues, first of all, oftener than not, into English.[4] But it seems unlikely that English-speaking students, American as well as British, flocked to the dissecting rooms of Laennec, Cruveilhier, and others primarily because they had read the French texts. Bichat's *General Anatomy*, or even Laennec's *Mediate Auscultation* alone, even though these particular works *were* part of a coherent text, did not lure hundreds of students to Paris from England after 1816.[5] Yet an exodus of such proportions was precisely the outcome once the close of hostilities between the two nations by early 1816 had made it possible for the scientific doors to open wide. The English students soon came by the score, and finally by the hundreds.

The importation of the French anatomicopathological tradition into England was thus not simply a matter of knowledge flowing through the funnel of a text tradition. Nor was it simply a question of "technology transfer" by which the stethoscope was taken to England. The process was rather one in which *experience,* from the dissection table and the hospital wards, flowed through the careers of multitudinous young Englishmen as they made the journey out and back. At stake for the historian in accounting for this flow is the attraction and fate of a tradition, its elaboration in France, and its reflection in English eyes. This reflection was to be found not solely in English eyes. The year in France was, far from a passive period of observation, a veritable *tour de main.*

THE CHANGING INSTITUTIONAL STATUS OF PATHOLOGICAL ANATOMY, 1816–1836

At first Britons who came to France to do pathological anatomy were not drawn to any one institutional locus. Such study was part of a much larger landscape of hospital-based subjects and didactic methods, spanning a large array of teaching hospitals, private courses and the Paris Faculty itself. This lack of discrete borders remained prominent in some respects well past the mid-1830s. It was characteristic in the late 1810s before Théophile Laennec had published and John Forbes had translated the landmark work of 1819 on pathological anatomy, that pressed physical diagnosis into the service of pathology.[6] Up to this point anatomy, normal and pathological, remained cognitively and institutionally a seamless whole.

Until the 1830s, neither England nor France could boast a single professorship of *pathological* anatomy. The Scot, Robert Carswell, while based in Paris, was offered the first such post in England in

1828. He accepted this position at the new University College of London, but did not return to assume the new teaching duties until after 1830. The first French chair, ironically, came even later. Laennec and Pierre Louis had taught Carswell and legions of others the expanding lore of pathological anatomy, but never from a securely institutionalized platform. Not until 1835 did the will of the influential and aristocratic surgeon–anatomist of the Hôtel-Dieu, Guillaume Dupuytren, create an official chair in Paris.[7]

Laennec, Louis, and their peers taught pathological anatomy as an adjunct of courses given under widely varying sponsorship and title. Some were offered privately, transiently, with ministerial blessing.[8] At the *Faculté de médecine,* François Chaussier and Bichat's disciple P. A. Béclard could profess ideas similar to Bichat's in pathological anatomy, as part of the ordinary anatomy course. So, too, could Baron Dupuytren include pathological anatomy in his surgical clinic or *clinique externe,* as did J. J. Le Roux, the Dean since 1810, in his internal medicine clinic or *clinique interne.*[9] Pathology itself, the ancient study of the "seats and causes of disease," was similarly divided into medical ("internal") and surgical ("external") subunits.[10] Under the Empire, pathology as taught at the Faculty included heady doses of pathological anatomy both in the *pathologie interne* courses of Philippe Pinel and A.-M.-C. Duméril, and, especially, in the *pathologie externe* courses of J.-N. M. Marjolin and P. J. Roux.[11] Hospital-based courses, given by them and others, routinely combined clinical instruction with frequent demonstrations of anatomical pathology based on postmortem examinations. Another who gave such a course was the future occupant of the first chair of pathological anatomy, Jean Cruveilhier. He collected the material for his influential 1821 treatise as well as for his magisterial two-volume folio atlas of organ-centered pathological anatomy by this means.[12]

While surgical practitioners primarily interested in an organ- or tissue-centered form of surgical pathology came close to dominating the teaching of pathological anatomy, there were notable exceptions, such as Jean-Noël Hallé, and especially his successor, Théophile Laennec, in the chair of medicine at the *Collège de France.*[13] When the first wave of English-speaking pilgrims arrived in the early 1820s, it was, in fact, the medically-oriented Laennec who indoctrinated them into the mysteries of the body and its morbid appearances. In his hands pathological anatomy cut across both domains, medicine and surgery. Until the mid-1830s it also cut across both anatomy and the clinic. Then, on the eve of the introduction of the microscope into pathology, the creation of new chairs began slowly to transmute this inchoate tradition into something like a discipline.[14]

The proximity of normal and pathological anatomy, cognitively and practically, was paralleled in France by the proximity of those two subjects in teaching exercises. The knowledge gleaned from the ritual and routine *ouverture des cadavres* was related, after all, to both the normal and the pathological.[15] What that knowledge was *called,* and which part of it drew special emphasis, depended on the somewhat arbitrary matter of the geographic location of the *ouverture.* The postmortem examining room of the hospital in which the patient died was one such location; here special pathology would be emphasized: of what lesion, the prosector might ask, did *this* patient die? The other primary locus of dissecting activity was to be found at either of the two officially sanctioned sites for anatomical teaching, the *amphithéatre* attached to the *Hôpital de la pitié,* or that of the *Ecole pratique de dissection* operated by the Paris Faculty. Private dissecting theaters were no longer possible alternatives to the official sites; in October 1813, fully ten years after an ordinance was first enacted enabling such an action, private theaters had been suppressed.

In the officially sanctioned *amphithéâtre,* general anatomy and elements of general pathology were emphasized. In neither case, that of the hospital postmortem suite nor the dissecting amphitheater, was there undue difficulty in obtaining bodies for dissection or demonstration. A large percentage of hospitalized patients died; under prevailing French law bodies were cheap enough to come by. Hospital *chefs de clinique* and the *chef des travaux anatomiques* at the *Ecole pratique* had equal access and an established routine for insuring a constant legal supply of human remains for teaching and research.[16]

In England, by contrast, there was a clear distinction between the practice of obtaining bodies for conducting teaching dissections and the practice of conducting the examination, as the necropsy was called in both countries. While the former was abhorrent to a sizable part of English society (an echo of the special fate awaiting the remains of hanged murderers), the latter was tolerated, at least in principle. But as long as anatomical teaching depended on the alliance, always an uneasy one, between anatomical instructors and the rough trade of resurrectionists and body snatchers, even the simpler practice of straightforward postmortem examination remained a sporadic, marginal activity. The eclipse (if never the total extinction) of postmortem dissection in England is difficult to delineate exactly, as are most liminal zones of medical practice. But traces of its decline may be found in contemporary complaints about the inadequacy of facilities for conducting postmortems and in the perennially hostile relations between hospital surgeons and private anatomists. Ironic traces of English resistance to dissection may also be inferred from the slackening of public revulsion toward orderly, legal postmortem examinations when, in the wake of the murderous body-snatching atrocities of the late 1820s, the intensity of antagonism toward illegal dissection swelled to new heights. [17]

What did the disparity between English attitudes toward the postmortem examination and toward dissection, illicit or not, mean in actual practice? In case records dating back to the period before John Forbes and his co-travelers went to France, there is little evidence that the examination was ever used, save on rare occasions, to go beyond descriptions of interesting anomalies. The elaboration of a cogent pathological system was not part of the program. At the simplest level, to have presented the description of the postmortem lesions *was,* in and of itself, to have satisfied the prevailing nosology, based on the taxonomic model of the eighteenth-century natural historian. Examination without methodical dissection was thus, like a suite of rooms with no view, morbid anatomy without pathology. It was a natural history museum of lesions, ordered according to a catalog that was merely a list and not a framework.

This is not to claim that dissection was never practiced. The gradual increase in the number of private anatomy schools in London, occurring since the 1790s, attests to the fact that it was. Nor can one claim that the practice produced no lasting imprint on the new pathological anatomy. The elaboration of a tradition around John Hunter and Matthew Baillie (Chapter 5) attests to such an assertion. But in the end there was, put simply, a relative dearth of new raw material and, hence, a dearth of the theoretical product. More damaging yet, the raw material, the supply of bodies, was at the best of times not only inadequate and hence exceedingly

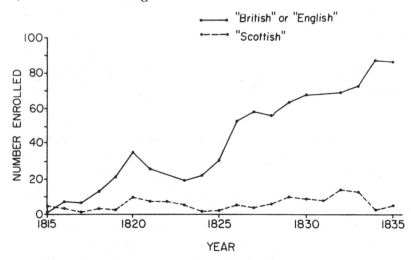

Figure 6.1. Number of students matriculated for a term or more in Paris Faculty.

dear, but also notoriously unpredictable: throughout the 1820s the noose of the law (and graveyard security) tightened around the scruffy suppliers; prices, accordingly, swung wildly.[18]

INCENTIVES TO STUDY NORMAL AND PATHOLOGICAL ANATOMY IN FRANCE

Why did British medical students come to Paris? Two groups of them are of interest: a large number who elected to do a stint at the Paris hospitals, and a subset of that group who enrolled formally for varying lengths of time at the *Faculté de médecine de Paris*. Figure 6.1 graphically depicts the curve of changing official British student enrollments in the Paris Faculty. This plot presents certain problems, since the greatest interest lies in gauging the movements (and motives) of *all* Britons who studied at the Paris Hospital, later to return to teach and practice in Britain.[19] The data nonetheless warrant discussion at this point for two reasons. The curve probably does represent a rough index of the rate of change in the size of the English swarm that made its way to Paris after the barriers of earlier bellicose relations had tumbled.[20] And for the critical initial sixteen years between 1816, the close of Anglo-French hostilities, and 1832, Parliament's passage of the Anatomy Act, the data are heuristically useful in structuring the argument.

If the appropriate assumptions are made about its significance, the curve suggests a rough division of the 1816–1832 period into segments roughly four years in length.[21] It then becomes possible to ask more discriminating questions about what induced English students to go to Paris during each quadrennium, and about how those motives themselves shifted over nearly two decades. It was inevitable that motives should have shifted subtly in this period because of the reflexive self-propagating nature of cultural migrations. While Paris teaching institutions prospered as a collective site for British medical education, the lessons learned by the British flooded back into England, both through their own verbal accounts and through the writings of their French mentors. In this manner, the interest of their slightly younger confrères was further stimulated, and eventually diverted into fresh channels. One such channel was physical diagnosis, which in turn developed into part of the lure of the French.

THE ANATOMY MARKET, 1816–1824

From the outset, the administrative arrangements of Paris medicine were attractive to the English in ways that differed markedly with the English situation. Foremost among those arrangements in promoting pathological anatomy were two particular functions: the regulation of the market in cadavers and the routine of the clinic.

The regulation of the body market was mainly economic rather than legal or moral. Postmortem examinations were of course outside this market. Even within the confines of such a market, however, the fact that cadaveric dissection was legal and orderly kept prices well within reach of students and teachers. Anatomy instructors, unencumbered by the nearly prohibitive costs that so weighed on their English counterparts, and fully tolerated by officialdom both within the Faculty and without, were at liberty to establish a variety of "free," that is, freelance, clinics and courses (*cours libres*) to supplement the official ones of the central faculty.[22] Dissection classes at the *Faculté* were the direct responsibility of the *chef des travaux anatomiques*.

Before Cruveilhier's 1835 appointment to the first professorship of pathological anatomy, the *chef*, it will be recalled, was the next closest thing to such a chair. The office of the *chef* also became a

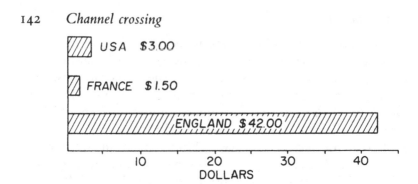

Figure 6.2. Price of cadavers in 1828.

sort of clearinghouse for the distribution of dissection material. The distribution network was the basis of a large, legally sanctioned market, derived from nine or more of the public medical institutions of Paris, and composed of the two public dissecting establishments plus the occasional *cours libre*. The existence of this market and network, along with its domination by a central officer whose responsibilities and credentials were both academic and public, assured a nominal and orderly price structure. That structure is difficult now to specify for the late 1810s, since *comptabilité* records were apparently not retained by the office of the *chef*. But some limiting notion of the relative prices in various countries is available for the time some ten years later when the issue had become so vexed that Parliament finally established a Select Committee to investigate the problem. Figure 6.2 indicates the prices of cadavers according to that report, for the period 1826–1828. Clearly revealed is the discrepancy in costs encountered by anatomists on the two sides of the Channel, even correcting for the upward creep in prices that the English experienced over the preceding decade.

The routine of the clinic represented another factor that furthered the integration of anatomy, pathology, and bedside medicine. Clinicians, physicians and surgeons alike, expected their students to follow them as they made the rounds from ward to lecture room to dissecting theater. Here those patients who fell into the one third or more of all admissions whose illnesses reached a *terminaison* in death, became the subject of the final lesson.[23] They became a part of the confirmation or discomfirmation of the clinician's diagnosis, and critically, the attempt to correlate antemortem external morbid appearances with the internal morbid appearances of tissues and organs in the postmortem state.[24]

The details are sketchy for the precise mechanism by which, in the first instance, both the ease of "anatomizing" in France and the anatomicoclinical method were brought to the attention of British medical men. It is possible to discern only in broadest outline how the earliest seeds were sown. But this much is clear: It was in Edinburgh, very early on, that the seeds were sown for Britons on both sides of the Scottish border.[25] Among Scottish medical educators of the late 1810s, longstanding pride in the indigenous educational traditions of Scottish medicine, cultural affinities for ideas and things French, and a fine disdain for London medicine combined to generate an atmosphere receptive to medicine as it was being taught in France.[26]

THE SCOTTISH CONNECTION

No single Scottish Moses led this new flock to the Gallic promised land. But two Edinburgh academicians in particular, Andrew Duncan, Jr. (1773–1832) and John Thomson (1765–1846), typified the attitude that pervaded medical education in the northern capital. Both were scions of families that carried on in the dynastic style of Edinburgh, typified by the Munros. In the late 1810s Duncan's better-known father (1744–1828), now enfeebled and dubbed "old Duncan" by the students, was still enshrined in the chair of the institutes of medicine. The younger Duncan occupied a lesser chair, that of medical jurisprudence, and from 1805 edited the *Edinburgh Medical and Surgical Journal*.[27] He joined his father in the medical chair in the year of the latter's retirement, 1819, and became professor of materia medica as well in 1821. Throughout his academic career, both by word and deed, Duncan, Jr., harbored two sentiments: a desire to see the profession expand in what he perceived to be the two critical fields of medical science, chemistry and anatomy, and an equally strong disdain for the quality of education available in those fields elsewhere in Britain. As early as 1795, while still a student, the younger Duncan had written his father from London:

I have seen almost no anatomical preparations made at Windmill St., but I believe there is no law against it. Warm weather is certainly unfavourable to the keeping of subjects, but frost is no less with regard to dissection. For the hands are so numbed that they cannot hold the knife. There is certainly a great deal of difference between Dr. [Matthew] Baillie's first and second course and every lecture of his is worth hearing till you have it by heart. Except seeing operations nothing is to be learnt at the hospitals here.[28]

The ideas that Duncan, Jr. expressed in 1795 on the relative merits of London hospital and private anatomy courses, ideas that remained with him into the 1820s, were prescient. They presaged later disputes between competing London surgeons that led scores of their would-be students to flee to Paris.

Over his first two decades as journal editor and professor, the younger Duncan's favorable attitude toward the Paris experience was sharpened both for practical reasons (he wanted students to anatomize) and for theoretical reasons related to the usefulness of a pathology of tissues and textures. This was particularly the case after Laennec introduced, in the service of his pathological anatomy, his new device, the *cylindre* or stethoscope, confirming and extending the Bichatian canon of tissues. Hence in 1823 James Clark, one of Laennec's most ardent English popularizers, could write the Frenchman in a postscript that:

You will see, on referring to page XX of the preface to Dr. Forbes's translation of your work, that it was at my earnest request that he undertook the translation. I have much pleasure in informing you that the translation as well as the original has been exceedingly well-received in England. At Edinburgh your work has also been much admired, particularly by Professor Duncan, a man of great talents and Editor of the *Edinburgh Medical and Surgical Journal*.[29]

Duncan's pathological theory was an eclectic one, amalgamating the Hunterian and Bichatian strains of tissue pathology. In Edinburgh that same July (1823), it was natural therefore, for him to step before a newly formed society of medical practitioners and teachers incorporating both physicians and surgeons to present a discourse on "inflammation of the cellular texture." He cited as his authorities both the chief exponents of the English tissue-pathology tradition, notably John Hunter and James Carmichael Smyth, and those of the French tradition as it was embodied in the early *Journal de médecine*.[30] Like his younger colleague, William Thomson (1802–1852), Duncan, Jr. became an early champion of the use of auscultation in anatomicoclinical science.[31]

Equally keen to promote French anatomical science was the professor of military surgery, John Thomson, a silk weaver's son who became the paterfamilias of a new medical dynasty. Keenly interested in the pathology of inflammation, Thomson looked to the pathology of textures as the best way to explain inflammatory affections. He was moved by the wish to see the new morbid anatomy practiced in a manner that seemed impossible in Britain, even in Edinburgh. Only in Paris were there enough hospital cases, and only in Paris did enough such cases come to the necropsy table. Thomson was perhaps the most influential of the Edinburgh faculty, therefore, as the source of direct, demonstrable admonitions to students to turn their sights across the channel. Like an American counterpart, John Collins Warren, Thomson sent his son abroad to attend the lectures of the medical luminaries of Restoration Paris.

Nine years before his son William made that journey, John Thomson published his own *Lectures on Inflammation,* a work that was well received and widely regarded as representing a perfection of the Hunterian doctrine of vascular pathology in inflammatory diseases.[32] The "influence of different textures" was considered one of the most important parts of these *Lectures.* Here, and again eight years later in the course of "extraacademical" lectures that he gave while an unsuccessful candidate for the University Professorship in the Practice of Physick, Thomson "put aside," according to one contemporary observer, "that arrangement of diseases which nosologists had adopted, in their desire to imitate the classification of naturalists, and substituted an anatomicophysiological arrangement . . ., a view . . . embracing as it did, the most recent researches of continental as well as domestic pathologists, and more especially those of M. Laennec."[33]

In the early 1830s, the aging John Thomson split his course on the Practice of Physick with his son William and moved up to a chair of General Pathology that he had been lobbying for years to secure for the University. Its creation, along with that of an additional surgery chair (both achieved with the help of Lord Melbourne) amounted to testimony both to his personal powers of persuasion, and to his intellectual convictions about the centrality of pathology. "It has been in this persuasion," wrote his elegist, "and with the knowledge of the want of proper opportunities in Edinburgh for studying pathological anatomy in particular, that Dr. Thomson has for a long series of years been induced to devote much of his time and of his professional income to the remedying, as far as has been in his power, of this most important defect in our medical institutions."[34]

Thomson would deliver his first course of pathology lectures in 1832–1833, only to fall ill two years later. Its founder absent, enthusiasm for the course tapered quickly. An assistant gave most of the lectures between 1835 and 1841, the year when Thomson finally retired at the age of seventy-six. As he grew older and more enfeebled, the university and civic authorities who had initially supported the chair threatened perennially to rescind that support. Thomson persevered, however, into the age of the microscope, and in 1842 a successor was appointed.[35] Robert Knox, the anatomist, would look back on Thomson's ability to turn science into bricks and mortar, and would dub him "the old chairmaker."[36]

John Thomson was interested in bringing French pathology back to Edinburgh in the most literal, material sense. Casting about for ways to accomplish this, he hit on Robert Carswell, a young Scot. Carswell (1793–1857) was from all appearances a superb artist and draftsman. Thomson suggested that Carswell, too, should go to Paris alongside the younger Thomson. This they did in 1822. Carswell made repeated trips to Paris, often for extended periods, spending what was doubtless the longest time of any Briton abroad in the 1820s. He left Paris in 1830 for the last time with a collection of hundreds of case descriptions, each minutely illustrated with richly detailed paintings and drawings. Drawn from virtually all of the major teaching hospitals of Paris, Carswell's paintings of cases in pathological anatomy survive to the present day. They never made their way back to Thomson's Edinburgh, however, but followed Carswell to University College, London.[37]

William Thomson and Robert Carswell arrived in Paris in the watershed years of the early 1820s, when Théophile Laennec was lecturing on pathological anatomy at the *Collège de France,* often drawing more auditors from across the sea than from his own countrymen. Laennec's classroom at the *Collège* was the central point around which many English students' activities pivoted. His English and Scottish students at the *Collège* would return to England within a few years to form the nucleus of a group, Thomson and Carswell as well as Thomas Hodgkin, John Forbes, and a number of other Laennec disciples, whose members proved most keen on bringing parts of the French tradition back to England.

Probably the most clinically oriented of those whom Thomson sent to Laennec was Charles J. B. Williams (1805–1889), whom Thomson took into residence in his home, in the custom of the time, along with six to eight other students. Williams later recalled that the anatomical lectures given by Alexander Monro *tertius*, written like the elder Duncan's lectures on the Institutes decades before, and "drawled forth . . . in a manner as dry as the bones he was demonstrating," were so lacking in immediacy that Thomson packed Williams and his fellows back off to private lectures. Not coincidentally, the private lectures were provided by two men: John Barclay (1758–1828) and Thomson himself.[38]

After 1820, with the publication of John Forbes's translation of Laennec's *Mediate Auscultation,* a potentially powerful new magnet was added to the attractive force of the Paris School: a technique, the stethoscope, designed expressly to discriminate between various antemortem clinical findings and to correlate them with changes disclosed at autopsy. Though partly intended as a way of extending the anatomicoclinical methods and theories of the Bichatian tradition, the new bedside technique of auscultation offered an enticing lure to those with purely clinical interests. The reception of the stethoscope, in England and elsewhere, has been studied at length by others. But it is noteworthy that hard on the heels of the publication of Forbes's translation came a spate of publications on pathological anatomy as well as on the use of the stethoscope.[39]

Alongside this upsurge in what one critic called "the thirst for inkshed," sprouted a clamorous reaction to all things medical and French, a reaction amplified in the rapidly expanding English medical journal literature.[40] The clamor was neither exclusively paean nor all protest, but it was conspicuous. No British medical student, unless unusually isolated from both the periodical literature and from the Scottish educational experience, can have failed to be inoculated with the insidious notion, fostered by many high-placed individuals, that the new Gallic methods were far superior to those available at home.[41]

INSTITUTIONAL DEVELOPMENTS, 1820–1828

By the early- to mid-1820s then, English medical students were well aware of the strong advocacy of their teachers toward the value of the Paris study tour. At the same time three further developments, one in French medical education, one in English medical education, and a third in English medical journalism, further prepared the ground for the accelerated pace of the student migration to Paris. This pace, as the curve in Fig. 6.1 suggests, continued to gather momentum after 1820, and did so particularly after 1824.[42]

The availability of Laennec's lectures at the *Collège de France* and his clinics at the teaching hospitals, coupled with the reception of the *Mediate Auscultation* in the 1819 original and (especially) in Forbes's 1821 translation, represented powerful factors promoting the influx of Britons. The weight of journalistic reaction was decidedly favorable, almost assuredly more favorable than the reception accorded Laennec by the bulk of England's medical practitioners. At first these practitioners tended to view even the work's most purely clinical element, physical diagnosis, with a jaundiced glance.[43]

Medical journalists, by contrast, tended to be among the most reform-oriented members of the professional groups they belonged to, having been drawn to journalistic careers when that field itself was taking off.[44] The sheer number of journals available, especially those explicitly intended to serve as guides to new developments abroad, was increasing rapidly as well. This fact no doubt also accentuated the sense that the new medicine depended heavily on French developments. A casual examination of any of these journals clearly discloses the two principal sources of this impression: to some extent a reaction to the new French chemistry and toxicology of Magendie and his collaborators, and, even more prominently, to the "medical Elysium . . . brought about by the extreme accuracy of French *Autopsia*."[45]

Those who determined to go to France before 1824 in order to attend Laennec's and his colleagues' lectures were faced with a second, potentially negative, influence on their decision. This was the parlous state of administrative affairs of the Paris Faculty, under the cold and stern gaze of the remarkable cleric who had recently assumed the newly reestablished post of *Grand-Maître de l'Université*, the Abbé Frayssinous. Caught between radical student and conservative government demands with increasing frequency, the *Doyen*, J. J. Leroux (1749–1832) had attempted stoutly, and with some success, to keep the Faculty on an even keel in the middle of stormy political seas.

But in the middle of the 1822 academic year his administration began shipping water badly. The final blow was the notorious *affaire Bertin* of June 1822. What began as a student heckling incident ended by bringing down the entire Paris Faculty. The purge was triggered when the hapless R.-J.-H. Bertin (1757–1828), designated successor to Jean-Noël Hallé in the Chair of Hygiene, lost control of his class on the fifteenth of June. The ensuing melee sent a shock up the administrative ladder as far as the Grand-Master, who returned the favor with shocks of his own. A full investigation and Leroux's best efforts at palliation were only partly availing.[46] The Faculty's critics had what they wanted: an excuse to reorganize it politically along less independent lines.

The effect of the *affaire Bertin* was the temporary shutting down of the Faculty. Dissolving it created an administrative nightmare for Leroux and his appointed successor, the caretaker dean Augustin-Jacob Landré-Beauvais (1772–1840). It also eliminated the possibility for most English students, just as their numbers were beginning to increase dramatically, of securing the linchpin experience of their foreign medical education.[47] It was entirely possible, however, to come to Paris and attend the courses and clinics run by Laennec and a host of others based in institutions other than the central faculty. So the 1823–1824 denouement of this unsettled state of affairs, with the settling (not to say clamping) down of the Faculty and its reopening under the stewardship of a new pro-royalist administration, may or may not have had a positive effect on the influx of foreign students. It certainly did have a positive effect on foreign registration at the Faculty itself.[48]

A third, hitherto little-noticed factor began in 1824 to militate more generally and precipitously for an increase in British anatomical study in Paris. Throughout the early 1820s, the antipathy between the hospital surgeons and the private anatomists of London had grown progressively more pronounced. The two groups gave similar courses. They competed for students, money, and authority. The dearth of dissectable bodies, in good shape, reasonably innocuous to the olfactory sense, at good price, let alone legally obtained, exacerbated this competition. By 1822 the hospital men were so exercised about the private teachers' encroachment that they impelled the Court of the Royal College of Surgeons to change its bylaws in hopes of ruining the competition. Henceforth certificates of dissection from summer courses would be unacceptable, ostensibly a measure safeguarding the public (and the students') health.[49]

The effect was in essence to squeeze the anatomy market into two-thirds to three-quarters of its original space at all the possible dissecting sites in London. But the Royal College's weapon proved to do relatively little damage to the private schools. They brought out the heavy armament two years later, in 1824, promulgating another new bylaw, stating that only "certificates in testimony of attendance on dissections would be received by the Court, except for the appointed professors of Anatomy and Surgery in the universities of Edinburgh, Glasgow, Aberdeen, and Dublin, or from persons who were physicians or surgeons to the hospitals in the recognized schools, or from persons unless recommended by the medical establishments of those hospitals."[50] The only "recognized" school of surgery in all of England was now the hospital base of the London surgical elite.

The College of Surgeons Court's 1824 move served to raise the stock of Paris as a dissection center while it substantially devalued that of the private London anatomists. In a period of rapid social change and particularly rapid growth in the learned professions, the overall number of medical students in London actually declined between 1823 and 1828 from roughly 1,000 to about 800.[51] Paris institutions, even after Laennec's death in 1826, derived a prolonged benefit from the weakening of the London private schools, explaining at least in part the point of inflection in the enrollment curve observed around 1824.[52] At the same time, this post-1824 increase in the Paris faculty's enrollment of Britons probably also reflected a more general flow of students from London to Paris, a "mass action effect."

In sum, the lure of pathological anatomy, well reported in the press and extended to include physical diagnosis, coupled with the stabilization of the Paris Faculty and the new requirements of the College of Surgeons, led to a striking increase in the English student population of Paris.[53] By 1828 there were about two hundred studying anatomy in the French capital, compared with perhaps four times that many in London and Edinburgh. It was enough to provoke a great deal of consternation at home.

THE PARIS EXPERIENCE, 1820–1828: CONFLICTS

A variety of contemporary observers remarked upon this rapid rise in the number of British students in Paris in the 1820s. Robert Carswell, for example, estimated that in 1822 the number had been in the range of thirty to forty students, increasing something like fivefold by 1828.[54] But crude figures supply only part of the story.

When the numbers are coupled with the sense of alarm voiced by the emigrés' countrymen at home, a central fact begins to emerge: Whatever *influence* the French may be said to have exerted, they had a striking *impact* on this suddenly large and rather cumbersome community of guests. That impact, moreover, seems to have been a mutual one.

This impression is reinforced by an examination of some of the details of the experience reported by members of the English community once they immersed themselves in the foreign milieu. They were a self-selected group, students and recent graduates mostly drawn from Britain's elite and far better off socially and economically than their French counterparts. Two separate gradients were established, therefore, a social gradient and an intellectual one. Both gradients separated the two communities. The Britons came with their own intellectual and social preconceptions and behaviors, forming the basis for a reciprocal relationship. The French setting affected their guests, while the English began, in turn, to make their impression on the French. This mutuality is best illustrated by a remarkable series of events that occurred in 1824 and 1825.

It was not unusual for groups of English students, borrowing a leaf from their French brethren, to rent their own dissecting rooms near the teaching hospitals and to organize their own courses in normal and pathological anatomy. James Richard Bennett (d. 1831) set up a course of this sort in 1822–1823.[55] He attached himself to the anatomy classes held on the premises of the officially sanctioned dissecting amphitheater of the *Hôpital de la Pitié,* offering instruction in English. Arousing considerable interest among his compatriots, he initially drew eighteen English students. His success was sufficient to impel him to repeat the course in the following academic year. This time forty-two English, or at least English-speaking, students signed up. The enterprise was a triumph of pedagogical marketing, purveying English and French ideas to Anglophones in their mother tongue, in a French venue and with French cadavers.

Needless to say, Bennett attempted to repeat the performance in the following year. At no point, he declared, was his enterprise more than "tolerated" by the French.[56] He noted that he had never attempted to practice medicine or surgery in Paris, but simply to teach anatomy. But in the middle of his third year of the course, academic 1824–1825, the forbearance of the French government suddenly evaporated. Hospital facilities formerly hired out for the purposes of private dissection and used, in this case, by the English students, were suddenly unavailable. (This was the tale that Bennett told on his return to England.)

Later Bennett was to recall the circumstances under which he was obliged to discontinue his teaching. He described harassment from French colleagues who "had the right of teaching at the *amphithéâtre de la Pitié*." He guessed that he "interfered with their interests." He appealed this treatment to the British Ambassador, Sir Charles Stuart, begging his intercession with the French government. Stuart felt that the matter was getting out of hand, and turned it over to the Foreign Secretary in London, George Canning. Bennett noted that he had been

led to expect [Canning's] concurrence; but on the subject being made known to the College of Surgeons in London, they waited on Mr. Canning and dissuaded him from granting my request; sometime after my return to Paris, the French authorities obliged me to desist from teaching.[57]

The traces of this incident in the correspondence of the Ministry of Instruction in Paris leave little doubt that, while the actors were the same, the account as seen from the other side would be shaded in a somewhat different manner. The official French view was ambivalent toward the English intruders: a mixture of arrogant receptivity, with all the implied superiority that this entailed, and consternation over the invasion from across the Channel. The dominant sentiment depended on whose ox was being gored. That there were considerable negative feelings, at least on the part of those who stood to gain less by the foreigners' presence, is clear. Equally clear is the manner in which Paris institutions, particularly the Paris Faculty, were willing to exploit the situation to their own individual internal ends.

Bennett's 1828 testimony, giving the English side of the story, was known to be slated for publication because of its venue in the Parliamentary Select Committee. The French side, unpublished and for internal consumption only, is the franker view, and from its pages, penned in early 1825, leap words describing the Anglo–French contretemps in terms of "menace" and "disorder." Landré–Beauvais had spent the last month investigating, at the behest of Frayssinous, the *dispositions malveillantes* allegedly harbored by the

French toward the English students. The latter had on January 6 received a letter from the Interior Minister that began:

M. the Ambassador of England has just written me that a rather large number of Englishmen studying medicine in Paris have addressed him to complain about the conduct of the French students toward them.

These foreigners claim that we have malevolent attitudes toward them, manifested by hostile language, and even by threats of personal violence; that we announce loudly the intention to force them, if at all possible, to abandon their studies. It would appear that it is particularly in the anatomy courses that these symptoms of *mésintelligence* have broken out.[58]

The Minister of the Interior announced his intention to hand the problem over to the attention of the education minister, leaving it with Frayssinous: "I am informing the English Ambassador that this affair depends now on Your Excellency." Frayssinous responded in kind by handing the problem down to the Dean of the Faculty of Medicine. He insisted that the latter help him discover the facts of the case and the measures that might appropriately be taken next by the Ministry. On 2 February, the dean wrote to the Minister of Ecclesiastical Affairs and Public Instruction that in his fact-finding about the "difficulties between the young English and French physicians,"

. . . [t]he French students have not viewed with indifference that the English, richer than them and making considerable financial sacrifices, were favored to their detriment[,] and [the former] gave themselves over to murmurs and threats. Nothing similar has happened in the dissecting amphitheaters at the Faculty.

I must, however, inform Your Excellency that since the beginning of the academic year it has been clear that the medical students have been less calm [at the Faculty] than in preceding years. In the dissecting amphitheaters they view the foreigners painfully and fear that the latter [will be shown] favoritism by payments to the subemployees. It is even probable that the same troubles occurring at the *Hôpital de la Pitié* were only prevented in the Faculty's amphitheaters by measures that we took to establish absolute equality between the nationals and the foreigners . . .[:] to admit to dissections only those French and foreigners who take out inscriptions at the Faculty; to allow the distribution of cadavers among students only to the *Chef des Travaux Anatomiques*, etc., etc.[59]

Landré–Beauvais announced to the Monseigneur that he wished to profit from the situation by defending the cause of the Faculty's students; the *Conseil Général des Hospices* was being entirely too generous with the dead bodies it delivered up to other institutions at the expense of the Faculty. The *Conseil* had indulged, in his view, in excessive generosity in connection with the teaching it had itself established at the *Pitié*. His Excellency would have to judge the delicate question, Landré-Beauvais declared, as to whether this teaching should be tolerated or whether it should all be concentrated at the Faculty of Medicine.

By February 24, when the Minister responded *in extenso,* the matter had already gone above him. His superior, the Interior Minister, had heard from the British Ambassador in the same outraged tones Stuart had employed in early January. Caught in the middle, Frayssinous asked the Dean to do some more fact-finding and to determine the validity of the complaints. "In the affirmative case, I invite you to interpose your authority efficaciously, . . . [and determine] what measures the University will be able to take in order to support you."

Four days later the education minister issued his report, in the form of a letter to the Interior Minister. It was for the most part a pastiche of earlier bits of information and correspondence that had posted up and down the administrative ladder. When he reached the final paragraph, Frayssinous dictated and then crossed out the phrase "Your Excellency will judge the measures appropriate to adopt to remedy the inconveniences [*inconveniens*] that have troubled the fine harmony between students in the *Pitié* anatomy courses." Substituted was this: "Your Excellency will think at least that it would be just that [the Faculty] not be deprived of the cadavers necessary to its work[,] and what is accomplished by [diverting them to] an establishment that may be considered in many respects illegal."[60]

The record does not make clear to what extent the teaching of normal and pathological anatomy was curtailed at the *Pitié* as the result of the Bennett fracas. It is unlikely that the Faculty was able to reestablish anything like a monopoly over this choice piece of pedagogical territory. What is clearer, however, combining the French and English evidence, is that, in this instance at least, the students from abroad became sacrificial lambs. So, too, did J. R. Bennett, who paid for the failed experiment with his own health. His reformist colleagues in London used the occasion of Bennett's sudden death in early 1831 to skewer the governing elites on both sides of the Channel for the "relentless tyranny" that had exacted "the last debt of nature . . . the dissolution of Mr. Bennett."[61] Though an inconstant supporter of anatomical reform, Thomas Wakley of the *Lancet* noted with revulsion the fact that the College of Surgeons had played the crucial role in staying the protecting hands of Canning and Stuart. Tellingly, noted John Armstrong (1783–1829), a physician and colleague of Bennett's in Little Dean Street, the surgeons had no real jurisdiction: seven-eighths of the English students in Paris were physicians, and the balance, who were surgeons, already had their diplomas. Yet the surgeons' "deputation succeeded in persuading Mr. Canning not to comply with Mr. Bennett's request." This was at a time, Wakley declared, "when there was, in London, not a subject to dissect." The *Lancet* editor reacted with indignation to the idea that, when "the conduct of the French students became so outrageous that [Bennett and his students] were obliged to withdraw, not one Englishman ultimately lifted a finger." The corporation's oligarchic use of power was surely, Wakley exclaimed characteristically, "the emanation of Satan."[62]

As for the long-range effects of the contretemps within the French system, the Englishmen's difficulties were to combine with the Paris Faculty's proprietary concerns and with a gradually mounting conservatism within the French populace to bring about the dismantling of the *Pitié cabinets* in the 1830s. An ordinance enacted in November 1834 prohibited dissection in all hospitals and related institutions. In its stead, and as a sop to those medical personnel used to dissecting routinely perhaps four out of every five patients who died in their care, the *administration des hôpitaux* were to build an *Amphithéâtre des hôpitaux*. It opened on the first day of November 1833, and replaced all hospital and private dissecting rooms. Though commodious (it was advertised to handle four hundred dissections simultaneously) it was inconveniently located near Montparnasse, on the southern perimeter, and posed serious logistical problems. The physician, the deceased patient, and the patient's records could seldom make the journey and arrive together.

THE PARIS EXPERIENCE CONTINUES

No social clash or administrative wrangling, not even new obstacles to morbid dissection, could entirely quench the desire to make the pilgrimage to the French capital. Ultimately neither the raw numbers of those making the journey, therefore, nor the tales of the difficulties some encountered, provide a complete story of that remarkable affinity dubbed "Gallomania" by home-town wags. To understand that magnetic pull one must look further, to the accounts of the texture of daily experience in Paris between, say, 1815 and 1833. No observer provided a fuller account of that experience, perhaps, than did another Laennec auditor, Charles J. B. Williams, John Thomson's Edinburgh protégé. In his *Autobiography,* Williams described his Paris sojourn in the mid-1820s.

Arriving in 1825, Williams became an habitué of Paris medical culture just in time to aim successfully for the same grand tour Thomas Hodgkin and Robert Carswell had lately completed. He sat in on courses, or paid personal visits, to Pierre Louis and Gabriel Andral (himself still a student), and Guillaume Dupuytren as well as Laennec, whose lectures he attended at the *Charité* and the *Collège de France.* Like many of his *compères* with interests in natural history and natural philosophy, he also visited W. F. Edwards, A. M. Ampère, Geoffroy St.-Hilaire, and Baron Cuvier, as well as a number of other French luminaries in general science.[63] His caricatures in ink of many such figures were mercilessly accurate.

The young Edinburgh graduate (M.D., 1824) entered Paris on a fierce midsummer day. He was astonished at the shimmering light that caught him as he approached the gilded domes of the chateau that stood in the place where the Arc de Triomphe now looms. But he soon entered the Paris of Honoré Daumier, contrasting the *grands bâtimens* with the squalor of the left-bank neighborhoods that harbored many of her medical institutions. In the shadow of Nôtre-Dame cathedral stood the Hôtel-Dieu, packed with disease and misery. Around it moved the brisk life of the grand boulevards and the Palais Royale, oblivious.[64]

Typically, Williams noted, a student settled in for a month or two, sampling the contrasts and contradictions of the French capital, perhaps even briefly studying astronomy or landscape painting. When the Faculty and the hospitals resumed their academic year, usually in October, Paris life became the medical life. Like many if not most Britons before him, Williams decided to make Laennec's lectures and clinics his educational centerpiece. The now-ailing Laennec would make his rounds of the wards of *Charité,* a clutch of polyglot students trailing behind, from ten to twelve in the morning, allowing time for auscultation demonstrations. Students placed hands on patients. At the bedside Laennec would lecture in Latin, afterwards in French. Postmortems would often, as the *terminaison* of a case dictated, take the place of didactic, vernacular clinical lectures. By now, unaware that he was himself dying of tuberculosis, Laennec was phobic about infection, brandishing long-handled instruments and vials of chloride of lime.[65]

Thin, vivacious, acerbic, Laennec was besieged by foreign students while "little valued," contended Williams, by their French counterparts, many of whom were more attracted by the "grand idea" and "sweeping hypothesis" of the "impetuous Broussais." By 1825, however, many of the Britons among Laennec's foreign adherents were clearly attuned almost exclusively to his ability to teach them auscultation. Indeed, like the better-known John Forbes, for his own purposes Williams also divided the clinical system of pathological anatomy into two parts, separating the physical signs from the morbid appearances.[66] Like many others, he had assimilated the one layer of the French synthesis that corresponded to his own image of medical expertise.

By now a stream of English medical students bound for Paris had been swelling for most of two decades. For the better part of a generation, British students had traveled abroad for their formative years of education in normal and morbid anatomy. Men like Robert Carswell, Thomas Hodgkin, John Forbes, Charles J. B. Williams, Charles T. Haden, and many others were now returning to England and hoping, in the early 1830s, to shape its new medical institutions and to reshape its old ones. The ideas and techniques that formed their shared concern were inevitably molded in turn by their French experience. Among the very few who returned, in fact, striving to sustain the synthesis fashioned by the school of Bichat and Laennec, and seeking to keep the French image of the body and its ills intact, were Thomas Hodgkin and Robert Carswell.

PART III

London

7

After Waterloo: Medical journalism and the
surgeon-apothecaries

Rampant xenophobia had preceded the end of hostilities between
France and England. After the Congress of Vienna those sentiments
could not be sustained at that early intensity. As malign feelings
receded, the new political atmosphere provided a framework in
which medical thought might be more freely channeled. The
emergence of a new genre of medical periodical, the review journal,
for example, had begun before the end of hostilities: the *Medical
Repository*, for example, was introduced in 1814.[1] But after 1815
there was a noticeable increase in both the number of competing
journals, and a concomitant desire to monitor Continental developments more closely. Suddenly in demand were the services of
Anglophile Europeans like the polymathic Italian Augustus B.
Granville, based in Paris, as well as the services of Continent-based
Englishmen like James Clark in Rome. In 1816 Granville, for example, began to send *résumés* of scientific activity in Paris to the
Journal of the Royal Institution, and of all medical proceedings to
the *Medical Repository*.[2] So began the process by which English
physicians' angle of vision began to be widened, and their images
of medicine abroad strengthened and focused.

At first this process, dependent as it was on stringers like Granville, was a desultory one. But there was a market for more systematic reviews of foreign literature, resulting in the appearance,
beginning in 1818, of several journals aiming to glean the best
from the Continental medical literature. The transition from a re-
liance on correspondents to a new, more systematic winnowing
mechanism represented a critical step for the flow of medical
knowledge between the Continent and the British Isles. It was still

an essentially passive step; the most active steps were taken by those with both the inclination and the resources to pursue French anatomy *in situ*.[3]

But in 1820 there was nonetheless much new information made available though the alliance between publishers anxious to capitalize on the new print economics, and physician–journalists anxious to capitalize on the cautious new internationalism beginning to take hold in medicine. The caution grew out of a desire to retain a readership, and to compete with others whose desires lay along similar lines.[4] From the outset, then, there was a gradient away from the more purely theoretical and the more resolutely anatomical aspects of French pathological anatomy, and toward its clinical and utilitarian aspects.

The first of these primarily "analytical" journals, the *Medico-Chirurgical Review,* illustrates the point nicely.[5] Aimed successfully at a wide circulation from its 1816 inception, the *Review* enjoyed the advantage of precedence. The first of its genre, it was soon represented by a regular overseas editor in the United States. Its founding editor, James Johnson (1777–1845), typified a career pattern that was to become common in the first quarter of the nineteenth century: Johnson was an individual who, professionally or geographically, was astir somewhere near the lower margin of the medical career pyramid, and then clambered his way to its top.

Born in County Derry, Ireland, Johnson was apprenticed at fifteen to a surgeon – apothecary. By the age of nineteen he found himself in London and, in the spring of 1798, was assigned to a naval vessel as surgeon's mate. He eventually became physician-extraordinary to King William IV, and part of the London medical establishment.[6] Johnson thus moved from Ireland – though ever capable of "his North Irish brogue and racy narrative" – to the London hub, and from surgeon's mate in the Napoleonic campaigns to physician-extraordinary.[7] Along the way he took time to study medicine in Paris, though for how long and in which subjects are matters that remain unclear.[8] Accordingly and not surprisingly he divided his interests between the climatology and balneology of his own publications and the Continental pathology that the *Review* now assiduously reported.

In late 1818 or early 1819, soon after James Johnson removed from Portsmouth to London to expand his journal, the medical booksellers and publishers Burgess and Hill induced another outsider, the peripatetic Augustus Granville, to take on the editorship of yet another new review journal.[9] Declaring his parental role in the *Review*'s creation with a characteristic want of modesty, Granville later recalled the birth of the *Medical Intelligencer:*

The length of time I had passed in Paris in reading and studying the various continental journals, whether medical or merely scientific, for the purpose of summarizing their contents, and in that state communicating them to societies in London, or to editors of certain English journals, had given me a certain facility, and at the same time a degree of pleasure and satisfaction in the doing it. No wonder, therefore, that I should readily accept a proposal made to me by a firm of medical booksellers, Messrs. Burgess and Hill, to edit a popular medico-scientific journal, the form and character of which I had myself suggested. Its object was mainly to be a monthly analytical index of the periodical literature of the day, of the transactions of medical and scientific societies, and, in fact, of all works, no matter from what country, connected with medical subjects. It was a small octavo, and in small type, so as to embrace much matter, and it was issued at a lower price than any other of the contemporary journals. Its title was *"The Medical Intelligencer,"* and it appeared twice a week. It served as a stimulus for the establishment of another weekly journal which, under the title of the *"Lancet,"* from the first commanded popularity, and next the esteem and approbation of the whole profession; while the same *"Intelligencer"* served to rouse the other, or second weekly contemporary, the *"Gazette,"* from the torpor that was overcoming it.[10]

In his memoirs Granville was to proclaim the importance of his review journal, which lapsed in 1823 after four years, as the stimulus for both the establishment of *The Lancet* and the revitalization of the *Medical Gazette*. He recalled also the sharply competitive temper of medical journalism in those years, noting that Burgess and Hill had firmly set their own sights on the *London Medical and Physical Journal*, the most successful general medical journal before *Lancet*. Accordingly, they recast the *Intelligencer* into the *Journal*'s precise format. Shortly thereafter, on the resignation in 1821 of William Hutchinson, Granville was offered and accepted the latter journal's editorship.[11] The year 1821 was to prove pivotal, not only for English medical publishing but for Anglo–French medical relations. In that year Granville was succeeded in the editorial post at the *Medical Intelligencer* by Charles Thomas Haden (1786–1824): former surgeon from Derby, early Laennec disciple, friend of Jane Austen, translator of Magendie, vice-president of the surgeon–

apothecaries, and now successful practitioner at the Chelsea and Brompton dispensary.[12]

Haden belonged in that small circle – it included among others Thomas Alcock, James Johnson, James Clark, and John Forbes – of reform-minded physicians who, born between the late 1770s and the late 1780s, came together in London just after Waterloo: English (and Irish) provincials become medical cosmopolites. Haden was perhaps the most literary of them all, in part because his failing health precluded an active full-time practice. He took a hand, usually a guiding one, in the editing of at least three journals.[13] Keenly interested in both of the research fields for which French hospital medicine was becoming known, chemistry and pathology, Haden translated François Magendie's influential *Formulary* in 1818.[14]

The next year, 1820, Laennec published his *Mediate Auscultation*. In its first number, the Medical Intelligencer responded with a note, by Granville or Haden, to the effect that this, the original, French edition, was "well worth the most attentive perusal." Haden was also provided a notice of his own plans for preparation of an English translation of "M. Laennec's excellent work."[15] An editor, probably Granville, excerpted a description of the *concours* for the *chef des travaux anatomiques* at the Paris Faculty, noting the "very severe examinations . . . superintended by seven commissioners chosen by ballot" and exclaiming, "How differently are the medical officers of English institutions chosen!"[16] The editor of the first volume also gave considerable space to Thomas Alcock for an advertisement, cloaked as a long letter in the March number, for his forthcoming book on inflammatory affections of the mucous membranes.[17] Suggesting that readers "desirous of more extended views . . . consult the works of Pinel, Bichat, Broussais, Bordeu and others," Alcock lamented that

. . . although much excellent information on individual diseases of the mucous membranes may be found in the works of practical men, yet I am not aware that any general view has been taken of this class of inflammatory diseases as a whole. It is not my intention to attempt to supply this deficiency, in all its parts, but after pointing out what may be considered to be the generalization of the subject, to confine my observations to the consideration of the inflammatory affections of that part of the mucous membrane which lines the organs of respiration.[18]

The organs of respiration were considered in great detail by Laennec in his *magnum opus*, casting Alcock's contributions into shadow. In the early 1820s, in fact, English medical men seem to have exhibited a general spurt of interest, judging from the journal literature, in the bronchial and catarrhal affections of the mucous membranes. John Abercrombie extended his observations from Edinburgh,[19] and Joseph Houlton, a London surgeon, published a digest of Bichat's work on the mucous membranes.[20]

THE "SMALL TALK BABBLE OF TEXTURE AND TISSUE"

As animosity between the two regimes subsided, Anglo–French medical relations reached a turning point in 1821. Without attempting to discriminate between cause and effect one can find several correlates of this change. The number of English students traveling to Paris for medical study increased sharply.[21] Forbes published his translation of Laennec. Haden, the ardent Francophile, took over the *Medical Intelligencer*. Houlton published his translation of Bichat on the mucous membranes. Confronted with the deluge of French pathology, James Copland (1791–1870), a physician contemporary with the Haden–Alcock circle but of a considerably more conservative cast of mind, said this in his own journal, the staid and established *Medical Repository:*[22]

Pathology has recently assumed a much more definite character than it possessed before the time of Bichat, and other investigators of vital phenomena, who, untrammelled by the supposititious and *terra incognita* philosophy formerly prevalent in the schools of medicine, have searched for truth in the anatomical peculiarities of the several organs and parts. . . .

There is another source of mischief connected with anatomical inferences, in medicine, carried out into an ultra extent, viz. the too great credit which it encourages to be given to the information of morbid anatomy. We often expect to see invisible things, – we are apt to suppose that pain *must* denote some condition of one or other of the tissues, that shall be traceable by the dissection knife, – we contemn the idea of functional without structural derangement; – and are thus often induced to forego leading facts and commanding views in physiological deduction, and therapeutic data, by attending to the small talk babble of texture and tissue. We gain in ingenuity, and lose in genius. . . .[23]

Haden was quick to respond in an "Analytical Review" published in the *Intelligencer* in December:

There can be no doubt of the advances made in pathology since the time of Bichat, but the reviewer is afraid we are now become too ana-

tomical and piece-meal in our medical notions and pathological inferences – foregoing leading facts and commanding views in physiological
deduction and therapeutic data, by attending to the small-talk babble of
texture and tissue. That it may not be suspected, however, that he is
unfriendly to minute anatomy and post obit investigation, it has been
thought not improper to introduce the present analysis (a very good one)
of a portion of Bichat's labours into this valedictory number of the *Repository*.

The importance of Bichat's views is now so generally admitted by
good judges, that we hope every medical man will take the opportunity
which [Houlton's] translation affords of becoming thoroughly acquainted
with their nature and tendency.[24]

By early 1822 the impact of Laennec's work as well as that of
Bichat was beginning to be widely felt among the new men of
English medicine, and they were beginning to disseminate it. In
the *Intelligencer*, an unsigned review, excerpted in part from the
London Medical and Physical Journal, and summarized by Haden,
declared that

The great merits and importance of Laennec's work, made known to
the public through the medium of the different periodical journals, seemed
to call for a translation of the original into the English language. This
duty has been performed in the most satisfactory manner by Dr. Forbes,
and a rich depository of valuable facts and observations is thus made
accessible to every one who is anxious to study or cultivate his profession.
That the translation has been executed with the utmost accuracy and
fidelity, we have the authority of the editor of the journal before us, who
must be allowed to be no mean judge on this point.[25]

Haden must, in fact, have been in France just about the time
that the review was being written for his journal; in mid-1822 he
traveled to Paris and studied for a time with Laennec, making clinical rounds at the *Necker*. In all probability he also became the
Frenchman's patient. By late summer, still in Paris, he would write
Laennec a letter of thanks

not only for the consolation which you have given me respecting my
health, but for the very valuable information which I have gained by
attending your practice. . . . I hope I may regard your acceptance of one
or two of my own attempts to improve the state of medical literature.
They are but humble performances. With respect to the Medical Intelligencer I can only lay claim to the first volume of the three last numbers;
& although the *Journal of Popular Medicine* may apparently savour of quack-
ery yet I hope you will believe that it was written in a very different spirit.[26]

Haden was in Paris at a heady time. The leaders of French medicine, especially Laennec, were surrounded by foreign students.
Among those Britons were the Englishman Thomas Hodgkin and
the Scot Robert Carswell, who would make the attempt on their
return home to institutionalize pathological anatomy. Haden left
no record of any contacts with his countrymen while in Paris. But
he did write to his friend Thomas Alcock back in London that, if
he should manage (presumably despite his illness) to reestablish
himself in London

I hope to place myself so as to be a nucleus for much being done by our
younger friends. One of the best parts of the French system is the mode
in which all the best of the Doctors, the working ones, are surrounded
by eager young men – not only the Doctors of hospitals, but such men
as Magendie; who works much, as Haller did before him, by the hands
of his numerous *protégés*.[27]

A few months later, at the end of 1822, Haden penned the "preface" for the third volume of the *Intelligencer*. It was in scope an
unusual essay, without precedent in the burgeoning medical review
literature. The readers of the *Intelligencer* and possibly his corre-
spondent Laennec were presented with "A disquisition on the state
of British medicine, as compared with that of foreign nations; on
the faults of English medical education [and] on the best mode of
studying medicine. . . ." In it Haden described the "beneficial impulse" the English had derived from "increased intercourse" with
foreign medical sciences. He spoke of how he had "frequently . . .
spoken of the defects of English medicine, and compared them,
not without offense, with more perfect plans as acted on by our
neighbours the French."

This Francophilia, declared Haden, did not blind him to areas
of excellence in English medicine. But English medical literature
lagged badly in all respects save the most practical treatises, a "peculiar defect" he was "ashamed . . . to confess" when asked what
English work was appropriate for translation into French. And
Englishmen were often oblivious to the defect: Too few foreign
works were translated, and what few were, sold poorly. "The
booksellers have well known that such works as Bichat's *General
Anatomy*, would not pay for the printing, much less for the translation; . . . even Dr. Forbes's Translation of Laennec's work, has
scarcely sold, although the whole [*sic*] of the English periodical
press has held the original work up to the public, as one of the

most important and perfect disquisitions of medical science that has ever appeared. . . .''[28]

Haden's enthusiasm for the French anatomicoclinical tradition did not go unnoticed by his contemporaries; many of them, indeed, considered it excessive. Soon after Haden died in 1824 at age thirty-eight, his compatriot Thomas Alcock noted that his friend's detractors had supposed his "partiality for the French Schools of Medicine" to be overzealous. As early as 1827 Alcock pointed out, however, that Haden "was one of the first to adopt in this country, the use of the stethoscope of Laennec, and his esteem for the now lamented Author of this great help to accurate diagnosis, has since been re-echoed by the general voice of the profession."[29]

Alcock's assessment of Haden's role in the advocacy of French ideas and techniques is not without touches of irony. Haden and Laennec both died young; each was eulogized on both sides of the Channel as the author of important unfinished agendas in both practical and theoretical medicine. Haden, had he preceded his colleague and competitor John Forbes in bringing out an English edition of the *Mediate Auscultation,* would probably have taken that work, disjointed it, and recast it much as did Forbes.[30] Even so, many Englishmen found their intellectual tastes more than a little piqued by the curious combination of pathological anatomy and physical diagnosis with which Forbes's reformulation confronted them.

The new English dress fashioned by Forbes for Laennec was marked, as acerbic reviewers were quick to point out, by "two deviations from the original."[31] The first such "deviation" was the "separation of the descriptive from the diagnostic part," an effort to disentangle pathological anatomy from physical diagnosis that Forbes defended emphatically.[32] The journals quoted him: In verifying and correlating physical findings, there was "only [the one] sure seal of merit, morbid dissection."[33] Forbes recognized that Laennec's "new diagnostic measures . . . are . . . immediately connected with, and necessarily dependent on the physical alterations which constitute the disease."[34] Yet he persisted in his aim of having "the work . . . restored to what I humbly [sic] conceive it ought always to have been, viz., two independent treatises, – the one on Pathology, the other on Diagnosis, – mutually adapted to each other, yet each complete of itself and not necessarily connected with the other."[35]

At first blush it is tempting to conceive of Forbes's move to segregate the study of thoracic percussion and auscultation in a discrete literary unit, apart from the pathology, as a way of appealing to an English market that he knew to be more clinically and less pathologically oriented in comparison with its French counterpart. To suppose this circumscribed his motives would be simplistic, however, for two reasons. In the first place, France was unique with respect to the cognitive style of its medical community. For many members of the French community, morbid dissection and bedside medicine were fused in the amalgam of routine tasks that were best addressed, considered, correlated, and completed in tandem. But Forbes felt that were he to retain Laennec's *mélange,* the two spheres might be self-cancelling instead of mutually reinforcing.

Second, and more specifically, Forbes expressed his own (since often quoted) misgivings about the potential acceptance of Laennec's physical diagnosis techniques: "That it will ever come into general use," he averred, "I am extremely doubtful; its beneficial application requires much time, and gives a good deal of trouble both to the patient and the practitioner; and because its whole hue and character is foreign, and opposed to all our habits and associations."[36] The journals' reviewers concurred,[37] Haden remarking on "the degree of formality which gives the operation [of auscultation] a somewhat ludicrous character."[38]

Within a very few years Forbes was to discover his pessimism over the stethoscope's acceptance to have been ill-founded. In time the instrument caught on with a vengeance. But the immediate response to his publication of Laennec's work, both the physical diagnosis and the pathology, was an accurate litmus of shifting, and divided, English attitudes toward French medicine. The *Mediate Auscultation* in English dress ended, in fact, by etching a deeper benchmark in the Anglo–French medical relationship than had any previous production of the Paris anatomicoclinical tradition, for two reasons. First, even though it was almost "two independent treatises," Laennec's work in English translation underscored the *clinical* importance of both the French style of pathological anatomy and the physical diagnosis with which it was alloyed. Second, and conversely, the work arrived on British shores at precisely the time that anatomical education in England was experiencing its own travails – difficulties that French institutions stood ready to exploit.[39]

THE SURGEON–APOTHECARIES LAUNCH A JOURNAL

There were, needless to say, those who stood at the ready in England as well to point out and exploit the defects in English anatomical education. Some of them went it more or less alone, seeking to point up their individual careers on the anatomical whetstone. That task could be accomplished either by wholeheartedly embracing the French system, as did Robert Carswell and Thomas Hodgkin (Chapter 9) or by rejecting it and insisting instead on an indigenous British pathological anatomy, exemplified by John Farre (Chapter 8). Others who perceived deficits in England's training of medical personnel were more organized. Not only careers but coalitions could be shored up by resort to pathological anatomy. Paramount among such groups as heralds of new pathological knowledge was the union of surgeon–apothecaries.

In 1823, just as the first wave of the impact of Forbes's Laennec translation was reaching its peak in both academia and the medical press, the surgeon–apothecaries ventured into the literary ranks with a journal of their own. Although it lapsed after a year, the surgeon–apothecaries' *Transactions* remains central to any understanding of the scientific aspirations of a group of men who found themselves at the near margins of the medical establishment. Their journal, in its one volume, survives as a remarkably clear window on those aspirations, the rank and file who embraced them, and the leaders who formulated them.

Principal contributors were by now familiar names in this discussion – James Johnson, Thomas Alcock, and Charles T. Haden – and the latter two were then active members of the Association's twenty-one-member General Committee as well.[40] The voluminous (137 pages) and self-justifying "Introductory Essay," was written by Alcock and Haden. They undertook to provide not only a historical précis of the Association's history and its role in fostering the 1815 Act, but also a program for reforming medical knowledge and hence medical practice in the 1820s.[41] The essay that Alcock provided "on the Education and Duties of the General Practitioner in Medicine and Surgery," in which he sought "to increase the usefulness and respectability of the general practitioner" by setting out criteria of his education, stressed "the investigation of disease [which] forms the very groundwork of rational practice."[42]

Haden and Alcock collaborated on the long manifesto that opened the pages of the *Transactions;* Alcock credited Haden with having conceived and executed most of it.[43] They summarized their tale of struggle against the College leadership, then launched into a diatribe against the sorry nature of "the true present state of medicine in this country," offering to render clear "its defects and their causes" and to propose "the best mode of obviating these defects, substituting for the existing limited views of medical science, such a more comprehensive system of study, as may at once tend to raise medicine to the rank it ought to hold, and will, at some period, hold among the exact sciences."[44]

The task at hand, argued the surgeon–apothecaries, was no less than the restitution of lost ability among English medical men to establish theory-as-truth, a faculty lost for "want of a necessary connexion between medicine and the accurate sciences."[45] Of the old guard they despaired. But if "the younger part of the profession [should] consider well what is the true basis of medical knowledge," then the general practitioner would arrive at "a subserviency to the principles of medical science" that would redress the imbalance.[46] Thus the rhetoric of the general practitioner was, in this guise, not that of succoring the masses, but rather one of high science. By shoring up his position intellectually, Haden and Alcock hoped to shore up the general practitioner's professional position. The G.P. was to be the steward of those new areas of knowledge for which the medical and surgical mandarins as yet had little use. Anatomy, physiology, and especially pathology would figure prominently in such an effort.

Pathology meant the study of derangements of structure, penetrating both medicine and surgery, it being "proper to consider surgery as only a branch of medicine," and based on an analysis of the elementary tissues in which those derangements reside. It was "necessary to pay attention as well to the fluids as to the solids," since many, having rejected a now-outmoded humoralism, had "run into extremes" with an excessive surgical solidism.[47] The "ardent and industrious student" must, declared Haden, examine the morbid parts and correlate them "with the symptoms which existed during life," in the manner of Etienne Serres on the brain and Théophile Laennec on the thorax. Therapeutics should similarly be subjected to scrutiny by systematically monitoring and recording patients' physical signs and abandoning the crude empiricism of the "majority of practitioners."[48]

Citing Gilbert Breschet's influential article on *"Anatomie pathologique"* in Adelon's magisterial *Dictionnaire de Médecine,* as "invaluable," Haden presented as the most utilitarian system of pathology that article's Bichatian hierarchy of tissues, organs, and "apparatus" (*appareils* or organ systems). A knowledge of the material alterations of each of these levels was critical, he maintained, to the general practitioner's ability "to avoid confounding organic lesions with their causes," an ability not well fostered by the "appreciation of exterior forms, and of their positions . . . *so useful to the surgeon* [representing] all that is usually taught in the English schools of anatomy. . . ."[49] Once "organic deviations" were understood, they might then be connected to "symptoms which characterize the lesion, and by which it may be known, although hid more or less from our view."[50]

From this program one cannot infer that either French-style pathological anatomy achieved a significant immediate impact among general practitioners, or that it was some mere window dressing for their pretensions to greater professional status. The notion of correlating external signs with internal derangements of tissue structure was, rather, a powerful mediating device. In the hands of the elite of the surgeon–apothecaries' coalition, the notion mediated on the one hand between claims about their expanded role in medical practice and claims about their expanded expertise in medical science. It also mediated between the otherwise distinct frames of reference of physicians and surgeons. Since the surgeon–apothecaries' association represented a coalition bound by its constitution to achieve a sort of professional suspension of outlooks, its leaders needed a theoretical base that would be commodious enough to accommodate both groups' cognitive habits as well. As it had done across the Channel, Bichatian pathological anatomy provided much of this mediating rhetoric.[51]

That this blueprint remained, however, just that – largely rhetoric, at least for general practitioners – has already been suggested. A crude but accurate reflection of its implementation as something more than a mere blueprint would have been the requirement of a display of competence in pathological anatomy on qualifying examinations. That was at least a decade away. Yet the blueprint, because of its mediating function, was by the mid-1820s already an important guide to an emerging self-image of the surgeon-apothecary as scientific clinician, and probably a clue to the motives of many who were actually making the journey to Paris.

Nowhere was the two-pronged function of science, as both edification and information for the general practitioner (especially pathological anatomy), better illustrated than in the surgeon-apothecaries' 1824 "premium." The premiums, or essay prizes sponsored by the Association, were to be awarded in early July 1824, for works on either of two subjects. The first was to cover "the subject of Medical Education, in which the relative importance of the various accessory sciences is ascertained, and the extent to which each separate science or branch of general knowledge should be cultivated, to afford the highest degree of usefulness in the healing art." The second was for "the best experimental Essay on Inflammation," beginning with an assessment of "the actual changes which take place in various tissues or textures of which the body is composed. . . ."[52]

Mainstream medicine was quick to take notice of the surgeon-apothecaries' aims, long before those aims were institutionalized. The author of the unsigned annual review for 1824 of "pathology" in the conservative *Anderson's Quarterly Journal of the Medical Sciences* presented the essence of the establishment response. The mood of that response ranged from ambivalent to flatly negative. Pathology, this journalist noted, seemed to be currently the most vigorously pursued of the medical sciences. This was fine unless carried to excess: "Morbid dissection is undoubtedly of high importance; but when it is performed, with the view of supporting some favorite theory as it most frequently is, particularly in France . . . we think that it is likely to be more productive of evil than good."[53] He then took aim squarely at Haden and Alcock: "The medical journals at home manifest a strong leaning to this deceptive field of speculation. In the *Transactions of the Associated Apothecaries* we have seen it carried to the highest point of visionary absurdity. We are happy that this dreaming system is more written about than practiced in this country, and we hope it will long continue so."[54]

Similarly, the same journal's reviewer of the year's progress in "the practice of physic" inveighed against "the French pathologists, and their imitators in England." English medical readers were at dire risk, by this account, of being "led by the absurd Frenchified system now vigorously attempted to be palmed upon them," into a state "which can only endanger their patients, and disgrace the profession."[55] In days gone by, said another, more congenial reviewer, many medical men had hoped "that pathological anatomy will become the polar star of nosology, and the surest guide of diagnosis." While their hopes had been dashed in the past, however, there was now perhaps reason to laud "the present rage for pathological anatomy. . . ."[56]

GALLOMANIA

So pervasive was the awareness of a French influence on English medicine in the mid-1820s, that it seems fair to say that ambivalence toward "the class of Gallomaniacs" became a central organizing principle in the institutionalization of pathology.[57] Those who spoke derisively of colleagues afflicted with Gallomania were moved to create a pathological anatomy that made sense in a native English idiom. Even so, the native brand was bound to be measured against the Continental product. John Farre, who attempted to establish one such idiom, forms the principal subject of Chapter 8. Still others, however, also substituted decisive action for ambiguous rhetoric. Anxious for exposure at first hand to the Paris experience, hundreds of young British students and practitioners found themselves drawn to the anatomical theaters and the hospital wards of the French capital. A much smaller number of them returned, afflicted with "Gallomania," to try embedding it in the very different soil of their native England.

8

Pathology and the specialist: The London Academy of Minute Anatomy

In 1835 Adolph Muehry, a Hanover physician and surgeon, followed time-honored custom with a Grand Tour of British and
European medical institutions. In the next year he published his
notes on the relative state of medicine in his native Germany
alongside that of England and France. Surveying the development
of pathological anatomy in England, Muehry identified a succession
of medical men who had been most active in furthering the traditions of English morbid anatomy. He singled out the work of
Matthew Baillie (1761–1823) and John Hunter (1728–1793) in the
late eighteenth century. He noted that they had been followed by
one individual, John Richard Farre (1775–1862), and that Farre in
turn had been more lately succeeded by a new group ascendant in
the 1830s. Among the latter group Muehry numbered Richard
Bright, Thomas Hodgkin, and Robert Carswell.[1]

Muehry's three groups, each separated from the next by half a
generation, provide appropriate guideposts around which to locate
the changing fortunes of English pathological anatomy in the early
nineteenth century. Only the first and third of these "generations,"
that of Hunter and Baillie and that of Bright, Hodgkin, and Carswell, are in any detail known to the twentieth century historian.
But if, over the critical half-century 1790–1840, each group of
physicians was disposed toward certain intellectual predilections,
social groups, and professional sensibilities, who was this "missing
link"? Who was John Farre?

John Richard Farre had practiced medicine in his native West
Indies before seeking to establish a London medical career. There,
in 1825, he announced his plan for an "Academy of Minute Anatomy." It was his hope, he said, that this new institution would
serve as an "incitement to the cultivation of Morbid Anatomy"

and as a model, "easy of execution, and admitting of extensive application in all the cities and principal towns of the empire."[2] His academy, though short-lived and never emulated by others, serves as a convenient focal point for a sketch of some of the issues associated with a particular, forgotten variant of British pathology in the early part of the nineteenth century. Growing out of a certain set of intellectual and institutional affiliations, this variant was, in important respects, the transition between the Baillie–Hunter and the Hodgkin–Carswell traditions. In other respects, as an approach to British pathology it was *sui generis* – ephemerally unique to the England of the 1820s. The context of medical science was itself changing so rapidly during this period that Farre's experiment barely got off the ground. His projected academy was left in the dust by more fully realized institutional forms, such as University College London, emerging in the 1830s and 1840s. But the Academy of Minute Anatomy, in its original conception and brief execution, remains, like some never-fully-realized architectural plan, an instructive guide to both the science of anatomy and the anatomy of science between Hunter and Hodgkin.

JOHN FARRE AND THE ENGLISH TRADITIONS OF PATHOLOGY

The careers of John Hunter, Matthew Baillie, and their immediate followers bring to mind tales of blood relatives (Hunter and Baillie were uncle and nephew), insiders, and well-placed patrons. They call up images of an increasingly elite cadre of surgical practitioners whose efforts put their immediate heirs, men like Astley Cooper and Benjamin Brodie, on a virtually equal footing with the aristocratically-minded and ever more otiose physicians of the Royal College in London. They summon, finally, afterimages of the natural historical sensibilities of the eighteenth-century collector: the classifier of medical cases, and the taxonomist of the remains and artifacts that might best illustrate those cases. This was a generation of medical men whose morbid anatomy revolved around a museum of organ-centered surgical pathology: The major bodily organs were to be found at the center not only of their nosological schemes but also of their illustrated texts and museum collections.[3]

By contrast, the generation of pathologists of the 1830s were outsiders and reformers both in medical science and in medical education. With the possible exception of Richard Bright, those who fell into this group were influenced by the histological images of body structure and function that they learned firsthand from French pathological anatomists in the 1820s.[4] Their chosen idiom for insuring the progress of pathological anatomy was a tissue-centered system of pathology. For a third of a century or more, such a system, rooted in both English and French concepts of the late eighteenth century, had bound a critical mass of physicians and surgeons together in common intellectual cause.[5] It was a system, to reiterate my earlier discussion, that comprised an ingenious array of compartments or body cavities, each in sympathy with the other. Each contained vital organs invested with surrounding membranous tissues – textures in the English idiom – that mediated the sympathies between the compartments and modulated as well the delicate balance, necessary to health, and vitiated in such pathological states as inflammation, between the bodily fluids and solids.[6] This complex image of the human body in health and disease was also an extraordinarily potent way of maintaining cohesion between the views of the physicians and surgeons in settings where such cohesion was institutionally mandated.[7]

As I have suggested, French pathological anatomy was by the 1820s beginning to have an important effect on British medicine.[8] Its impact was mediated through the assimilation of both French tissue pathology and the physical diagnosis that was in part its offshoot. In the 1830s Carswell and Hodgkin were to become the leading exponents of the morbid anatomy wing of this third generation, Gallicised pathology. Understandably, this process of accommodation to foreign ideas did not take place without friction. The preceding chapter only hints at the irruptions of many and various reactions to French pathology, ranging from the rapt to the phobic, that adorn the pages of the several English medical journals founded in this period.[9]

It is thus with some curiosity that one turns to John Farre, Muehry's second and intermediate cohort of one. In some sense, Farre was both a transitional and a pivotal figure. His arena was the London of 1828, two years before the introduction of the achromatic microscope by J. J. Lister, four years before the Anatomy Act, six years before Parliament investigated the need for reform in medical education, and about ten years before Hodgkin's major publications on tissue pathology. Why in this year was Farre trying to launch an Academy of Minute Anatomy?

In his *Apology for British Anatomy* (1827), the abstract of an introductory lecture delivered at the Academy in the previous year, Farre outlined his view of the proper method of advancing medical science. His academy was intended "to cultivate the Anatomy of Structure, as contradistinguished from the Anatomy of Relative Situation, which chiefly occupies the attention of the Schools." He was, that is, concerned with "the disorganization of textures" rather than traditional surgical anatomy.[10] Farre did not belabor the distinction, clearly one that was obvious enough to him. He favored the pathology of normal and deranged tissue structure over that of the old pathology of organs. The surgical anatomists teaching in the new, quite numerous private schools of anatomy (12 in London by 1826) were confined, he felt, to a narrow and limiting perception of the body.[11]

Farre, after abjuring the "Anatomy of Relative Situation," nevertheless located his anatomy firmly in the tradition of John Hunter, whom he declared to be the discoverer "of those changes which take place at the extremities of the arteries . . . which constitute the basis of pathological science."[12] Yet was not Hunter the surgical pathologist of "relative situation," *par excellence?* The resolution to the contradiction emerges in three parallel streams each related to an area of emphasis and detail within Farre's pathological system. First Farre saw Hunter as embracing the pathology of both organs and textures in his overall system of morbid anatomy.[13] While Hunter had not, in the 1794 *Treatise on Blood, Inflammation, and Gun-Shot Wounds,* emphasized tissue inflammation as much as Xavier Bichat would soon do in his *Treatise on Membranes* (1799) and *General Anatomy* (1801), Hunter's work did nevertheless include a sophisticated analysis of the "surfaces taking on inflammation."[14] Farre evidently incorporated both aspects of the Hunterian system of pathological anatomy when he gave his own view of inflammation, explaining that

when the capillary arteries are in a state of active congestion, effusion commences from their extremities. This condition of arteries is called inflammation; and although the action be morbid, it often preserves the life of the part, which, under the various circumstances exciting congestion, would die, if this process did not take place. The first effusion is a mere increase of the fluids which are separated from exhalent or secreting arteries. Thus, when cellular membrane, or the investing membranes of internal cavities are feebly inflamed, it is serous; but when the membranes which line external surfaces, or those which are exposed to irritating matters, are inflamed in the like degree, the effusion is simply an increased quantity of the mucous fluid with which those parts are naturally covered.[15]

The passage indicates also a second element of Farre's self-perception as a Hunterian: his concern with the relations between the solids and the fluids of the body. The hydraulic state, as it were, of both the local parts and the cardiovascular system as a whole was of paramount importance to Hunter and hence to Farre. The latter's early interests in pathological anatomy were in fact centered on the morbid structure and function of the heart and great vessels, culminating in the first essay of his *Pathological Researches . . . on Malformations of the Human Heart.*[16]

The third and last part of Farre's system was his image of the eye, which he related to each of the first two components, the membranes and the cardiovascular system. His institutional links with the London Ophthalmic Infirmary, discussed at some length later, provided him with the impulse to make the eye increasingly his primary concern. Most of the noncataractous diseases that he and his colleagues were to see at the ophthalmic hospital involved inflammatory affections of various types: "Under any arrangement," Farre noted, "of the morbid conditions of the eye, which we may choose to form or adopt, inflammation must be the chief object of our consideration."[17] The eye, in turn, was nothing more than a remarkable assemblage, a microcosm in fact, of the various tissues comprising the rest of the body.[18] And finally, to understand inflammatory or any other affections of the eye, one must correlate its state with that of the cardiovascular system. The most obvious instance of this relationship was pointed out by Farre in considering the effect of rapid changes in the "congestion" of the blood vessels: "It is not unusual under a sudden loss of blood, for the patient, previous to fainting, to exclaim, 'I am blind.' "[19]

By the 1820s, then, John Farre had created a surgical pathology infused with tissue theory and inflammation theory, and focused on the ophthalmic and cardiovascular systems and their interrelations. He combined these elements into his own system of pathology, a system that he could then legitimately label as Hunterian. Farre held up Hunter's nephew, "the illustrious Baillie" as the "finest medical example of the excellence of [this] doctrine; and the best model that can be held up to the young physician for his pursuit of pathological anatomy."[20]

Up to this point Farre's approach to a science of pathological anatomy – his cognitive style, as it were – has been characterized in terms of his own self-perceptions as Hunterian. There were, however, other features within his immediate cultural context that shaped Farre's program and style of pathological anatomy. Three such points were particularly important in determining Farre's conception.

The first spurred Farre's emphasis on the need "to cultivate the fine Arts of Drawing and Modelling, as far as it is desirable that they should be connected with Minute Practical and Morbid Anatomy." He declared that "it is indeed highly desirable that all persons who cultivate Medicine from a love of the Science, should study Painting" and insisted that "every student of the Academy, over whom he may have control or influence, shall both Dissect and Sketch." Farre's own works were carefully illustrated, usually with colored plates. It is easy to understand as well as to trivialize his insistence on this point, but an important implication should not be overlooked. A variety of techniques for the publication of accurate illustrations were being explored during this period. Some uniformly entailed a rather substantial expense, though the economic circumstances of publication by the various methods were very much in flux.

The anatomist frequently relied upon the professional artist to model and draw his preparations, or the skilled engraver to prepare them for the press.[21] The results – for example, John Dalrymple's *Pathology of the Eye* (1852) – were often beyond the pocketbooks of many medical men.[22] Hence the physical form in which this pathological anatomy was presented – and Farre had good reason to see to it that it was so presented – in many instances insured exclusive access by a well-off elite. This was especially so in the face of severe limitations on the use of libraries: The library of the Royal College of Physicians was, for instance, generally unavailable even to its own licentiates.[23] In contrast, the format of much of the journal literature of the period was more readily accessible and lent itself to popularization of new ideas and techniques beyond elite circles.[24] Farre evidently wished to have it both ways, because by the mid-1820s he was projecting the publication of a new *Journal of Morbid Anatomy* that would convey to the public his own image of native English pathological anatomy.

Furthermore, Farre's stated intentions were explicitly and intensely nationalistic. "Great Britain," he admitted, "has been reproached that her Medico-Chirurgical Schools have no pretensions to Anatomy; as having done little either in the way of discovery to advance it, or of practice to cultivate what had already been discovered." But he declared that "amidst this confessed deficiency, Great Britain, in particular, has produced the anatomists, whose discoveries, doctrine, and mode of instruction, have advanced medicine to the dignity of a science." He regretted the "undue preference" of medical students for the schools of France, and found it "necessary to give the student a caution on the subject of the morbid anatomy of the French School. Their writers confuse the subject by a verbose and inflated style, which is very seductive to young minds."[25]

In retrospect this sounds like special pleading since at least some of Farre's own research seems derived from French pathology; his protégé Dalrymple actually cited Bichat, although Farre apparently did not. Whether Farre acquired French concepts and methods through the filter of Matthew Baillie and John Hunter, and whether he was unaware of their source or unwilling to admit it, probably represents a cluster of problems that allows no resolution. What seems most important, though, is the perception that Farre had of his system. He clearly wished to see it distanced from the attribution of French influence.

Farre's search for an English national style of pathological anatomy could rely, however, neither on the production of new sorts of illustration nor on xenophobic pieties. He needed to tap what was recognizably, quintessentially, British in the range of possible pathologies available to him. This he found in the peculiarly clinical, functional approach to disease that had been a hallmark of much of English and Scottish medicine since the eighteenth century. Hence, in addition, Farre emphasized the "physiological" character of British anatomy, which he traced to the "genius of the British nation, and . . . the peculiar character of its mind, which requires utility as the object of its pursuit, brevity in expressing it, and energy in applying it to useful purposes."[26] In his own *Pathological Researches* of 1814 he explained that the title was

intended to express chiefly a purpose of tracing the diagnostic signs of the imperfect functions or structures of organs, and of endeavoring to discriminate between the conditions which admit of curative, and those which admit only of palliative means. If some attention has been bestowed on a physiological subject in this Essay, it is due to its importance, and to the interest which that subject has excited.[27]

By "physiological" one should clearly read "clinically useful assessment of functional disturbance." Thus, Farre emphasized that the combination of clinical observation of the course of disease combined with anatomical observation "affords the only means of distinguishing between diseases of function and diseases of structure . . . and the lapse of the former into the latter." This was "the professional method of investigating disease, which we call Clinical medicine."[28] He had been "forcibly impressed with the importance of this combination" in the work of Baillie, in contrast to the study of morbid anatomy "considered only as a part of natural history" by Morgagni.[29] Morbid anatomy was too theoretical, insular, and fanciful on the continent, whereas his own, native version had practical, "physiological" utility in the diagnosis and treatment of disease.

By the late 1820s, when he published his *Apology* and began the *Journal of Morbid Anatomy,* however, Farre was no longer content to sit quietly by siding with English clinicians against French theoreticians. Though his own opinions had not shifted, his perception of the opposition had. At that time anatomy in England, normal and morbid, received far less than its due. He cautioned junior members of the profession

that they exceedingly undervalue its services, when they limit them to a sepulchretum, or mere depositary of the ultimate and immutable forms of structural disease, which are hopeless either to the curative or palliative powers of medicine, and inseparable from death; that Morbid Anatomy, for the legitimate purposes of Medical Science, is to be viewed as a retracing of organic changes, from the final to the most incipient alterations of structure . . . [S]tudents should seek with avidity, not only the symptoms which mark the first transition from disordered function into diseased structure, but also the means which can avert, while there is opportunity, the impending fatal change.[30]

Farre was here arguing both *pro* and *con*. He was *for* a renewed English effort at "anatomizing." Such a surge of effort was, ironically, to come within a very few years, but without Farre's participation. He was *against* the "seductive" body of French work that he continued to disparage as overly theoretical. Probably his most strenuous objection was reserved for John Forbes, Laennec's translator and a man whose seduction, in Farre's view, seemed complete.[31]

At all events, the perception of an excessive emphasis abroad on structural damage may explain Farre's choice of the "physiological" appellation in describing British morbid anatomy, although it does not yet explain why he saw French work to be so antithetical. That question may simply be unanswerable in intellectual terms. What then does become significant is that Farre, an English medical student during the period just after the French Revolution and during the Napoleonic wars, propounded a view of pathology that joined organ and tissue pathology into a system that was avowedly both utilitarian and *English*. It was also a system that was heavily dependent on an institutional experiment of the 1820s, an early example of the specialty hospital.

THE INSTITUTIONAL LINK: THE LONDON OPHTHALMIC INFIRMARY

Farre's Academy of Minute Anatomy was to be an offshoot of the London Ophthalmic Infirmary, founded in 1804–1805 by John Cunningham Saunders with the encouragement and support of Astley Cooper.[32] The establishment of the Infirmary is worth examining both because of its importance to Farre and because of its value in illustrating the ways in which ideas and institutions helped shape one another. Farre's cognitive style, as it related to pathological anatomy, and Saunders's institutional ambitions, as they related to the development of a new type of hospital, were in this case drawn together by a common interest in reform and innovation. Then, and only then, did the question of interaction and of mutual "fit" become important.

Born in Devonshire in 1773, Saunders was educated at Tavistock and Southmolton, and apprenticed in 1790 to John Hill, a Barnstable surgeon. After the customary five years he came to London, without friends or introduction, and "walked the wards" at Guy's and St. Thomas's Hospitals. There he became a dresser for Astley Cooper, the consummate surgical practitioner, patron and kingmaker of the early decades of the nineteenth century. In

1797 Cooper helped him obtain the post of Demonstrator of Anatomy at St. Thomas's.[33] But this was as far as Cooper could take Saunders on the basis of his evident and growing merit as a surgeon.

By the end of 1800 it was clear that Saunders stood little chance of professional advancement in the metropolis. The friendly conspiracy between governing boards and elite medical men, whose hold on power was secure, and was securely based on nepotism, raised a clear-cut bar to the progress that Saunders's merit might have warranted. It was in this way, as M. J. Peterson notes, that the "grammar of social history" was applied to professional connections in early nineteenth-century Britain.[34]

But by the same token, this system, in which nepotism reigned and patronage bested merit, was slowly becoming porous. While family or other connections could still negate the impact of incompetence, genuine competence could nevertheless at times be recognized and, where it did not clash with other imperatives, be rewarded (if often only deviously) even by the likes of Cooper or Benjamin Brodie. Cooper's next two moves on behalf of Saunders are best viewed in this context. His was a traditional apprenticeship, followed by a distinctly untraditional move to establish and farm the younger surgeon out to an unproven new institutional genre: the specialty dispensary.

Farre later recalled that Saunders had been possessed of great talent but that this was insufficient to secure him a hospital post:

> It was impossible: they were shut against him. He could only be admitted in one way; talent could not admit him. He must be admitted by money; by entering as an apprentice to one of the surgeons of those hospitals.[35]

Saunders therefore left St. Thomas's in the spring of 1801 to begin private practice in the country. But Cooper, dissatisfied with Saunders's replacement, induced the younger man to return only months later to resume his old post.[36]

At about the same time, an epidemic of eye disease swept across England, originating among the troops returning from Egypt and quickly spreading to the civilian population.[37] In the words of one observer, "as the general body of surgeons did not understand diseases of the eye, the public necessarily resorted to 'oculists,' " regarded by respectable medical men as quacks.[38] Saunders saw in this situation a unique opportunity to attempt private practice in medically untilled fields. In 1803 he launched forth as a specialist in diseases of the eye and ear.

Cooper, weighing the possibilities in such a situation, suggested an extension of the idea: the creation of a London Dispensary for Curing Diseases of the Eye and Ear. Saunders seized the idea and began efforts to bring it into being. Farre later explained the proceedings:

In 1804, John Cunningham Saunders proposed the establishment of an infirmary for curing diseases of the eye. No such establishment existed in the British Empire at that time; and I know by my surgical education at the principal London hospitals . . . that the practice of ophthalmic medicine and surgery could not be acquired in those two schools, simply because there were no patients to be seen. A certain degree of manual dexterity had enabled the oculist to carry off the rich; and the poor always follow in their train. The poor, therefore, would not consult the profession on diseases of the eye; and the establishment of the Eye-Institution became the means of restoring diseases of the eye to the profession.[39]

Saunders, explained Farre, was unwilling "again . . . to undergo a novitiate of seven years," and therefore, "this institution was established for him. . . . By virtue of that effort, the diseases of the eye have been restored to the profession, both to physicians and surgeons."[40] Recognizing the necessity of obtaining the support of the medical elite for this enterprise, Saunders, again acting on Cooper's advice, successfully solicited the endorsements of both the medical and surgical staffs of Guy's and St. Thomas's Hospitals.[41] The self-conscious attention that he and his colleagues at the Dispensary paid to pathological anatomy both enhanced the respectability of the project and justified the emphasis on a tighter alliance between medicine and surgery in the enterprise.

The institution, in effect, had not one, however, but three cofounders. The managerial leadership of the Dispensary was soon swelled to an entrepreneurial *troika* with the addition of John Richard Farre and Richard Battley, both of whom had known Saunders around 1798, when the three were together at St. Thomas's under Cooper's supervision.[42] Like Saunders, both Farre and Battley were outsiders in the medical aristocracy of London. Farre was born in 1775, the son of a provincial physician in Barbados, where he received his early education and studied medicine with his father. Arriving in England in 1792, he studied at the United Borough Hospitals and became a dresser at Guy's.

A year later the eighteen-year-old Farre joined the Corporation of Surgeons in order to qualify as an assistant staff surgeon in the army, a major employer of medical personnel throughout the warring nations of Europe. He divided the next few years between France, England, and the West Indies, practicing both medicine and operative surgery. By 1800, when Farre permanently returned to Britain, his interests were narrowing to internal medicine and pathology. Because the College of Physicians proscribed dual membership with the Surgeons, he was forced to choose between the two.

Farre would later describe the College's exclusion principle as "a suicidal act." But fortunately for Farre, the dissolution of the Surgeon's Company provided him an almost unique opportunity to "cross over" without heavy financial penalties, although he still could have practiced generally on the strength of his surgical qualifications. He thus acquired a Glasgow medical degree in 1802, a procedure which entailed no residence requirement, and little more than a single oral examination and two Latin dissertations. Farre next resided in Edinburgh for two years to fulfill the requirements of the College of Physicians, and became a licentiate of the College in 1805. In later years Farre defended this course of study, arguing for the superiority of the physician with surgical training, and of London over Oxbridge for a medical education, "preferring," he said, "knowledge to honour." It is perhaps ironic to note that Farre sent his own sons, both eminent medical men in later life, to Cambridge.[43]

Richard Battley (1770–1856), the third member of the original dispensary triumvirate, was a still more unlikely associate of Astley Cooper's. The son of a Wakefield architect, Battley was educated at the Wakefield Grammar School, studied with a local physician, and then became medical attendant to the collieries at Newcastle-upon-Tyne. Ambitious to further his medical education, he attended the medical schools of the London hospitals before enlisting in the navy as an assistant surgeon. Settling down as an apothecary in London, probably around the turn of the century, Battley came to be known for his innovations in pharmaceutical technique, and for the museum of materia medica that he maintained, first in his home and later in Farre's institution, and which he allowed London medical students to use freely.[44] When the Dispensary was established in 1805, Battley became its secretary and supplied its medicines, while Farre assumed the post of Consulting Physician.

While the eye infirmary provided an institutional base for these three "outsiders," it never posed a real challenge to the London surgical establishment. After Saunders's untimely death in 1810, in fact, his heirs elected to close ranks with St. Thomas's, the mainstream institution. Farre and (presumably) Battley remained secure in their posts, while their institution drifted, indeed bolted, back into the Cooper orbit. It had never, in fact, strayed very far. Thus Cooper himself served as acting surgeon until Benjamin Travers, Jr., Cooper's house pupil, whose father had chaired the organizational meeting of the Dispensary, was appointed to replace Saunders. In the following year the practice of the Infirmary was opened to medical students, a clear-cut expression of the closer links that had recently been forged.

A formal series of lectures was undertaken. Travers was succeeded in 1817 by another pupil of Cooper, Frederick Tyrrell, who was elected explicitly on the basis of his connections with St. Thomas's. William (later Sir William) Lawrence was meanwhile elected as a second surgeon in 1814. The institution's commitment to the cause of moderate professional reform was formalized in 1817, with the imposition of new requirements for its officers: The physician would have to be a Fellow or Licentiate of the College of Physicians, or a Bachelor of Medicine from Oxford or Cambridge; the surgeons would have to be members of the College of Surgeons and, significantly, would have to have served a hospital apprenticeship. In like fashion, the apothecary must needs be a member of the College of Surgeons as well as a licentiate of the Society of Apothecaries.[45]

The incumbents at the eye Infirmary appear to have all met these criteria though Saunders, the *primus inter pares* of the founding trio, clearly would not have done so. The routinization of credentials reflected in the move also relates to general efforts under way in the 1810s in England to achieve medical reform. Medical reform meant rationalizing medical licensing and medical education. It dealt with the several ragged fissures between the classes of medical practitioners, fissures traditionally widened by the obduracy of the royal colleges. It meant upgrading the role and the status of a group whose interest in pathological anatomy has been discussed: the surgeon–apothecaries, who were coming consciously and publicly to think of themselves as general practitioners.[46] Each of the overlapping elements of medical reform represented a perceived threat and a genuine thrust against existing norms and structures. One of the strongest of these elements that aimed at upgrading the apothecaries' station within the profession was an organization already discussed in these pages, the Associated Apothecaries and Surgeon–Apothecaries of England and Wales that began meeting in July of 1812.

The passage of the Apothecaries Act of 1815 for many reasons was only an ambiguous success. But the Act did serve to legitimate and consolidate the credentialling authority of the Society of Apothecaries. It also insured that the trend toward seeking double credentials in surgery and the apothecary's trade would continue and accelerate.[47] Two points growing out of the 1815 Act bear emphasis here. First, the requirement at the Ophthalmic Infirmary that the apothecary also be trained as a surgeon was entirely consistent with the stated objectives of the surgeon–apothecaries, as well as the realities of power in their formal organization.[48] Second, and perhaps more important, was the fact that the surgeon–apothecaries seized with a vengeance on the inadequacy of British anatomical training in the 1810s. They contended that enhancing the emphasis on pathological anatomy, because it was clinically relevant yet grounded in the new anatomical science, might go at least part of the way toward meeting that inadequacy.[49]

In 1810 John Saunders died unexpectedly, leaving a few published papers, a mass of unpublished case reports, an impecunious wife, and no will. At the request of the Trustees of the Infirmary, and after the resolution of the legal issue of literary rights, Farre undertook the task of editing the *Treatise on Some Practical Points Relating to the Disease of the Eye* (1811), which Saunders had projected. When she remarried, the proceeds of the publication – originally intended to provide an annuity for Mrs. Saunders – were diverted to a "Saunderian Fund" established by Farre, with a large contribution of his own, as a memorial to the Infirmary's founder. The Fund was later used to finance the Academy of Minute Anatomy, which also came to be known as the "Saunderian Institution."[50]

The *Treatise* set the tone for the scientific work of the Infirmary during the 1810s. Saunder's essays on "Inflammation of the Iris" and "Inflammation of Conjunctiva in Infants" were reproduced with few changes. But Farre, as editor, departed self-consciously from the nosology used by Saunders in his annual reports. Farre's own classification, based on Hunterian principles, made a major division between diseases of structure (subdivided mainly into types of inflammation, but also including tumors) and those of function (amaurosis).[51] As Farre later pointed out, ophthalmic anatomy offered an excellent field of study for pathologists with a physiological orientation, since morbid phenomena of the eye were observable throughout the course of ocular disease. For the same reason such studies could contribute also to the "theory of therapeutic medicine."[52] Travers's *Synopsis of Diseases of the Eye* (1820), dedicated to Farre, adopted the same approach.[53] In his view of the eye as a sort of microcosm or laboratory of pathology and therapeutics, Farre may have also realized that its study circumvented the problem of obtaining whole bodies to dissect. This, however, he never stated in print.[54]

According to Farre's scheme, then, ophthalmic anatomy was especially significant as an instance of the unity that could be forged between physicians and surgeons on the basis of pathology. "Whilst the manual department of the Profession distinguishes the Surgeon from the Physician," he announced in 1826, "Pathology unites them, the science being one; and, consequently, by a careful record of the morbid changes which take place in the respective organs submitted to their management, each will enlighten the department of the other, and thus contribute to the perfection of the whole."[55]

Explaining the position in greater detail in 1834, Farre contended that the treatment of eye diseases was more precise than almost any other branch of medicine because of the "physician and surgeon coming directly into contact with the disease" and collaborating in its treatment. Thus was illustrated the necessity of the two branches being "more intimately united": In fact, there should be "but one profession," although the extent of the subject made a division of labor advantageous. Citing the example of iritis, he explained that the physician could follow the morbid action through the cornea "as through a glass," and could also watch the structural changes produced as the administration of mercury effected a cure. "I am now supposing," he noted, "that a physician is learning medicine, by studying the surgical treatment of a disease of the eye. He sees the morbid action, and the countervailing action of the remedy; and he learns in what way he can arrest the same process of adhesive inflammation, on the heart, on the lungs, on the brain, on the liver, and, in short, on every organ and texture of the body."[56]

The importance to Farre of the combination of medicine and surgery is also suggested by the pieces of Saunders's work that he chose to assemble in the *Treatise*. While most of its text concerned the Hunterian explanation of inflammation, comprising a subtext of internal medicine, Farre also paid substantial attention to the techniques employed in ophthalmic surgery. The significance of these techniques, especially the dramatic procedure for the relief of cataracts in young children, may perhaps be gauged by the frequency and intensity of priority disputes over their development, a subject that provided much of the material in Farre's preface to the second edition (1816) of the *Treatise*.[57]

Morbid anatomy, which Farre interpreted as stemming from the tradition of Hunter and Baillie, was hence a bridge between academic knowledge and technical expertise in a nascent specialty that transected medicine and surgery. It could be used as well to forge links between disparate and perhaps even apparently contradictory aspects of medical science itself. Farre was capable of enthusiastic advocacy of the new clinical medicine, while adhering to the older view of the essentially unitary nature of most disease. "In investigating diseases by anatomy," he wrote in 1814, "the author chiefly proposes to contribute to the diagnostic part of medicine. The study of symptoms, without regard to the organic changes which gave rise to them, leads to a confused knowledge of the genera, species, and varieties of internal diseases."[58] But Farre also said that

physicians in treating of Nosology, have thought fit to multiply the genera of diseases in an artificial manner. They teach us, that inflammation, instead of being a single genus, consists of as many genera as there are organs in the body; but nature manifests by similar phenomena in all textures, that although it may vary in its seat or degree, yet it constitutes only one disease.[59]

For Farre, then, the combination of bedside observation with the autopsy did not inevitably lead to a multiplying of individual disease entities, nor a radically new view of illness. In an implicit slap at the younger generation returning from Continental education in pathology and crowding his territory – a crowd derisively labelled "Gallicised" by those of his own generation – the aging Farre rejected their far-fetched theoretical transports. Pathological anatomy for Farre, despite his advocacy of the "pathology of textures," had more a formal than a substantive role in revolutionizing medicine. Pathological anatomy was a tool for the perfection of existing diagnosis and nosological accuracy. There is much to suggest that Farre saw the true and proper nosology as a return to the principles of Sydenham, rather than a turn toward Gallic novelty.[60] Yet, as the above passages suggest, he could at times sound remarkably like his French counterparts.

With the opening, late in 1822, of new facilities at Moorfields, an ambitious program of lectures was launched at the Infirmary. Farre was to offer a course on "Morbid Anatomy, illustrative of the Practice of Physic in general, as well as Ophthalmic Medicine in particular." Lawrence was to lecture on "Anatomy, Physiology, and Diseases of the Eye," and Tyrrell promised clinical lectures. Battley was to instruct students on "the chemistry of light" and materia medica, while the Reverend T. Gill was to lecture on optics. Lawrence stressed in the introduction to his *Treatise on Diseases of the Eye* (1833) that instruction at the Infirmary was "intended to impart to physicians and surgeons a knowledge of ophthalmic disease, and not merely to make oculists."[61]

The ambitious plan was not an unqualified success. Gill resigned after only a few months, while Battley, finding the laboratory and museum inadequate, refused for a long time to give any lectures at all. Lawrence's lectures, on the other hand, were published regularly in the *Lancet* in 1825–1826, perhaps without his permission, and later formed the basis of his textbook. One of Farre's lectures was also published, and while it may have appeared unimpressive in later years, it drew praise from Lawrence as a mirror of his teaching prowess. The Saunderian Fund provided the means to expand the facilities: The new Academy of Minute Anatomy was built adjacent to the Infirmary building. Battley donated money of his own for a new laboratory: Hence "Pharmaceutical Analysis," another nascent science that was yet to find its institutional niche, was incorporated into the scope of the Academy. (This branch of pharmaceutical chemistry would also become part of the purport and the title of Farre's new journal in 1828.) Farre donated eighteen volumes of the *Philosophical Transactions* as the nucleus of a library for the associated institutions. The inclusion of the transactions of the Medico–Botanical Society in Farre's new *Journal* suggests yet another connection as well.[62]

Though medical historians have dated the beginning of scientific ophthalmology to the introduction of the ophthalmoscope in 1851, the Infirmary and Academy were unquestionably important in promoting the specialized study of eye disease a quarter of a century earlier.[63] By 1828 Farre could justly boast that the more than one thousand students who had been instructed at the institution had spread out over the world; six years later he estimated the number of alumni at over twelve hundred. The first student, R. Richardson, established an eye infirmary at Madras on the model of the London Infirmary, while other former students did the same at Calcutta and Bombay. Some of the earliest students were the Americans Edward Delafield and J. Kearney Rodgers, later key figures in the development of ophthalmology in the United States.[64] The thousands of students who took advantage of Battley's instruction testified to the accuracy of Farre's estimate of "the difficulty often experienced by Medical Students of obtaining Pharmaceutical Knowledge."[65] In this respect, too, the Infirmary and Academy seem to have filled a gap in contemporary medical education that was characteristic of the first third of the nineteenth century.

Of the men trained by Farre and his colleagues in the tradition of the Infirmary/Academy, John Dalrymple (1803–1852) was perhaps typical of the nexus of ophthalmology and pathological anatomy. After an apprenticeship with his father, William Dalrymple, a surgeon at the Norfolk and Norwich Hospital and a former Astley Cooper pupil, John Dalrymple continued his medical studies in Edinburgh. After several years in the north, he came to London and became a member of the College of Surgeons in 1827. In that year he also arrived at the Ophthalmic Infirmary, where he served for over twenty years first as secretary and demonstrator at the Academy of Minute Anatomy. He attempted in this capacity consciously to base his research on Farre's model of pathological anatomy in the service of the clinic.

After 1832 Dalrymple was given the post of surgeon to the Infirmary, along with one of Farre's sons, revealing rather typically the manner in which a pathologist's post was to become a stepping-stone to a more purely clinical one. His connection to the institution was reinforced by the marriage of his sister to Richard Battley. On the strength of his *Anatomy of the Human Eye* of 1834, as well as several minor papers on topics in general pathology and natural history, Dalrymple was elected a Fellow of the Royal Society in 1850. His lavishly illustrated *Pathology of the Eye,* dedicated to James Clark, appeared two years later, a short time before his death.[66]

During the 1820s the Ophthalmic Infirmary also achieved prominence (or notoriety, as the case may be) as one of the main targets of Thomas Wakley's *Lancet*. Perhaps reformers of different hues may be expected to behave with mutual suspicion toward one another. In any case the Infirmary, as far as Wakley was concerned, epitomized, not without reason, the exclusive and elitist nepotism of the Cooper circle. Moreover, Tyrrell and Travers were two of the three culprits most obviously responsible for the attempts to suppress Wakley's publication of clinical lectures delivered at St. Thomas's, not to mention his actual exclusion from that hospital. Wakley further charged that Tyrrell's 1825 text was plagiarized from Cooper's lectures as they had been transcribed for the *Lancet*. (Tyrrell thereupon sued Wakley for libel – of necessity as his name and honor seemed at stake. Though he won the case, Tyrrell found his victory a Pyrrhic one, when the damages awarded were nominal.)

William Lawrence, whose path through the medical politics of the period was vacillating, cooperated with the publication in the *Lancet* of his own lectures, and probably blocked passage of a by-law prohibiting note-taking at the Infirmary. Such a by-law had already been passed at St. Thomas's in an obvious attempt to thwart the heinous dissemination of unauthorized knowledge to Wakley's journal-reading public. When Lawrence resigned from the Infirmary to accept a mainstream hospital position, however, open warfare erupted between Wakley and the Ophthalmic Infirmary.[67]

The first intimation of Farre's plans for the Academy of Minute Anatomy coincided, ironically, with the outbreak of these hostilities. Even more ironically, Farre probably associated Wakley's political radicalism with the abominable foreign influences in pathological anatomy, with their overemphasis on structural lesions and the multiplication of entities. Both Farre and Battley had been military surgeons during the Napoleonic conflict, and Farre recollected that Saunders had wished not to enter medicine but "to have distinguished himself in the service of his country."[68] Wakley, on the other hand, very likely associated the London Ophthalmic Infirmary with the sort of halfway measures toward medical reform that in his view had left the traditional elite more firmly in control than ever.[69]

Farre pressed on, however, and in 1828 brought out the first volume of his new journal. In his "Advertisement," he noted that his original intent had been to publish what would have been Britain's first journal devoted exclusively to pathological anatomy, "a Journal of Morbid Anatomy, embracing researches physiological, pathological and therapeutic."[70] But the final product incorporated, as I have noted, a potpourri of several scientific and professional elements that had collectively provided the impetus for growth in the parent institution, the Infirmary. Farre, for his own part, clung tenaciously to the notion of pathological anatomy as the intellectual cement between those elements, citing his own recent lectures on the morbid anatomy of the cardiovascular system in 1826 and 1827. But in the pages of the *Journal* one also finds a range of concerns inherited from earlier generations, ranging from humoralism to medical climatology.[71]

THE FATE OF THE ACADEMY OF MINUTE ANATOMY

In the end Thomas Wakley had the last laugh. That end was not long in coming. The quiet demise of Farre's Academy is, as one would expect, more difficult to trace than its well-publicized inauguration. Only one volume of the *Journal of Morbid Anatomy* saw the light of day, and the Academy faded back into its parent institution. The Infirmary received the royal warrant in 1837 and was renamed the Royal London Ophthalmic Hospital. Both Farre and Dalrymple retained their association with it until their retirement from practice. Indeed, Farre remained on the staff, a physician attuned to surgical pathology among the medically-minded surgeons until 1856, when he retired at the age of eighty-one.

From 1828 until his death in 1862, Farre published no further pathological research, nor did he again become engaged in editorial work. He was by now active in an extensive private practice, having carved out a profitable niche as a consultant on surgical and obstetrical cases, and not a few medical cases as well.[72] It is perhaps to this period and to figures like Farre that one may look for the archetypal role of the consulting internist. In this capacity Farre may have also devoted some of his attention to the passage of the Anatomy Acts, though he was not called to testify before the 1828 Parliamentary Select Committee convened to study the advisability of such legislation. Even in his introductory article for the *Journal,* Farre commented defensively that the Academy was

mainly intended to cultivate a spirit of inquiry on the part of the profession, *with the consent of the Public,* into the seats of disease, and the lapses of functional disorder into those changes of structure which are destructive of organised life. Its projector hopes, that . . . the two-fold purpose will be accomplished of cultivating Medico–Chirurgical Science on its true basis, and promoting the desirable spirit of peace and good will between the members of the profession and the public, on this delicate, yet most important research.[73]

On 17 April 1834 John Farre appeared as a witness before the Select Committee on Medical Education that Parliament, after years of provocation, had finally convened. Farre's testimony can be seen as a converging lens for the two parallel reform elements – the moderate reform of the profession through conventional, established channels, and the moderate reform of medical science through a particular genre of pathological anatomy – that he had supported for a third of a century. His program for medical research remained fundamentally unaltered: He still lauded John Hunter as the author of works on pathology that "form the basis of all the improvements which have taken place in the cure of disease" where their users had troubled themselves to make them "perfectly understood." He added, characteristically, that "at present they are not at all understood on the Continent."

Farre lamented the decline of physicians relative to surgeons, which he attributed directly to the disregard of anatomy by the College of Physicians since the time of William Harvey. In more recent times, he said, "by neglecting anatomy they have lost their strong hold on professional knowledge. They have struck out the basis of it, and have disregarded it. Baillie helped them a little, by becoming a teacher of anatomy, and by extending the study of morbid anatomy. We are much indebted to Baillie." Farre proposed that physicians could recover their position by appropriating the study of surgery as part of their own training, the course he had taken (though probably not with a great deal of premeditation) some forty years earlier. In this way they could overcome the natural advantage of the surgeon: "The subject of his inquiry being external, he sees it, he handles it, he submits it to his senses. The physician, on the contrary, the subject of his inquiry being internal, must become acquainted with it by signs." He here interpolated the example of iritis, discussed earlier, apparently to the great confusion of the Committee. Perhaps by 1834 they would have better understood if Farre had used the example of auscultatory signs in chest disease. But such could hardly be the case. Only a younger generation would have been capable of that next step.[74]

Farre's criticisms by no means constituted an unmitigated attack on the beleaguered leadership of the College of Physicians. Himself the holder of a Licentiate in the College, he declared nonetheless that he would not accept Fellowship were it offered to him. The reason he gave for refusing (or threatening to do so) was personal: he "could not consent to be placed at the feet of men whom I had contributed to educate." He had no grievances with the Fellows, and thought that they enjoyed no real advantage over the Licentiates, either in practice or in other respects. He had not signed the Licentiates' petition of grievances "because I think professional matters should not be submitted to any tribunal but their own." He declared, in concluding his testimony, that the public "are pretty well satisfied" with the present medical system. Farre, in any case, was not unsatisfied.[75]

JOHN FARRE AND THE EVOLUTION OF PATHOLOGY

The conclusions that Adolph Muehry, the German physician-traveler, drew on the basis of his 1835 wanderings, the year after Farre gave his testimony, were buried in bare-bones description. Implicit, however, in his statement about pathological anatomy in England was the notion that the kaleidoscope's image had shifted twice, from Hunter and Baillie to Farre and thence to the new men of the 1830s. If indeed this was Muehry's contention, he was right. There seems to have been a genuine shifting of frameworks as each generation gave way to the next, although each attempted avowedly to base its formulation of the best pathology on that of its forebears. What is of greatest interest to us, however, is the nature of these shifts and what propelled them.

Each of these shifts need not have been purely cognitive, nor need they be seen simply as accommodations to changing institutional and professional circumstances. Rather, each was a seamless mesh of profession, nosography, and technique evolving down a common path. John Farre's ideas and techniques, however short-lived, were one way station. Certainly his professional circumstances, as a surgically educated physician practicing among surgeons, influenced his view of disease. Conversely, his knowledge of pathological anatomy, and in particular the pathological anatomy associated with ophthalmic disease, influenced his views on the proper path that the medical profession, writ large, should take.

Farre's affiliation with a nascent specialty gave him license to advocate moderate reform, as he was marginal in major respects throughout his career by virtue of that affiliation. But he was still a member of the generation that was trained during the Napoleonic wars. He saw the virtue of tissue pathology, both in ophthalmology and in general pathology, but he could only see it in its most Anglicized and clinically relevant form. He was the most traditional of the new men, and the most daring of the Hunterians. But his ideas in fact represented neither the cutting edge of the first nor the trailing edge of the latter. He was an eighteenth-century man who confronted and accommodated himself to nineteenth-century realities of professional change, patterns of disease, and images of the body.

9

Propagation

Crummles: "Invention! What the devil's that got to do with it!
Nicholas: "Everything, my dear sir."
Crummles: "Nothing, my dear sir. Do you understand
French?"
Nicholas: "Perfectly well."
Crummles: "Very good," opening the table-drawer and giving
a roll of paper to Nicholas. "There, just turn that into English,
and put your name on the title-page. Damn me, if I haven't
often said that I wouldn't have a man or woman in my
company what wasn't master of the language, so that they
might learn it from the original, and play it in English, and by
that means save all this trouble and expense."
  – Charles Dickens, *The Life and Adventures of Nicholas Nickleby*
                                                            (1839)

In the 1820s and 1830s the heart of power in medical London still
lay in the alliance of laymen and medicosurgical elites. The power
to act as arbiters of medical truth and its clinical use in correct
social circles continued to reside in large measure in the hands of
those who held key posts. To physicians and surgeons the Royal
Colleges' ruling councils and the major hospital teaching posts offered such access to power.[1] Behind them, conferring patronage,
sat the lay hospital governors and financial officers, shoring up
the medical men's authority or, on occasion, severing it.[2]
  Ringing this innermost circle of medical opinion leaders and their
lay patrons were men like John Farre and his colleagues at the
Academy of Microscopic Anatomy and London Ophthalmic Infirmary. While they could hardly ignore the powerful activities of
the hospitals and examining bodies, Farre et al. were set apart by
their origins in the English provinces and their position as a sort
of inner circle, as near marginals. That position was echoed in the
views they put forward on scientific culture. Hence Farre's attempt

through pathological anatomy to fuse traditional, Hunterian intellectual forms of explanation with a novel institutional form, the specialty hospital, rested on a fundamental inclination toward preserving the cultural values of English medicine.

Farre and his circle, their sensibilities tempered by the Napoleonic struggles, still xenophobic, represented a negative, reactive response to the French challenge. But in the 1820s another, perhaps more peripheral, circle of medical men began to reveal warmer, more organic connections with the Continental experience. Scots, Quakers, and dissenters from other quarters converged on London as rank outsiders who remained disposed, to one degree or another, to remain so. Those who had trained in medicine or surgery had often completed their training in Paris. Returning now, they were as hospitable toward ideas and values from abroad as they felt toward those emanating from the traditional center at home.

In this chapter I will examine two experiments informed by this new attitude. Each involved an attempt by a particular figure to fit ideas about pathology into a career shaped by the interaction of those ideas and others'. Each career was interwoven with the development of a particular institution, and in different ways each pointed away from the traditional power center. In the case of Guy's Hospital, Gallic influences moved the Quaker physician, Thomas Hodgkin, to attempt the institutionalization of pathological anatomy. Ultimately, however, the inwardly directed, parochial views of the hospital bureaucracy defeated his reform efforts, with pathological anatomy only one of his reform ideas. To those in power, French pathological anatomy was far from the most threatening of Hodgkin's interests, which ranged from health promotion for the poor in the Mechanic's Institutes, to the protection of aboriginal tribes abroad, from the reform of medical education to its establishment at the new University College London, from the abolition of slavery to the development of the microscope.[3] Hodgkin's was therefore, at best, a qualified success at importing the French tradition.

More apolitical but little more successful was the Scot, Robert Carswell, who in 1829 became the first professor of pathological anatomy in England at London University – a new school for students from families of religious dissenters. Neither his Scottish education and birth, nor his years of yeoman service in the dissecting rooms of Paris, endeared Carswell to the London medical establishment. Even the distinctly nonestablishment leaders at the new University of London turned to Carswell only after they had offered the pathology professorship to a German, J. F. Meckel, who was ultimately unwilling to essay the risky new post.

Robert Carswell achieved far less renown in subsequent years than his Guy's Hospital counterpart, owing at least partly to Hodgkin's adventitious discovery of a disorder of the absorbent glands to which Samuel Wilks would later assign the eponym "Hodgkin's disease."[4] But Carswell actually fared at least as well as Hodgkin in his attempt to institutionalize pathological anatomy. When he, too, ultimately failed at University College, it was not the politics of social reform that defeated him as, at least in part, it had Hodgkin. Ironically, it was instead the narrow-gauged politics of medical curriculum reform that pushed aside Carswell and his field at the University of London.

Normal anatomy gradually came into its own in the wake of the Parliamentary inquiries of 1828 and 1834. Pathological anatomy, having been separately organized in the late 1820s for the first time in either country in the context of curricular innovation at London University, now became displaced as the study of normal anatomy increasingly became the standard for both education and accreditation.[5] At the end of the decade of the 1830s Carswell would leave university and metropolis to practice medicine among Belgian royalty, while Hodgkin began diverting most of his energies to a broad array of reformist causes. Outsiders to the end, Carswell died in Brussels in 1857, Hodgkin in Jaffa in 1866.[6]

LIFE IN PARIS

There is little to suggest that Carswell and Hodgkin were acquainted with one another in the early 1820s. By 1832, however, after both morbid anatomists were established back in London, Hodgkin could describe Carswell as "my friend." Indeed, he was to diagnose one of the cases of what later came to be known as Hodgkin's disease directly from one of Carswell's "unrivalled" Paris drawings.[7] It seems unlikely that the two men, dissimilar in tastes and backgrounds, were acquainted a decade earlier in Paris. What is clear is that they were both part of the swelling migration of Britons who arrived in Paris in the early 1820s. When Hodgkin and Carswell reached French shores they confronted the scene that, several decades later, their near contemporary, the clinician Charles J. B. Williams, would later characterize (Chapter 6) so fully and colorfully.[8]

Thomas Hodgkin's medical education began in 1819. After a classical education at the hands of his pedagogue father and, beginning in 1819, between one and two years in London at Guy's Hospital, the young Hodgkin proceeded (in 1821–1822) to Paris to learn pathological anatomy and physical diagnosis. After a final year, 1822–1823 in Edinburgh, where he gained the M.D. degree, he traveled for two years, spending the second year again in Paris before his 1825 return to London. In Paris Hodgkin cut an odd figure indeed. Here was an intellectually adept, inquisitive student, completely fluent in French and in the Latin in which Laennec was used to lecturing, traversing the riotous neighborhoods between the *Necker* and other Paris hospitals, between the *Jardin du Roi* and the Paris Faculty, clad in the severe garb of the birthright Quaker.

Hodgkin arrived in Paris closer to the beginning of term than would Charles Williams. Through friends' local introductions, he "procured a very comfortable little room in the *Jardin des Plantes*." Writing to his brother, John Hodgkin, Jr., he lamented his distance from the hospitals and Faculty, but was pleased to have ready access to the library and museum of the *Jardin,* as well as to the *Pitié,* "where through the influence of William Cullen I hope to dissect."[9] Six weeks later he was settled into a routine, which he described in a letter to his mother: "Up at six and away at seven; at the *Charité* by 7:30; rounds with Boyer, clinical lectures or operations followed by breakfast at ten in the Place St.-Michel; an anatomy lecture at the Faculty or dissection until four at the *Pitié*."[10] Despite the bustle, he felt isolated: "The Medical Professors may make a polite speach [sic] on opening a letter of introduction but seem to take no further notice. . . . I have few or no French acquaintances wh [sic] for the sake of the language I should like myself avoid the French élèves who interrupt by their noise."[11] Hence his progress in perfecting his already serviceable French was painfully slow.

Hodgkin was the source, in letters to his family, of an endless stream of complaints on subjects ranging from his own predicament over making ends meet in Paris to the predicament of African natives over the slave trade. (He found both appalling in equal measure.) Throughout, however, he endlessly scrutinized the

French academic scene. By the beginning of 1822 he was again altering his routine, embarking on an important new course. On January 5 he wrote:

> I discontinued going to la Charité at the end of the year and now attend Lanec [sic], the inventor of the stethoscope. . . . I prefer Lanec to any French practitioner I have yet seen. I have once had the advantage of going round with him almost with great ease and fluency. I have also [attended] Broussai [sic] but with much less satisfaction.[12]

Later that winter, in a letter to his cousin in Worcestershire, Hodgkin recorded some of his early impressions of Paris and its denizens' reactions to the eccentric in their midst. "[T]he spot where I am now living [close by the Jardin du Roi] thou hast no doubt often heard of in conjunction with the celebrated naturalist Buffon who once resided on it," he noted, though it was "not without its inconveniences[,] being situated at one of the extremities of the city."[13] He had to spend long hours, therefore, on the "bad pavements" swinging back and forth between the "remotely situated" hospitals, the Faculty and the Collège de France. He inscribed his name – few English students oriented toward pathology did so – on the rolls of the Faculty in 1821 and 1822.[14] At about the same time Laennec recorded his name on the 1822 list of pathological anatomy *lecteurs* at the Collège. With his reserve and his linguistic facility, Hodgkin became a favorite of the conservative Breton physician.[15]

Writing to his cousin in the depth of the Paris winter of 1822, Hodgkin urged his relative to join him once warmer weather arrived, noting that "[Quakers] are very little known here," and that his appearance, "which excites much attention," led many to mistake him for an American, since "they would not conceive that so strange a costume could be produced at so short a distance."[16] Touching on events that dimly reflected the conservative backlash at the Medical Faculty, he fulminated against the revival of Catholic religiosity he found growing about him in Paris, gaining ground by the hour and "offensive to many of the Catholics themselves." Hodgkin concluded the body of his letter with a characteristic remark on the "uphill work" that the Paris Bible society was facing in the execution of its mission.[17]

Hodgkin continued to travel extensively through his *Wanderjahre* of the mid-1820s, though he returned, as I have noted, to Britain long enough in 1823 to obtain the Edinburgh M.D. degree.[18] Tellingly, his M.D. dissertation was dedicated to Andrew Duncan Jr., and dealt with the functional role of the absorbent glands.[19] His concern with the humoral concepts of absorption and secretion, coupled with his concurrent interest in morbid dissection of the solid tissues, led as inexorably to his adoption of the Bichat–Laennec model of tissue pathology as it did to his 1832 description of the lymphoma that subsequently bore his name. As he himself began, in the mid-1820s, to ease into the role of morbid anatomy curator and instructor at Guy's Hospital, he naturally gravitated to the anatomy of the serous and mucous membranes, moving them to the center of his system of pathology.[20]

There is little question, then, that Laennec's and others' pathology – both the morbid dissection and the theoretical histopathology – exerted a profound impact on the young Hodgkin in the 1821–1825 period. The impact of the freewheeling French system of medical education was no less substantial. Returning to London and undertaking the museum curatorship and a series of lectures in morbid anatomy at Guy's Hospital, Hodgkin quickly became active in two distinct circles: professionally, in the scientifically-minded Guy's Hospital Physical Society, and socially in the tight network of London Quakers peopled by figures like William Allen and J. J. Lister.[21] On occasion the two spheres overlapped. They did so, for example, when Hodgkin collaborated with Lister (Lord Lister's father) in using the latter's new achromatic microscope to attempt a refutation of the globularist notion of tissue structure.[22]

THE PHYSICAL SOCIETY

The Guy's Hospital Physical Society, when Hodgkin joined it first as a student and later, in 1826, as a lecturer, was already a venerable and thriving institution.[23] Dating its foundation to 1771, the Society united medically oriented scientific enthusiasts in the hospitals south of the Thames.[24] Its membership indeed extended beyond this core of Thomas's and Guy's men to those, like Alexander Marcet, Edward Jenner, John Lettsom, and Richard Bright, who were eager to embrace the new scientific intellectual culture.[25] Some, like the physician–accoucheur Charles Locock,[26] most likely kept their membership current in order to add luster at decent intervals to the patina of scientific sophistication that they wished to sustain in their well-placed private practices. But even Locock would on occasion dip in to indulge in bursts of more active participation.[27]

For Thomas Hodgkin, the Physical Society formed the natural context in which to display most clearly his predilection for French medical education. In an essay read to the Society in the autumn of 1827 and published in the following year, Hodgkin expounded on the means of best promoting medical education, by borrowing leaves from the notebooks of his brethren in foreign schools. In his reckoning, the balancing of medicine and surgery, of physiology and pathology, which characterized the French systems, were to be specially prized:

Though I am convinced that, in this City, the study of internal Pathology is injuriously sacrificed to the more captivating branch of Surgery, I am by no means desirous of running into the opposite extreme. The Physician without that knowledge which the public is wont to consider as the peculiar province of the surgeon, is little else than a dignified Empiric – but, I am very sure that my Surgical Friends will be one in sentiment with me, when I say that, without Physiology and Pathology, internal, as well as external, their art, though it might be more excellent in degree, would still be one in kind, with that with which it was formerly associated. We are indebted to Surgeons for some of the most valuable additions which Pathology has received; and be it also remembered, that some of the most important anatomical facts have been brought to light by Physicians.[28]

Hodgkin next expatiated on the value of the formulation of general anatomy that had served so well in Paris as a sort of cognitive hinge between medicine and surgery. "I would place Anatomy as the first and most important object to which the commencing Student can devote his attention. He cannot too soon, or too thoroughly, become acquainted with it, both theoretically and practically. . . ." Hodgkin believed that the subject of Descriptive Anatomy was well-served in the London anatomical schools. But general anatomy, or the anatomy of tissues, was unfortunately neglected. The French schools recognized the particular importance of this subject "through the labours of the great Bichat. The late lamented Beclard devoted to it a considerable portion of his course; and the crowd of pupils . . . amply attested the interest and importance attached to it." Hodgkin suggested that comparable changes be made in the London curriculum, by entering more fully into the subject of general anatomy.[29]

HODGKIN'S PATHOLOGICAL ANATOMY

By 1830, long before he was to lock horns with the lay administration at Guy's Hospital, and some months even before Robert
Carswell returned to London from his long sojourn in Paris,
Hodgkin began to experience problems in sustaining his student
audience. Though self-deprecating in his willingness to shoulder
the blame, he was more likely in a situation where his subject was
simply being squeezed aside:

For the three years that I have filled the unprofitable thankless post of
lecturer on Pathological Anatomy I have been cut short not by the termination of the subject but by the desertion of my audience. I am painfully
sensible how strongly this bespeaks the want of talent in the lecturer.
But . . . By the recent acts of an important body you are recommended
not to neglect this study and what is more it is rendered incumbent upon
you to become acquainted with legal medicine. Now morbid anatomy
is to legal medicine what mineralogy is to Geology – I might almost say
what letters are to language.[30]

He nevertheless launched into the system of classification that
he considered most appropriate to a fundamental understanding
of diseased structures.

I shall have no hesitation in adopting the plan of Bichat and founding
the classification on the basis of general Anatomy.
    I shall commence by speaking of the characters which mark the morbid
appearances of a particular tissue in whatever part of the body it may be
found, and shall afterwards notice the modifications which these characters
present in different situations. I shall begin with the most simple and
elementary structures, such as the serous, the cellular, and the mucous
membranes, and proceeding to the more complicated, shall subsequently
take up the consideration of the derangement of particular viscera such
as the spleen, the kidneys, and perhaps the lungs; unless, as will probably
be the case, I shall deem it more expedient to speak of these last in conjunction with the mucous membranes with which they are most naturally
and intimately connected. . . .[31]

In the next lecture he fulminated against Broussaisism, the "*soi-
disant* physiological doctrine" whose disciples "will see nothing
but inflammation, and see inflammation everywhere."[32] Despite
his annoyance over the inconstancy of the student market for his
morbid anatomy lectures, and despite the more general antipathy
he felt toward the Broussaisist heresy (contracted no doubt from

his French mentor) Hodgkin continued nonetheless throughout the early years of the decade to develop his system of morbid anatomy. He did so concretely through the Museum, which he catalogued extensively. He did so theoretically by means of his consistent emphasis on the serous and mucous membranes, a formulation that he developed further between 1827 and 1840, placing him squarely in the Paris tradition of Bichat and Laennec.[33]

In 1836, both in his lecture series and in print, Hodgkin commented explicitly on the continued resilience and the persistent utility of the French model of membrane pathology. Early that year he published the first of his magisterial two volumes on the *Morbid Anatomy of the Serous and Mucous Membranes*.[34] The first volume, dealing with the serosal tissues, was well-received by the medical journals;[35] in its preface Hodgkin explained his choice of focus:

Although, in different seasons, some other subjects have been taken up [in my lectures], I have invariably found that the important objects first enumerated [i.e., the serous membranes] have unavoidably occupied the best part of the course. I have therefore felt disposed to yield to the suggestion of some of my friends, who have been led . . . to recommend the publication of the Lectures.[36]

Hodgkin then proceeded to give, in the first lecture, perhaps the most articulate expression yet voiced of the difference between morbid anatomy as pathology and as special, meaning local surgical, anatomy. In a critically important section headed by the marginal notation, "good special anatomists not necessarily Pathologists," Hodgkin explained that "the special anatomist may give us a minute account of the wound or to throw light on very many of the effects of disease. . . . The changes which disease effects . . . may be regarded as experiments in animal chemistry, performed by nature herself; . . . with this view, morbid appearances, which may be regarded as trivial, either in themselves, or from their being situated in parts of little moment, as regards treatment, sometimes acquire a new and important interest."[37]

Hodgkin now surveyed the history of pathology from the standpoint of the emergence, only lately become clearly visible, of general anatomy – the global, organismal pathology of textures and tissues whose outlines "were faintly sketched by Dr. Carmichael Smyth." He added immediately, however, that Bayle, Pinel, and, especially, Bichat and Laennec deserved "the higher praise" for developing the subject to its fullest extent.[38]

But why select, in particular, the serous and mucous membranes for closest scrutiny? This question, Hodgkin knew, lay at the heart of the matter, just as these tissues were collectively the pivot of his articulation – indeed, of any fully explanatory articulation – of the French model. The answer, as before, lay in the notion that, when he sought to use anatomical substrates to teach not about regional anatomy but about *disease,* "I shall bring under your notice the morbid alterations of certain pervading tissues which present the same characteristics throughout the entire organismus, although they enter into relations with organs widely distinct in function and locality."[39] In the serous and mucous tissues in particular, the overwhelming frequency of disease in them and their "very general distribution throughout the economy" made them ideal to this purpose.[40]

He continued, in his second lecture of this series on the serous membranes:

Nature seems to delight in the production of reflected membranes – a form which many of the serous membranes present. We not only have them in the more familiar examples, the arachnoid, the pleura, the pericardium, the peritoneum, and the tunica vaginalis, but they are also seen in the eye, in the pulps by which the teeth are formed, in the synovial capsules, which are slight modifications of the serous membranes, and, as I shall hereafter more fully explain to you, in very many adventitious formations.[41]

He further noted that these tissues were among the earliest to declare themselves during embryological development, and, most important of all, "the large extent of surface presented by some of these membranes affords the best opportunity for observing the varieties in the modes of inflammation, in the products to which they give rise, and in the stages through which they pass."[42] He concluded this lecture, a general overview of this class of animal textures, with an enumeration of characteristic properties well known within the Bichat–Laennec tradition: Of particular importance were pathological changes referable to vascularity, innervation, convertibility into mucous membranes, excess of secretion, inflammatory tendencies, false membrane formation, and effusion.[43]

In the new version of these lectures that he prepared for the medical students in 1836, Hodgkin alluded again to the reason for their publication and the importance of that event:

> The great facilities afforded by the serous membranes for exhibiting and explaining the phenomena of morbid changes have hitherto induced me to commence my course by treating of them. I have therefore repeatedly gone over this ground, and the time which they have occupied has prevented my treating of several other subjects of great interest and importance. I am this year relieved from the necessity of taking up the serous membranes by my having printed [published] those lectures which relate to them, to parasitical animals, and to that class of adventitious structures which possess the type of adventitious serous membranes. . . . I would advise such of you as propose to attend my present course, to make yourselves acquainted with them, as without this step some of my observations and views must be but imperfectly intelligible.[44]

Doubtless the notion of projecting the image of a "professional pathologist" was the furthest thing from Hodgkin's mind. As yet the notion hardly conveyed any real concrete meaning, absent the disciplinary trappings that the field would take on in ensuing decades. Rather, he sought to project a form of pathological anatomy as a tool of the clinician's trade, but a tool of sufficient versatility, of sufficiently global application to nosology and pathophysiology, that its use would spread to every stratum of the profession. In the introductory lecture of 1836, bordering on the key question of "fit" between the profession's social and cognitive resources – How do surgeons and medical men develop appropriate funds of knowledge? – he made the point explicit:

> Although I strongly recommend to you the study of pathological anatomy as the very cornerstone upon which alone the fabric of sound medical and chirurgical knowledge can be raised and desire to impress you with the importance of becoming practically acquainted with the fenomena [sic] which it presents, and, as far as our present state of knowledge admits, to understand their mutual relations to each other, yet I am far from recommending you to seek these acquirements to the neglect of other objects no less important. London has long been justly distinguished for a succession of Surgeons of the highest order, and I believe that that circumstance has had a powerful influence on those who have sought their medical education in this city. It has inspired them with zeal and perseverance in the acquisition of those branches of their education which

are most conspicuously essential to the Surgeon, whilst there was often a lamentable deficiency with respect to many others. I confess that I am not so devoted an admirer of the past as to shut my eyes to the manifest improvement which has already been made in the course generally pursued by the students of the London medical schools.[45]

Finally, Hodgkin identified one of the critical elements of the social system of medicine that, between 1815 and 1834, had been changing shape most rapidly.

The improvement to which I alluded has consisted in the effort which has been made to raise other departments to a proportionate and true relative degree of importance, the effect of which has been to render the body of medical students not only more generally informed but more constantly industrious, and therefore I trust less dissipated than formerly – a change no less happy for themselves than satisfactory to their friends and advantageous to the public. This improvement, which I trust is still progressive is, I believe, very much to be attributed to the improved regulations and increased zeal of the Apothecaries' Company. . . .[46]

Two aspects of Hodgkin's clinical outlook as a physician deserve further emphasis, as a way of understanding and explaining his focus on the general and pathological anatomy of the tissues. The first feature of his approach that provides such a clue relates to his discussion of effusions. The exudation – today one would say exudation and transudation – of fluids, into cavities created by membranes that "Nature dearly loved to reflect," was an occurrence observed every day in every hospital physician's or surgeon's practice. Bellies filled up with ascitic fluid, distending the abdomen, compromising patients' digestion, impeding their breathing by pushing up the leaves of the diaphragm. Chests filled with pleural fluid, preventing expansion of the lungs.

In England as in France, the physiological interface between bodily solids and fluids was not merely a theoretical construct separating two dogmas – medically-oriented humoralism and surgically-oriented solidism – but a clinical reality with considerable impact on the course of patients' illnesses.[47] The pathology of serous effusions was thus the most direct link between theory and observation, binding together the pathological anatomy of the solid and the fluid elements of the body, and yoking speculative questions about pathological theory to practical clinical questions of management.[48]

Hodgkin saw, as had the French, the importance in this scheme of the technique of paracentesis, the procedure by which fluid was drawn off through a hollow trochar inserted through the skin into the affected cavity.[49] Paracentesis could be, as Hodgkin was well aware, a life-saving maneuver when the serosal cavities involved were, in turn, anatomically constrained within other, largely fixed or immobile spaces. Paramount among such potential catastrophes were galloping empyema or hydrothorax involving the pleura and compressing the air-expanded lung parenchyma, and tamponade of the heart as the result of hydropericardium or pyopericardium.[50]

Similarly, though usually more slowly, effusions into the peritoneal cavity, both infectious and noninfectious, could distend the belly to the point that respiratory, absorptive, or bowel function was compromised. Dramatic relief could be afforded patients by surgeons and physicians who dared invade body cavities with the paracentesis needle, knowingly risking sepsis. But the knowledge required, discussed in the Guy's Hospital Physical Society, was based as soundly in medicine as it was in surgery. In the first place, the trochar's point of entry into the cavity might be at a considerable distance from either the predominant source of symptoms or the local affection that constituted the original insult. Such an insult may have initiated a "sympathetic" reaction elsewhere in the affected, fluid-filled body cavity or, indeed, in an altogether different cavity in which yet another fluid accumulation might occur.[51]

In paracentesis, another reason why both the technique's rationale and its effects bridged the traditional English scission between surgery and medicine was the potential for shock.[52] Clinicians were keenly aware that patients with dropsy or serous effusions could rapidly lose consciousness if the excessive amounts of fluid present in their serosal cavities were too rapidly evacuated. Great care had to be taken to preserve the entire "body Economy" in such situations, and not merely to protect the often concurrent local site of injury.[53] Thus of renewed importance was an old, eighteenth-century (or older) notion: the metaphor of the body economy.

Finally, the physician's use of the economic metaphor was a highly appropriate image for a certain therapeutic style that Hodgkin shared with other environmentalists and meliorists: the use of "airs, waters, and places" – baths and salutary physical conditions – to intervene in a variety of such disorders.[54] The metaphor of the body economy was another way of thinking about morbid occurrences that related observed (or prescribed) alterations of the patient's environment to changes in the fine structure of the body. In this way one might tie together the meliorist approaches of environmental medicine with the impulse, in an anatomical age, to atomize – to *anatomize*. Like many of his contemporaries, Hodgkin exhibited both impulses, meliorist and atomistic. A belief in the body economy, coupled with a commitment to the tissue pathology articulated in the *Serous and Mucous Membranes,* represented a strategy for keeping the two sorts of impulse consistent.

HODGKIN LEAVES GUY'S HOSPITAL

In the summer of 1837 Hodgkin became embroiled in an episode that has been cited ever since as a classic case of the blocked career, and of bureaucratic meddling tainted by favoritism. It has also been cited as a classic illustration of the persistence of lay control in early Victorian medicine: The Guy's Hospital treasurer, Benjamin Harrison, was clearly the source of Hodgkins troubles.[55] When the physician, James Cholmeley, died and Thomas Addison was nominated to succeed him in the post of Physician, the Assistant Physicianship was freed for new candidates. The by now well-published and acclaimed Hodgkin was considered a worthy candidate, but so too was his well-placed, if somewhat less scientifically accomplished rival, Benjamin G. Babington.[56] Despite an intensive (and, to the self-effacing Hodgkin, exceedingly embarrassing) lobbying effort by Hodgkin's family and friends, a General Court of the Guy's officers and governors appointed Babington to the Assistant Physician position on 6 September 1837.

It should be recalled that Hodgkin, already curator of the museum of morbid specimens, was not angling for a position in pathological anatomy. A professorship and department of pathological anatomy would not be created at Guy's until the twentieth century.[57] Hodgkin was seeking, rather, to move into a clinical post from which he might derive the student-paid emoluments that routinely accrued in such a post. One might argue that Hodgkin, even had he succeeded in securing the post, had already burned his bridges. He had, after all, already resigned the curatorship to set his candidacy forth as starkly and credibly as possible. He had already chosen to divert his career from pathological anatomy. Hence Hodgkin's midcareer crisis might seem to have little to do with his pathological anatomy program.

But the opposite case can be equally made. Though the 1837 episode had little bearing on the content of his tissue pathology, it had much to do with the broader question of Hodgkin's attempt to instill part of a new scientific culture, with which pathological anatomy was mutually constitutive, in the Guy's Hospital milieu. It is reasonable to suppose that if in the 1830s the graft would not "take" in the most receptive of the old line hospital medical schools – Guy's with its Physical Society and its emphasis on the publication of carefully culled case reports – then it was all the more unlikely to take in the others.

That this has not been the commonly accepted view owes to a perception of Hodgkin and of the 1837 episode as atypical. His failure to gain the post then becomes the unfortunate interaction of two strong, eccentric personalities. The episode becomes an anomaly with little bearing on the culture of British medicine in the mid-1830s. Some elements of the account will probably remain unquestionably idiosyncratic, with little bearing on the content or context of Hodgkin's work. But recent interpretations of the process of medical professionalization in Victorian London, of the role of Quakers in the culture of medical science in general, and of the particular role of this particular Quaker in this particular episode, all suggest that the analysis is more complex.

A birthright Quaker in the traditional style, Hodgkin was a severe man who "thee'd" and "thou'd" his betters and lessers, a meliorist who joined cause with any number of social reform movements. Who could take seriously, ask proponents of the received wisdom, a man who drove around with a half-naked American Indian in his hansom carriage?[58] Thus it was hardly unexpected when the remarkably powerful lay Treasurer of the hospital, Benjamin Harrison, either on a personal whim or in concert with the Governors of the institution, responding in either case to the bizarre behavior of this most peculiar individual, wielded the hatchet.

But Harrison's antipathy toward Hodgkin was neither a litmus of general sentiment nor merely the expression of some stylistic eccentricity or personal animus.[59] Rather, the animosity grew out of Harrison's aversion to Hodgkin's meliorism, triggered by a series of events between 1833 and 1836. Harrison was one of the seven members of the influential Committee of the Hudson's Bay Company. Hodgkin's meliorism already extended to the status of the aborigines of North America.[60] His entreaties to Harrison to use his influence to change the Company's policies in the interest of the Indians' welfare were to no avail. Indeed, Hodgkin's supplicant posture, full of sincerity and righteousness, backfired badly when Harrison expressed intense annoyance. The relationship continued to sour and Harrison was henceforth an uncompromising foe. Hodgkin's 1837 reversal, and his move later on to St. Thomas's, where he published on the pathology of mucous membranes, seemed almost foreordained from 1833 onward.

In the mid-1830s Hodgkin's meliorism further expanded into a number of different channels. He corresponded at length with John Herschel, both before and during the latter's long sojourn at the Cape of Good Hope in Southern Africa, on the welfare and the ethnological niceties of that region's "native race."[61] He had become deeply interested in education as process: He was simultaneously and equally involved in addressing the mistreatment of Cape aborigines, the improvement of the English system of educating physicians, and the education of the British masses in the "means of promoting and preserving health."[62]

As early as the late 1820s Hodgkin had begun lecturing, in Spitalfields, to the local Mechanics' Institute on the preservation of the public health through temperance, moral management, environmental salubrity, and the education of the nation's youth and honest workingmen.[63] With J. J. Lister and other members of his Quaker circle he lobbied for the establishment of two institutional experiments, one that failed and another that succeeded. The first was the Southern Retreat, an attempt ca. 1839 to bring the principles of the Tukes' York Retreat, favoring the moral treatment of the insane, to the south of England. The second, begun some ten years earlier, was the University of London. From 1836 on, Hodgkin was an active and vocal member of its Senate.

For Hodgkin the meliorist, then, medical education, health education, and health care reform were to pathological anatomy as form was to content. The several elements of his meliorist stance – improvement of the lower orders, of the air and light of London or Calcutta, or of medical studies – were parts of an important, larger configuration of interests that he shared with many other marginal and provincial medical men. Whatever the personal and idiosyncratic reasons for his failure to advance at Guy's Hospital, Hodgkin's pathological anatomy was just as much a part of a growing activist attitude regarding social and scientific change as was his ethnology. He was part of a new scientific culture that both provided social roots for his ideas on pathological anatomy and medical education, and at the same time relied on those ideas as resources.

Hodgkin's championship of pathological anatomy is but one example of a range of technical and theoretical resources that were available – if sometimes, like Hodgkin's tissue pathology, not very successful – for reform-minded medical men in the rapidly changing 1820s and 1830s. One might equally point, for example, to some practitioners' attempts to get cholera patients during the 1832 outbreak admitted to hospital for intravenous saline injections.[64] Such attempts also foundered, but in doing so again illustrated broader cultural and professional tensions between conservative practice and risky reform. Viewed in this way, Hodgkin's approach to clinical medicine and the new morbid anatomy, to the extent that they were linked with a much larger system of beliefs, reflect a broad set of tensions within the medical profession in the second quarter of the nineteenth century. It is hence in the new culture of reform and scientific change that one finds the most appropriate context within which to locate and understand Hodgkin's pathology and indeed his whole career.

LONDON UNIVERSITY

The University of London and its founders also sought to embody the new culture of science, and of science in medicine. But it was a far remove from Guy's Hospital. In his interests, Thomas Hodgkin in fact more closely resembled the early stalwarts of the University of London than he did most of his peers at Guy's. Edinburgh-educated Englishmen, Quakers and other Dissenters, even the occasional Jew – the fathers and sons of the new "middle rich": these were its leaders, with names like Henry Brougham, Charles Bell, George Birkbeck, John Conolly – and Thomas Hodgkin.[65]

In the early 1820s a number of early educational reformers, including the figures just mentioned, met frequently in private to discuss the redesign of higher education in England. Beginning in July of 1825, their private gatherings led to public meetings to discuss a plan for an institution combining medicine, law, and arts education. The Duke of Sussex laid a cornerstone in Gower Street, Bloomsbury, for what is now University College London in April, 1827. On the first of October 1828 Charles Bell, Professor of Surgery and Physiology, gave the inaugural lecture opening London University.

Leonard Horner, F.R.S., was named Warden of the University in May 1827, and with the help of Council and friends, set about finding suitable faculty. As early as July 1827 a published Statement of Aims listed some tentative faculty appointments. Among the names in various areas of clinical medicine were Bell, Granville Sharp Pattison, John Conolly, and Anthony Todd. Along with Pattison and Bell, in one of the chairs of "surgery, anatomy, and physiology" appeared the name of Johannes Meckel of Halle.[66] The highly regarded German pathologist was their initial choice, but by December he was to write asking to delay his arrival. The Council, sensing irresolution, determined to press him for a final answer to their invitation. In the same meeting of 22 December a letter of interest from Robert Carswell, a Scottish artist–physician well known to Andrew Duncan and John Thomson of Edinburgh and now residing in Paris, was referred to the Education Committee pending Meckel's decision.[67]

CARSWELL IN PARIS

Robert Carswell was, as a colleague was to recalled years later, "a man of singularly unobtrusive and retiring disposition with a soft voice [and] a melancholy expression of countenance."[68] He exhibited almost an artist's sensitivity to his work, and preferred the deadhouse to the lecture platform and the sickbed. He had been in Paris off and on since the 1821–1822 term, attending and performing dissections at virtually every one of the major teaching hospitals.[69] Throughout, he studiously engaged himself in the preparation of what he called his "Coloured Delineations." As pictures, Carswell's representations appeared to lean to the localistic, macroscopic tradition of Jean Cruveilhier in France or the Hunters and their followers in England more than they did the more theoretical and less representational Bichatian mode.[70] But his descriptive notes on the cases he rendered amply reveal the influence of Laennec and the *pathologie tissulaire* of the French tradition.[71]

On December 21, 1827, hearing of a post to be made available at the professional level at the newly established institution in Bloomsbury (whether his informant was Hodgkin or someone else in the continuous stream of Englishmen entering Paris is not revealed) Carswell wrote a letter to Horner and the University Council, detailing his own program for the development of a pathological anatomy chair. It was this letter that the Council sent to Committee while they waited for Meckel to make up his mind. He proposed to create a Museum consisting of his own delineations, "together with diseased organs preserved in spirits, and accurate histories of each individual case."[72] A course of lectures on pathological anatomy would be built around this ensemble, with an eye to eventual publication.

But to round out this project and the collection it was based on, he averred, two further years in Paris were required, during which time "any connexion which I might form with the University could only be nominal." In the meantime, however, he could send materials to London. For these services and the eventual deposit of the materials with the University he requested a subvention of £300–400 per annum, reserving to himself only publication rights. The final condition was not only the museum curatorship but the role of Professor of Pathological Anatomy.[73]

The minutes of Council indicate that Carswell's proposition moved along rapidly in the winter of 1828. In March Carswell was invited to come from Paris to interview after a number of "eminent professional men" gave testimony to his acumen. On March 25 the Education Committee recommended to Council that they appoint Carswell to the chair, stipulating tight arrangements for acquiring the delineations – purchase at £1.48 each – and pathological preparations. In the same meeting the question of responsibility for the institution's dissecting rooms, an innovation by their very existence and centrality, also arose: J. R. Bennett, lately the cat's-paw in Anglo–French anatomical politics, was named as one of the two ideal candidates. Four weeks later the

Council appointed Carswell and Bennett.[74] Carswell immediately
responded, accepting with pleasure, expressing the "hope that I
will be able to justify the choice you have made . . . and that I
will also be enabled to . . . ultimately contribute to the general
prosperity of the University," and promising "redoubled zeal" in
his efforts.[75]

Bennett would be dead and gone before Carswell had the opportunity to establish himself at the University, for the roster of
classes in the College Record Office discloses no instruction in
pathological anatomy for 1828–1829, 1829–1830, or 1830–1831.
For nearly three years Carswell remained abroad working on his
delineations. He kept up a steady stream of chatter by correspondence, writing Horner in June that he was discovering good material. He anticipated over one hundred delineations within three
months. Bennett's appointment pleased him especially, Carswell
wrote, and he hoped to see the beleaguered anatomist in Paris.[76]
A month later he reported a total of 93 delineations and about 50
wet preparations to date.[77]

Documents generated on both sides of the Channel disclose little
programmatic content for the academic years 1828–1829 or 1829–
1830, other than a certain testiness between Faculty and Council
concerning Carswell's appointment – no doubt reflecting in part
the former's reaction to the small subvention being supplied Carswell as part of his agreement with Council.[78] Carswell's letters
dwindled to entreaties in the main for more time and more money.[79] One of those letters, however, written in mid-spring, 1830,
articulated clearly his views on the role of pathological anatomy
in medical education:

I am disposed to make many sacrifices to secure, if possible, the success
of this branch of medicine. I was well aware at the time I engaged with
the University that attendance on a Course of Lectures on Pathological
Anatomy is not required of the Student in order that he may obtain a
License to practice medicine or Surgery, and that therefore I could not
expect to derive much emolument as a teacher at the commencement.
But I have good grounds for believing that this obstacle will not exist
long; and even should it, you have it in your power to render it ineffectual
by a very simple process, and of securing at the same time the advantages
of such a course to the Medical Student. The study of Pathological anatomy has become too general to be considered as not constituting an essential part of a medical education – the objects which it embraces, too

numerous and too important not to demand the special consideration of the Pathologist. Such is the opinion of medical men in general, and of those in particular who have acquired the greatest share of public favour.[80]

Carswell continued in a manner that bore the hallmark of an agenda for professionalizing medical science: the confounding of career goals and a cognitive program.

[A]nd therefore I feel persuaded, that my time has been and will be well employed, and that the efforts which the Council have made or may still make to promote this branch of medical Science, will give to it an impulse which it has not, hitherto, received in England, and which, if properly directed, cannot fail to give to it the rank which it ought to hold in Medicine and Surgery. The cooperation of the medical Professors of the University will no doubt contribute much to the accomplishment of this object, and it is very agreeable to me to know that they have expressed themselves to this effect. In the meantime, I must repeat, that the principal element of success lies with myself – It is by means of a sufficient number and a good choice of delineations that I can hope to simplify the study and communicate a knowledge of the material conditions of diseases, and thereby obtain the attendance of students on my lectures.[81]

In the spring and summer of 1831, with his return imminent, Carswell began filling in the details. He reconfirmed his intention to give a lecture course.[82] Several weeks later, in mid-June, Carswell was proposed as physician to the Dispensary – later North London Hospital and still later University College Hospital – the Council resolving "that the Warden ask Dr. Carswell whether he will undertake the duties of one of the Physicians of the Dispensary."[83]

At the end of May, 1831, Carswell arrived in London and wrote Horner announcing his intentions to begin his course using the 900 to 1000 delineations that he now had in hand. The lectures would, he noted, cover

the History and Description of all those perceptible modifications of organization which constitute either a deviation from the normal type of organs, or a real state of disease. They will constitute a great part of what is called the theory of Medicine or the whole of the theory of Organic Diseases, in as much as the Pathologist, in order to determine the Seat of Nature of these diseases – which, indeed, is the principal object of his researches, requires, besides teaching the Student how to know each diseased state, product, or formation in particular, to point out to him all those conditions of Structure, and function, whether healthy or morbid, under the immediate influence of which they are produced.[84]

ROBERT CARSWELL AND PATHOLOGICAL ANATOMY AT THE UNIVERSITY OF LONDON

Beginning in the first regular term of 1831 Carswell set out on an experiment to institutionalize pathological anatomy on a par with other teaching subjects; he was soon beset with problems. His difficulties fell into two main categories. The first grew out of what would, over the next century, become a classic defining tension in medical education: the tension between bedside and bench.[85] Here was one of the earliest examples of this perennial tug in physicians' minds and careers: but for Carswell, unlike some of his intellectual progeny, the problem was rooted, at least partly, in straightforward financial concerns. One simply could not finance a salary out of museum-keeping the way one could with a practice, hence his nomination to the dispensary staff. (One of the graver ironies of Carswell's ten-year career at the University was the fact that a fully financed and staffed affiliated hospital, capable of supporting a pathological anatomist in both ways – at bedside and bench – did not open its doors until halfway through his decade in London.) The tension was also based on issues of professional control and access to resources, such as the specimens Carswell sought and could only partially attain.[86]

The other main difficulty Carswell faced related to the necessity of locating a market among the students for the sort of global, histopathological system that he stressed in lectures on "the various morbid conditions of the body, . . . the changes they undergo. . . ; their termination and cure [as well as] those modifications which they present in the different tissues, systems and organs in which they are found. . . ."[87] But those who heard him lecture on pathological change remembered his exposition as interesting and instructive, presented without oratorical flourish but with the keen attention to detail determined by his Paris experience and the "delineations" that enshrined it.[88]

It appears that Carswell did not arrange to get his course under way until the 1832–1833 winter term.[89] As soon as he did so his agenda for developing pathological anatomy, clearly stated in his

Table 9.1. *Enrollments, by faculty, in University of London, 1829–1839*

Subject	Year				
	1829	1832	1833	1838	1839
Medicine	165	232	283	470	474
Arts	269	168[a]	148[a]	137	146
Law	123			n.a.	n.a.

[a]Combined arts and law.
Data given for all years in which specific figures are supplied in
University of London *Annual Reports*, 1829–1839.

early correspondence with Horner, ran afoul of the larger medical
education reform program enunciated by Charles Bell and other
participants in the 1834 Parliamentary Select Committee on Medical Education. It is in this context, and that of medical education's
special role in London University, that Carswell's efforts must be
understood.

A glance at Table 9.1 reveals enrollments within each faculty
during the 1830s at the institution. It is clear that the medical faculty
was no mere appendage but, in fact, the institution's backbone.
During the course of the decade the ratio between medicine and
arts students increased, for example, from about 3:2 to more than
3:1, with student ticket fees increasing accordingly: By 1839 receipts were £6444.10.0 for the Faculty of Medicine *versus* £2278.12.3
for the Faculty of Arts.[90] The asymmetry was, in fact, a cause for
considerable alarm among the general faculty: As early as 1833 a
group of them could write, in an unsigned letter on the "present
crisis of affairs of the University," of their belief that literature
and general science classes could still catch up with their medical
counterparts, and that "the whole University will participate in
the advantages which will accrue from the reputation which it is
rapidly acquiring as a Medical School."[91]

Hence a well-placed course in the medical curriculum at London
University would have enjoyed an "amplifier effect," in terms of
its content, much as a well-placed scientific article would have had
in a medical journal in the decades immediately preceding. This
is precisely what occurred with respect to some other branches of
anatomical instruction, as displayed in Table 9.2. It is clear, how-

Table 9.2. *Enrollments, by subject, in University of London Faculty of Medicine, 1833–1839*

Subject	Year						
	1833	1834	1835	1836	1837	1838	1839
Anatomy	203	204	260	321	338	367	371
Practical Anatomy	187	138	257	326	354	374	384
Morbid Anatomy	9	11	13	18	36ᵃ	31ᵃ	—
Practice of Medicine	122	167	196	202	207	206	210
Comparative Anatomy & Zoology	25	13	26	34	49	30	26
Medical Jurisprudence	19	38	44	33	19	70*	57*

ᵃSummer session.
From University of London *Annual Reports*, 1829–1839.

ever, from the same data that pathological anatomy had virtually no role in bringing about the new state of affairs in which medical education as a whole, as well as certain of its constituent subjects, played an increasingly dominant role in the institution.[92]

What befell Carswell, essentially, was a case of relative deprivation. Any opportunity he might have found to enhance his own position, based on the growing place of medicine within the University overall, was outweighed by others' agendas. The teaching of pathological anatomy, in order to accommodate disproportionately expanding courses like practical anatomy, had to be progressively written down. In 1833–1834, during the most vigorous ferment over curriculum changes, Charles Bell was recommending the extension of curriculum beyond the fifteen months demanded by the Royal College of Surgeons in its latest set of requirements.[93] After the Anatomy Act the normal anatomy subjects taught by G. S. Patterson and perhaps others at London University were increasingly becoming the scientific funnel through which one needed to pass in the process of certification. Few students took more than the core of courses required for the surgeons' or the apothecaries' examinations. Pathological anatomy was conspicuously absent from those requirements. By 1836 the morbid anatomy course, as the *Annual Report* for that year noted, had had to be moved to the precarious status of a summer course "by the new regulations of the Apothecaries' Company."[94]

Table 9.3. *Receipts for medical courses in University of London, 1832–1833*

	Year			
Subject	1832–33	1833–34	1834–35	1835–36
Morbid Anatomy	£32	£32[a]	£36	£54[b]
Normal Anatomy	£766	£1067.10.0	£1054.16.8	£1270.6.8
Materia Medica	£528	£699	£640	£789
Comparative Anatomy & Zoology	£37	£90	£93	—[c]

[a]"Carried forward."
[b]Summer term.
[c]Receipts for Practical Anatomy (formerly "Demonstrations") = £1235.6.8 in 1835–1836. From University of London *Annual Reports*, 1829–1839.

The results of the course shifts in the mid-1830s may be discerned graphically in the receipts of the respective courses (Table 9.3). With his course drawing even fewer students and smaller fees than the other summer course, medical jurisprudence, Carswell was compelled to deflect his energies partly elsewhere – into clinical work and into the curatorship of the museum of normal anatomy.[95]

The erosive effect of competition with other courses on pathological anatomy at University College, especially the competition with the normal and practical anatomy courses, was exactly the reverse of the amplifier effect discussed earlier. A well-known phenomenon (the "Matthew effect") among sociologists of science,[96] this effect made for an ironic turn of events for Carswell. In Paris, where he had learned most of what he knew on the subject, pathological anatomy before 1835 had not been dependent for its support on the elaboration of a distinct disciplinary identity. Indeed, the fact that it had been in a fluid state and not cleanly separated from either anatomy or the clinic had served it well.

But Carswell, spreading his efforts too thinly, could find no single secure mooring for his career: not the deadhouse, not either of the two museums, not the lecture-room, and not his private practice. With the help of Sir James Clark he obtained the rather undemanding post of personal physician to the king of Brussels. He left London in 1840 and remained in Belgium, his own health slowly fading, until his death in 1857.[97] In 1837 he published his delineations, marking, according to one observer, the "highest

point which the science of morbid anatomy had reached before
the introduction of the microscope."[98]

Carswell's concerns with respect to both his science and his career
in pathological anatomy were nevertheless those of a new professional culture. Those concerns, pertaining as they did mainly to
the development of a rigorous curriculum, and to his efforts to
establish means of support for himself and for a body of knowledge
and teaching, were less tightly linked to the general scientific culture in which Thomas Hodgkin remained an active participant.
His inability to stay the course makes the experiment no less interesting, however, especially since pathology would again display
a sort of cyclical pattern of vogue and decline later in the century.[99]
Eight years after Carswell's death, Richard Quain, the successor
to J. R. Bennett in the chair of practical anatomy, viewed the ap-
propriation of French skills and ideas into the English idiom, and
shed more light than anyone could (in the event) on the context
of that effort:

The young physician found in Paris much to learn, especially in diagnosis
of disease, and morbid anatomy. Percussion, Auenbrugger's discovery,
was then adopted by us from France; and Laennec was busy teaching his
great method of Auscultation. The very careful examination of bodies,
in order to verify diagnosis, was another characteristic of the Parisian
hospitals. . . .

It must be admitted, however, that the condition of things in the
schools, I mean the teaching places of Paris and London, was at that time
very different, as regards the completeness of their organization. But
while the fact is admitted, it should not be forgotten how that everything
here was the work of single persons, unaided by the Government, or by
the Public; while all in France was provided by the State.[100]

Conclusion: A language of morbid appearances

I have tried in this account to provide evidence for the proposition that ideas spread unevenly. Medical traditions are influenced by chance and by context. How, for example, can one account for the differential reception of Bichatian pathology in France and England? And how did pathological anatomy become entrenched in different degrees and ways in different parts of Napoleonic Europe? Various explanations suggest themselves. Perhaps, for example, the science of pathology took different turns on opposite shores of the channel because the material biological reality itself differed between London and Paris.

According to this explanation, patterns of disease would offer sufficiently disparate stimulus to the medical imagination to create ultimately quite different explanatory frameworks. Tissue pathology, for example, might have emerged where there was an isolated superabundance of disease of the serous and mucous membranes, a state of affairs known to exist in the Paris of 1800. Or the new laboratory discipline of toxicology and its sibling, experimental physiology, might have emerged where there was a conspicuous excess of poisoning and newly discovered poisonous materials.[1] This sort of material argument, though attractive, fails finally to persuade. There is too little evidence to suggest that patterns of morbidity and mortality varied significantly between Paris and the urban and military concentrations in Britain or elsewhere. And there is at least a modicum of evidence, both textual and epidemiological, that the contrary may have been true.

A different sort of explanation of historical change would be near-randomness, for the truth is that many events result from circumstances that are contingent and indeterminate, when not entirely unaccountable. Examining the problem at a higher level of magnification, one might thus ask how a single text like Laennec's could look so different and be appropriated in such a different manner in each of the two contexts. How "determined" can such a change have been? Evolution offers an analogy. Not every differentiation, not every added characteristic of an organism in a given habitat can be shown to have evolved because of the selective advantage it confers. An element of caprice intrudes. Historical change, including that occurring in scientific medicine, need not always satisfy functionalist canons of explanation.[2] Thus one might quite nihilistically suppose that Théophile Laennec's *magnum opus* was shorn of most of its pathological anatomy for reasons of local fashion almost randomly applied.

Yet this begs the question. In the complex skein of historical change, few events are so random or unrelated that one cannot infer certain conditions of change. There must be some sort of residue of causal relations between events and their antecedents. Hence a third sort of explanation for the uneven spread of Bichatian pathological anatomy is that two different professional cultures fostered two quite different pictures of the body and its morbid appearances.

It is not sufficient, however, to focus on context without balancing it with an understanding of content. Sometimes it may help, after all, if the ideas themselves are good ones. Pathological anatomy was a good idea. Its novel features were intrinsically positive ones. Otherwise there would have been no issue surrounding an idea's differential success. Of course, neither novelty nor goodness has much to do, it turns out, with an idea's ultimate origin. Recent scholarship has indeed shown that tissue pathology did not even originate, necessarily, with Bichat or anyone else in the French circles preceding and succeeding his brief career.

Perhaps, rather, the meaningful moment is that point at which the new system begins to reach a receptive audience, to find staunch and forceful champions. This view makes possible a clearer grasp of the importance of Xavier Bichat's contributions, given that the young physician–anatomist's ideas, and hence his career, found little immediate success in the main stream of French medical culture. What Xavier Bichat, the Mozart of medicine, and after him Bayle and Laennec, offered was an alternative scheme for thinking about the body and its morbid appearances. They created a new landscape of disease. It was a landscape derived, perhaps, from native French elements, or perhaps from elements found elsewhere.

In either case it proved in time to be particularly consonant with the new professional realities of Napoleonic France.

Two different sets of determinants then shaped the evolutionary fate of the new scheme of pathological anatomy. The first, undoubtedly, was irreducibly physiological, harking back to the issue of the goodness of ideas and their continued "truth value." If tissue pathology had not successfully explained and predicted certain disease outcomes in individual cases, and if it had not lent itself to a fruitful fusion with physical diagnosis, then no amount of cultural bias would have insured its continued longevity. The new landscape of pathology did, in fact, provide a lucid guide for physicians to explain the course of disease and to predict its outcomes. Yet even so, it met with greater success in France than in England. The disparity suggests a second set of factors important in shaping the fate of pathological anatomy, namely the evolution of the profession and its institutions. Specifically, the continued separation of medicine and surgery in Britain did not select in the same way for ideas already popular across the Channel.

To be viable, a model for understanding the reception of ideas must account for both their flux across national or cultural boundaries, and the differential fate they may meet once put in place in the new setting. The two processes, the translocation and the implantation of ideas, are related but distinct. The move abroad is characterized by its own peculiar dynamic, involving the unique experiences of individuals who are exposed to new ideas in an alien setting. Such was the case with the "Gallomaniacs" who trooped onto the shores of Brittany and Normandy after 1815. Those expatriates, men like Robert Carswell and the ill-starred James Bennett, were first-line translators who began the work of processing foreign knowledge for home consumption.

A second wave of translators might be termed the domesticators. They took pains to adapt and, where necessary, to bowdlerize the foreign tradition in such a way as to insure its fit with the norms and customs of the local intellectual marketplace. One style of domestication, exemplified in my discussion by John Farre, emphasized the indigenousness of ideas and techniques claimed to be new and superior. Another style, perhaps typified by Thomas Hodgkin, was characterized by invidious comparisons to the superior lot enjoyed by those just beyond one's own shores. In the case of pathological anatomy the purest example of the domesticator might, ironically, be the very individual who discarded much of Laennec's tissue pathology, John Forbes. Forbes, in essence, domesticated a dog until it became a cat.

    ★   ★   ★   ★   ★

As one commentator has noted recently, there is a peculiar disjunction in the historiography of modern medicine. Historians of medicine and of health care "from the bottom up" derive their analyses from discussions of Latin countries, as might be expected given the French origins of the *Annales* approach. Historians of the professions meanwhile emphasize Anglo-American traditions.[3] But the benchmarks of actual historical change in the professions happen to have differed markedly between continental Europe, Britain, and English-speaking America. Between 1800 and the present, at the same time, the clinical medical communities of each western nation saw profound scientific shifts, while assimilating theoretical and technical innovations in a variety of ways. That assimilation occurred in waves, the first and in some ways the most important occurring in the Napoleonic era when medical men adopted a new language of the body and its morbid appearances.

To conceptualize the interrelationships of these waves of professional and scientific change requires a comparative analysis of medical discourse. Physicians, surgeons, and apothecaries functioned as might tribes or subcultures, each with its own codes and symbols – virtually its own dialect – for the body. Just as agrarian cultures develop their own refined language of the earth and its fruits, and as communities of the bazaar elaborate their own complex language of commerce, so too have practitioner communities each developed their own languages of the body. When such communities coexisted within a single national context, each with its own system for educating and certifying its members, it was possible for different dialects, sometimes overlapping and sometimes not, to arise. Each group's representation of the body and its morbid appearances evolved in a manner best adapted to and best accounting for the day-to-day activities of the clinician who used it to explain what he saw in the diseased patient, to prescribe appropriate interventions, and to predict the outcome.

To surgeons in France and England the body was a mosaic of individual parts, differing from one species to another according to the canons of comparative anatomy, each part susceptible to characteristic disease entities. Most surgical illnesses were related to diseases, like inflammation, or scirrhus, or gangrene, that were amenable to one of the paradigmatic surgical interventions, extirpation or amputation. For physicians the code of the body was different, involving an ecologic conception of interdependent regions, bound together by circulating humors that carried medicaments, poisons, or other substances that might explain the prosperity or weakening observed in the body economy.[4]

But what happens when two tribes, once in proximity but with disparate conceptions of health and disease, suddenly find themselves forced to make common cause? Precipitously, institutions and professional groups must grasp for means of accommodation. Intellectual resources must be discovered or created to help adjust to shifts in worldly resources. Covering explanations must be found. New habits of mind must be developed to permit the rupture and rethinking of old, exclusive roles and relationships. All of these things are accomplished through education and communication, through the assimilation and dispersion of symbols and ideas. In France those ideas formed a new grammar of the body, creating a new *lingua franca* amongst practitioners who found themselves forced to share a common educational trunk.

Philippe Pinel's metaphor thus looms up again. Before the Revolution – and before Bichat elaborated his system – the two languages of the body were separate root-and-trunk systems, each with its own intellectual apparatus for explaining the body and thereby sustaining its practitioners. By the early 1820s the pathological anatomy of Bichat and Laennec gained strength and prestige, ultimately becoming the common root and trunk supporting what were now simply branches of the same profession. In this manner advocates for a united profession produced what one historian has felicitously termed the "double product": a body of knowledge and a corps of practitioners, the inseparable cognitive and professional unities. At least until the advent of microscopy, pathology would not be a discipline, subject to the laboratory-based *Methodenstreiten* of the sort physiology and other fields would soon confront. But the autopsy suite and the clinicopathological correlative method were near ancestors of the scientific laboratory, itself to become the "crucial intermediary" in the formation of the cognitive and social "double product."[5]

Hence pathological anatomy seeped into the French medical consciousness by a process not unlike the adoption of a new linking language. Elements of tribal dialects, heretofore deemed incompatible, were pulled together. Means to enhance the commensurability of medicine and surgery were sought and found in pathological anatomy. In Britain, on the other hand, physicians and surgeons collaborated in more constrained circumstances, and for the most part only among their most elite members. Only in a few cases, notably those of Hodgkin and Carswell, returning from their French pilgrimages full of zeal for the new language's explanatory power, were there attempts to spread its usage abroad. The apothecaries, rather than the physicians or the surgeons, stood in the end to gain from such a shift. The apothecaries did not grasp the reins of educational power, however, and were not to become coequal with the elite physicians and surgeons for generations yet to come. So the new language of the body did not achieve the prominence in Anglo-Saxon medical cultures that it had come to enjoy in France. In the former it functioned as a distinctive flourish, in the latter as intellectual currency.

This conclusion, despite its antitriumphal tone, suggests intriguing implications for the history of medical ideas. Not only historians of science, but historians in general have argued vociferously in recent decades about the importance of ideas – especially nonutilitarian ideas – in men's affairs.[6] What the story of morbid appearances in the early nineteenth century suggests, in fact, is that ideas have a life that cannot be accorded an incidental role in understanding what moves men. Under the right conditions ideas like those of Bichat and Laennec become linchpins of cultural change. As much as anything it was the idea of pathological anatomy that permitted the intellectual center in France to hold fast.

Pathology in England was an active and useful pursuit, at least within the thin stratum of its medical élite, despite the exodus to France of many of its brightest medical students after peace broke out in 1815. But it was utterly different than what was evolving in the radically different intellectual and cultural climate of the French capital. What emerges in the foregoing, then, is not so much a story of the emergence of dynamism out of stasis, but the growth and development of new forms in altered circumstances.

Appendix

Transcription and translation of Figure 1.1

N° *Deux:* ouverture de cadavre du 27 Prairial an VIII Républicain:

Inflammation lente et générale du péritione—le malade éprouvit depuis longtemps une douleur dans l'abdomen à la suite d'une péripneumonie. Il avoit un toux habituel et un crachat comme purulents. Le ventre étoit tendu et météorisé.

[Système d'] exhalation et absorption:

Membrane séreuse du péritoine rougeâtre parsémé dans toute son étendue de tubercule blanchâtre [,] serosité abondante dans la cavité[,] flocon[s] blanchâtre[s] nageant dans cette serosité[.] Epiploon changé comme masse dure et consistante[,] présentant une infinité de petit[s] point[s] blanchâtres. Plèvre et péricarde intact.

La maladie étoit absolument dans le péritoine qui était augmenté d'épaisseur. Et avant la plèvre offre cette [?réponse]—les flocons blanchâtres n'étoient pas copieux mais comme fibreux et par filamens.

★ ★ ★ ★ ★

12

Ouverture d'un cadavre [avec] inflammation du péricarde, anevrisme de l'aorte péctorale

Réspiration et circul[on]:

Coeur dans son état ordinaire[;] poumon entrera de la aorte dilatée. . . .

Exhal[on] et absor[on]:

Péricarde opaque[,] épais[,] rougeâtre[;] beaucoup de serosité purulent[;] flocon purulent adhérent à la surface interne du péricarde[;] adhérences diverses dans les deux plèvres; péritoine adhérent dans diverses parties[.]

Secretion:

Foie rien[;] rate[,] pancréas intact[.]

Digestif:

Estomac dans l'état ordinaire[;] intestins grèles et gros contenant beaucoup de sang qui paroit avoir suanté de la membrane muqueuse laquelle extrèmement rouge. Ça explique le vomissement de sang qui a eu lieu devant la mort; la malade a rendu beaucoup de la fluide.

N^o *two:* autopsy on the cadaver of 27 Prairial, Republican year VIII:

Slow, generalized inflammation of the peritoneum—for a long time the patient experienced abdominal pain following a peripneumonia. He had a chronic cough and purulent sputum. The belly was tight and distended.

Exhalant-absorbent system:

Peritoneal serous membrane reddish, throughout its extent studded with whitish tubercle; abundant serous fluid in the cavity, whitish flecks floating in this serosity. Epiploon transformed into a hard, homogeneous mass, with an infinitude of small whitish specks. Intact pleura and pericardium.

The disease was absolutely in the peritoneum which was augmented in thickness. And before the pleura offered this [?response]—whitish flecks were not copious but as though fibrous and filamentous.

★ ★ ★ ★ ★

12

Autopsy on a cadaver [with] inflammation of the pericardium, aneurysm of the thoracic aorta

Respiration and circul^{on}

Heart in its ordinary state[;] lung coming from the dilated aorta . . .

Exhal^{on} and absor^{on}:

Pericardium opaque, thick, reddish; a great deal of purulent serous fluid; purulent flecks adherent to the internal surface of the pericardium; several adhesions between the two pleural surfaces; peritoneum adherent in various places.

Secretion:

Liver nothing; spleen, pancreas intact.

Digestive:

Stomach in its ordinary state; large and small intestines containing a large amount of blood appearing to be stimulated by the extremely red mucous membrane. That explains the vomiting of blood which took place before death; the patient gave up a great deal of fluid.

Notes

INTRODUCTION

1 Othmar Keel, *La généalogie de histopathologie: une Révision Déchirante: Philippe Pinel, Lecteur Discret de J.-C. Smyth (1741–1821)* (Paris: Vrin, 1979). Keel has usefully expanded his theme in "La formation de la problématique de l'anatomie des systèmes selon Laennec," in *Commemoration du Bicentenaire de la Naissance de Laennec, 1781–1826: Colloque Organisé au Collège de France les 18 et 19 Février 1981* (Paris: Revue du Palais de la Découverte, No. Special 22, 1981), pp. 189–207.

2 On the sepulchral events related here see: Raphael Blanchard, "Sur la tombe de Bichat," *Bulletin de la Société Française de la médecine* (1902), 1: 261–68; Frederick Brown, *Père Lachaise: Elysium as Real Estate* (New York: Viking, 1973) pp. 9–57; "Procès-verbal d'exhumation des restes de Bichat," *Journal des connaissances médicales pratiques et de pharmacologie* (1845), 13: 119–20; Jacques Leonard, *Les médecins de l'ouest au XIXᵉᵐᵉ siècle* (Thèse, Université de Paris IV, 1976) pp. 798–99; "The strange adventures of an anatomist's head," *British Medical Journal* (1 Dec. 1900), ii: 1601. Most accounts state, with varying degrees of archness, that Roux simply kept the skull as a souvenir. This seems a reasonable assumption since Roux performed the postmortem examination on Bichat and disciples of well-known teachers at the time often retained such *memento mori*. Why Roux kept the group in suspense before producing the head for reattachment remains mysterious.

On France's loss of prestige see Joseph Ben-David, "The rise and decline of France as a scientific center," *Minerva* (1970), 8:160–79. Ben-David's analysis, it should be noted, typifies the now standard "declinist" account of mid- and late-nineteenth century French science. This account has been called into question by recent work in the area by Robert Fox, George Weisz, and others. Their revisionist view is nicely summarized, with supporting references and documentation, in "The institutional basis of French science in the nineteenth century," in a volume edited by them: *The Organization of Science and Technology in France 1808–1914* (Cambridge: Cambridge University Press, 1980). While it is inappropriate here to recapitulate in detail their cogent argument, suffice it to say that at mid-century there was clearly a *perception* of decline, similar to that obtaining a generation earlier in England (cf. Chapters 4 and 6), emanating from central Paris institutions. While Ben-David et al. may now have simply reified that perception into the historical record, the perception alone may be sufficient to explain the fact that the stream of foreign students was diverted to other locales, mainly the German-speaking countries, in the period after 1845.

CHAPTER 1

1 One answer, partly at odds with that proposed here, is found in John Pickstone, "Bureaucracy, liberalism and the body in post-revolutionary France: Bichat's physiology and the Paris school of medicine," *History of Science* (1981), 19: 115–42. Pickstone's intriguing contention is that Bichat's work, representing "the

fulfillment of [the Paris medical community's] collective aspirations," maps the organization of the body politic onto that of the body human. Pickstone's view is not wholly inconsistent with mine, but depends rather more heavily on a programmatic "social constructionist" argument. For an appraisal and further examples of this general approach, see Peter Wright and Andrew Treacher, eds., *The Problem of Medical Knowledge: Examining the Social Context of Medicine* (Edinburgh: Edinburgh University Press, 1982).

2 The standard account of the events of 1789–94 remains that of Erwin Ackerknecht in *Medicine at the Paris Hospital* (Baltimore: Johns Hopkins University Press, 1967). In his more recent appraisal of the role of the surgical profession in fostering these events, *Professionalizing Modern Medicine* (Westport, Conn.: Greenwood Press, 1980), however, Toby Gelfand provides considerable added insight and detail on the role of certain key actors. On the importance of military needs see David Vess, *Medical Revolution in France, 1789–1796* (Gainesville: Florida State University Press, 1975), and Dora Weiner, "French doctors face war, 1792–1815," in C. K. Warner, ed., *From the Ancien Régime to the Popular Front: Essays in the History of Modern France in Honor of Shepard B. Clough* (New York: Columbia University Press, 1969).

3 Dora Weiner, in a forthcoming monograph, examines the genesis and fate of the notion of a right to health care in this setting.

4 On the former see Ackerknecht, n. 2, and Weiner, n. 3. On higher education there is a much larger literature. See, e.g., Louis Liard, *L'enseignement supérieur en France,* (Paris: 1888) and *L'Université de Paris* (Paris: Renouard, 1909); Ackerknecht, *Paris Hospital* (n. 2), is a reliable guide to allied, quasi-academic medical institutions (such as journals and societies); on the most important cognate *scientific* institutions see Roger Hahn, *The Anatomy of a Scientific Institution: the Paris Academy of Sciences, 1666–1803* (Berkeley: University of California Press, 1971). On the reform of clinical instruction see Ackerknecht and Gelfand (n. 2); the latter author's "A confrontation over clinical instruction at the Hôtel-Dieu of Paris during the French Revolution," *Journal of the History of Medicine,* (1973), *28:* 268–82; and, for useful comparative material, Ramunas A. Kondratas, *Joseph Frank (1771–1842) and the Development of Clinical Medicine: A Study of the Transformation of Medical Thought and Practice at the End of the 18th and the Beginning of the 19th Centuries* (unpublished doctoral dissertation, Harvard University, 1977).

5 Gelfand (n. 2) argues lucidly that, precisely because of the surgeons' success over the course of the entire eighteenth century in improving their own lot, the groundwork was laid for a tradeoff between professional power and markets: the physicians yielded the former in return for the surgeons' yielding the latter. Each group stood to gain in the transaction: the physicians foresook their citadel, forestalled the possibility of becoming an insular elite, and gained some valuable real estate, argues Gelfand, while the surgeons bridged the final gap in prestige. My contention here is that this conjunction found its cognitive analog in the new pathological anatomy since physicians' and surgeons' outlooks could now be merged.

6 This seems an appropriate point at which to expose my preconceptions about the relationship between novelty in intellectual versus professional structures. I posit neither to be necessarily antecedent to the other. I will argue neither that Bichat conceptualized his tissue pathology "because of" the need for a cognitive adhesive between medicine and surgery, nor that his ultimately producing such an adhesive "led to" the unification of those two professions. Indeed, as Toby Gelfand has shown, quite another sort of interprofessional dynamic was involved in their coalition. I wish to argue, instead, for a reflexive relationship between the two parallel processes. Each reinforced the other. This contention gains strength when one considers the necessary reinterpretation of "innovation" in this context. In a carefully reasoned *analyse du texte* Othmar Keel has demonstrated the notion that Bichat and his *compère,* Philippe Pinel, do not necessarily deserve priority for establishing the tissue theory of disease. Uncovering textual evidence consistent, he believes, with a major revisionist break (*révision déchirante*) in his-

torical understanding of the period, Keel shows that, from the standpoint of the "earliest-statement" criterion, priority should be accorded to James Carmichael Smyth, a Scot who anticipated the tissue theory in his 1790 consideration, *"Of the Different Species of Inflammation, and of the Causes to which these Differences are to be Ascribed."* Compare O. Keel, *La généalogie de l'histopathologie, une révision déchirante: Philippe Pinel, lecteur discret de J.-C. Smyth (1741–1841)* (Paris: Vrin, 1979). The problem, of course, arises in defining what is meant by the establishment of theory. If mere adumbration is enough to accomplish this, then Keel's assessment is truly *déchirante*. If, on the other hand, the establishment of theory also depends on its implantation and survival in an appropriately receptive context, Smyth's work does not itself impel us to "tear up" or discard previous historical accounts.

7   Medical men in the still all-physician Paris Faculty were already taking a cue from their surgical counterparts by the 1770s with respect to the centrality of practical hospital training in basic medical education; see Gelfand (n. 2), pp. 132–33.

8   By convention, when I discuss the "medical" community here I shall mean those practitioners and educators trained in the medical faculties, excluding both surgeons and *officers de santé.*

9   Among the surveys of this material are Jacques Léonard, *Les médecins de l'ouest au XIX*ᵉᵐᵉ *siècle*, doctoral thesis, Université de Paris IV, 1976 (Paris: [Diffusion] Librairie Honore Champion, 1978); Paul Delaunay, *D'une révolution à l'autre, 1789–1848: l'évolution des théories et de la pratique médicales* (Paris: Editions Hippocrate, 1949); Ackerknecht (n. 2), chs. 1, 3, 5, and passim. In what follows, my account accords most closely with that of Léonard, pp. 305–20, although he is more exclusively concerned with the state of medical (as opposed to surgical) science in the early nineteenth century, i.e., as it stood at the beginning of the Napoleonic era.

10 This is a matter of emphasis. Surgeons certainly could – and many if not most did – simultaneously harbor a neohumoralistic notion of health as a state of balance, and its absence as a state of imbalance. See Owsei Temkin, "The role of surgery in the rise of modern medical thought," *Bulletin of the History of Medicine.* (1951), *25*: 248–59.

11 A physician, by contrast, particularly in the eighteenth century, would have stressed the constitutional effects, such as the febrile response, in maladies of this sort.

12 The choice of an example from Desault is not accidental. In addition to being the most influential figure of the late eighteenth century in the training of young Parisian and French surgeons, Desault was Bichat's mentor. At Desault's death Bichat became his widow's choice to collate and edit the master's posthumous collected works. See F. M. X. Bichat, ed., *Oeuvres chirurgicales de Desault*, 3 vols. (Paris, 1798–99; 3ʳᵈ ed. Paris: J.-B. Baillière, 1830), article *erysipèle*, p. 581.

13 On this general question see Georges Canguilhem, *On the Normal and the Pathological*, trans. C. R. Fawcett ([orig. ed. Paris: Presses Universitaires de France, 1966] Dordrecht, Holland: D. Reidel, 1978), esp. pp. 17–28.

14 On recurrences in medical thought of self-styled Hippocratic revivals amidst attempted reform, see Erwin H. Ackerknecht, "Recurrent themes in medical thought," *Scientific Monthly* (1949), *49*: 80–83.

15 On Laennec, see Chapter 4; for De Mercy's views see his *Demande du rétablissement d'un chair d'Hippocrate, année 1821: Mémoire pour la Commission de l'Instruction Publique.* (Paris: n.d.)

16 On the particular complexion of Bichat's vitalism, and the relationship it bore to his physiological predecessors and successors, see W. R. Albury, "Magendie's physiological manifesto of 1809," *Bulletin of the History of Medicine* (1974), *48* and "Experimentation and explanation in the physiology of Bichat and Magendie," *Studies in the History of Biology* (1977), *1*: 47–131. A classic paper on the subject is Owsei Temkin, "The philosophical background of Magendie's physiology," *Bulletin of the History of Medicine* (1946), *20*: 10–35. A more recent monograph

that places Bichat's sensualist physiology squarely in its eighteenth-century context is Elizabeth Haigh, *Xavier Bichat and the Medical Theory of the Eighteenth Century, Medical History* Supplement No. 4 (London: Wellcome Institute, 1984). Like Keel (n. 6), Haigh adheres to a historical framework that is strictly conceptualist in emphasis and interpretation. The most balanced recent treatment of these issues is John E. Lesch, *Science and Medicine in France: The Emergence of Experimental Physiology, 1790–1855* (Cambridge, Mass.: Harvard University Press, 1984); compare esp. ch. 3, "Bichat's two physiologies."

17 The first to point out this link was in fact Bichat's eulogist: see A. F. T. Levache de la Feutrie, "Eloge de Marie-Francois-Xavier Bichat," *Memoires Société médicale Emulation* (1803), *5:* xxvii–lxiv.

18 For general biographical information see Louis Dulieu, "Bordeu," *Dictionary of Scientific Biography,* II, 301–302, and Paul Delaunay, *Le monde médicale Parisien au dix-huitième siècle,* 2nd ed. (Paris: Rousset, 1906).

19 A brief note on the family as hydrotherapeutists is found in Paul Delaunay *D'une révolution à l'autre, 1789–1848: l'Évolution des théories et de la pratique médicales* (Paris: Editions Hippocrate, 1949), pp. 76–77.

20 Théophile de Bordeu, *Recherches sur le tissu muqueux, ou l'organe cellulaire* (Paris: Didot le jeune, 1767), pp. 22, 32–33, 65, 79–80, 85–89, 173–74.

21 Bichat's comment is in Faculté de médecine de Paris (hereafter FMP) MS 46, Brouillon 5^u, f. $18r^o$; for the anachronous identification see A. P. Cawadias, "Théophile de Bordeu: An eighteenth century pioneer in endocrinology," *Proceedings of the Royal Society of Medicine* (1950), *43:* 93–98.

22 Théophile de Bordeu, *Sur l'usage des eaux de Barèges,* published in multiple editions, including that bound in with his *Recherches sur le tissu muqueux* (n. 20).

23 On the impact of *idéologie* – its importance for pathological anatomy now partially called into question (see Toby Gelfand's review of Keel (n. 6) in *Annals of Science* (1981), *38:* 248–49) – the most useful sources begin with George Rosen, "The philosophy of ideology and the emergence of modern medicine in France," *Bulletin of the History of Medicine* (1946), *20:* 328–39 (the classic article); more recent works that extend Rosen's analysis and provide a broader institutional context for late Enlightenment medical philosophy are: Martin Staum, *Cabanis: Enlightenment and Medical Philosophy in the French Revolution* (Princeton, N.J.: Princeton University Press, 1980), and John E. Lesch, *Science and Medicine in France,* n. 16 above, esp. ch. 2, "Context for change: the 1790s."

24 Compare Lester King, *The Medical World of the Eighteenth Century* (Chicago: University of Chicago Press, *1958); and Georges Canguilhem, On the Normal and the Pathological* (n. 13).

25 On French adherents compare Léonard (n. 9), pp. 310–311.

26 To test this assertion further one could examine the contrasting manner in which late eighteenth-century surgeons and physicians employed the perennial therapeutic tactic of phlebotomy or bloodletting.

27 On solidism see Pierre Huard, "Quelques idées sur la structure de la matière vivante au XIXème siècle; leur incidence sur la pratique médicale," *Clio Medica* (1974), *9:* 57–64.

28 A notable exception is the now-classic account of the response to infectious disease in nineteenth-century America, *Cholera Years* by Charles E. Rosenberg (Chicago: University of Chicago Press, 1962).

29 On this point see Michel Foucault, *Naissance de la clinique,* 2nd ed. (Paris: Presses Universitaires, 1972), trans. *Birth of the Clinic* (New York: Pantheon, 1973), chs. 5–6.

30 Early nineteenth-century nosologies, besides being incommensurable with their twentieth-century successors, might be termed also preparadigmatic and hence multiple, lacking consensus between contemporary groups. In the case of the dominant public health problem of communicable diseases, the paradigm that finally "took" after 1880 or so was the Pasteur–Koch theory of pathogenic microorganisms. Hence, after this point syphilis, say, could be agreed to be that which was characterized by invasion by the spirochete. (See Ludwik Fleck, *Genesis*

and *Development of a Scientific Fact* (Basel, 1935; English edition: Chicago: University of Chicago Press, 1979). Put more simply, "phthisis" or "scirrhus" meant different things to different people. Disease categories, to an extent far greater than a century later, were unstandardized. Thus to attempt systematic analysis of records such as those mentioned here would be hazardous, if one wished to be more than merely impressionistic.

31 On fever in the eighteenth century, see ch. 5 in Lester King, *The Medical World of the Eighteenth Century*, (n. 24). On fever theory in the sixteenth-through-eighteenth centuries see W. F. Bynum, ed., *Theories of Fever From Antiquity to the Enlightenment, Medical History Supplement No. 1*, (London: Wellcome Institute for the History of Medicine, 1981).

32 Hôtel-Dieu: *Registre pour inscrire les entrées, sorties et décès des malades reçus au dit hôtel-Dieu*. Archives de l'Assistance Publique, Liasse 518.62.

33 On another set of causes of mortality in this period see the interesting recent work by Richard Cobb, *Death in Paris: 1795–1801* (Oxford: Oxford University Press, 1978). Conventional nosologies of the last two decades of the eighteenth century had important consequences, not least of which was the arraying of patients with disparate conditions (but common admitting diagnoses such as "fever") side by side. Since the practice included those unfortunates afflicted with puerperal fever, the maternal death rate at the Hôtel-Dieu at the turn of the century hovered around six percent. Redistributing patients according to more refined diagnostic entities, according to the reformer Jacques Tenon, halved that number in two decades. See Giorgio Pons, "Essai de sociologie des malades dans les hôpitaux de Paris pendant les années 1815 à 1848," *Zürcher medizingeschichtliche Abhandlungen*, N.R., No. 63 (Zürich: Juris, 1969), p. 23 and passim.

34 Most of the materials used in this section are in FMP MS 5150, Bte. VII.

35 The former was completed and published posthumously by Buisson (t. III–IV) and Roux (t. V). Some autopsy reports were set down in what was doubtless great haste, probably well warranted in certain times of year when bodies decayed rapidly. In such cases at times the protocol was abridged.

36 Xavier Bichat, *Anatomie générale, appliquée à la physiologie et à la Médecine* (Paris: Méquignon, an IX [1801]), p. xcix.

37 FMP MS 5150 – 6°. At the turn of the century the term "serosity" denoted a much wider range of fluids than it has for the past hundred years. On the *tissu cellulaire*, or loose stromal connective tissue, not cellular tissue in the modern sense, see J. W. Wilson, "Cellular tissue and the dawn of the cell theory," *Isis* (1944), *35:* 168–73.

38 FMP MS 5150 – 9°, f. 11; this was undoubtedly a case of tuberculous peritonitis with miliary spread.

39 Ibid. Noteworthy in this case was the manner in which local affections in individual tissues were correlated with antemortem and postmortem signs of pathological change elsewhere in the body.

40 The standard accounts of Bichat's life remain those of the family Genty, *père* and *fille:* much of the material published over many years in *Progrès médicale* has been compiled in "Xavier Bichat," in Pierre Huard, ed., *Biographies médicales et scientifiques* (Paris: Dacosta, 1972). See also G. Nicole-Genty, *Bichat: Médecin du Grand Hospice d'Humanité* (doctoral thesis, Faculté de médecine de Paris, 1943). Also useful are P.-E. Launois, *Xavier Bichat: Sa vie, son oeuvre, son influence sur les sciences biologiques* (Paris: Naud, 1943) and J. Coquerelle, *Xavier Bichat (1771–1802): Ses ancêtres et ses arrière-neveux* (Paris: Maloine, 1902). The best recent analysis of his career in its scientific context is in John Lesch, *Science and Medicine in France*, ch. 3, "Bichat's Two Physiologies" (n. 16).

41 On Desault as pedagogue see Gelfand, *Professionalizing Modern Medicine.* (n. 2); P. Huard and M.-J. Imbault-Huart, "Pierre Desault (1738–1795)," in Huard, "Biographies médicales" (n. 40), pp. 119–180, and "L'enseignement de chirurgie à l'Hôtel-Dieu d'après une lettre inédite de Desault à l'Assemblée Nationale (1791)," *Revue d'histoire des Sciences* (1972), *25:* 55–63; Charles Daremberg, *Histoire des Sciences Médicales*, 2 vols., (Paris: Baillière, 1870), II, 1286–95; and P. A. Rich-

mond, "The Hôtel-Dieu on the eve of the Revolution," *Journal of the History of Medicine* (1961), *16*:335–353.

42 Xavier Bichat, "Discours préliminaire," *Mémoires de la Societé médicale d'Emulation* (an V [1797]), *1:* iv–v.

43 On the importance of the private courses see Chapter 7, and Lesch (n. 16), pp. 29–30, 55. On Desault's teaching see also Gelfand, "Confrontation" (n. 4).

44 Xavier Bichat, "Mémoire sur la membrane synoviale des articulations," *Mémoires de la Societé médicale d'Emulation* (an VII [1799]), *2:* 350–70; pp. 350–351.

45 The term, part of the English medical idiom as well at the time, was coined around 1541 by Paracelsus, and applied to all serous fluids; only later was its meaning narrowed to refer only to the joints. Bichat ultimately regarded it as one type of serous fluid: all synovia was serous fluid to him, but not all serous fluid was synovia.

46 Bichat, *Mémoire* (n. 44), pp. 354–66. He remarked (p. 368) that the synovial membranes were slightly anomalous in that the hydropsy so frequently seen in other serous membranes was hardly ever observed in the joints.

47 Xavier Bichat, ed., *Oeuvres chirurgicales, ou exposé de la doctrine et de la pratique de P.-J. Desault* (Paris: Citoyenne veuve Desault – Méquignon l'ainé, an VI [1799]), II, 304–307 [3rd ed., 1830].

48 Ibid., pp. 368–69. On these *mémoires* see also Maurice Genty, "Xavier Bichat (1771–1802)," pp. 181–318 in Pierre Huard, ed., *Biographies médicales et scientifiques: XVIIIème siècle* (Paris: Dacosta, 1972), esp. pp 242–43.

49 *Mémoires de la Société médicale d'Emulation* (an VII [1799]), *2:* 371–85.

50 See, e.g., J.-L. Moreau de la Sarthe, "[Extrait et analyse du] Traité des membranes en général et des diverses membranes en particulier," *Recueil périodique de la Société médicale de Paris* (an VIII [1800]), *7:* 321–342, 457–462. One voice in opposition came from the figure who came as close as anyone to becoming Bichat's arch-rival: see A. B. Richerand, "Réflexions critiques sur un ouvrage ayant pour titre, Traité des membranes," *Magazine encyclopédique* (an VIII [1799]) *5:* 260–272.

51 Jean Monteil, *Le cours d'anatomie pathologique de Bichat: un nouveau manuscrit* (Grenoble: Guirimand, 1960); a distorted and personalized version was brought out by another disciple, Pierre Béclard: *Anatomie pathologique: dernier cours de Xavier Bichat* (Paris: Baillière, 1825).

52 Leon Elaut, "La théorie des membranes de F. X. Bichat et ses antécédents," *Sudhoffs Archiv* (1969), *53:* 68–76.

53 MS notes on anatomy, FMP MS 5145 – 3°.

54 FMP MS 5145 – 3°, f. 45.

55 See Albury (n. 16) on Bichat's vitalism, and Lesch, (n. 16) for an overall summary. Bichat's sensualism is emphasized in Michael Gross, *Function and Structure in Nineteenth Century French Physiology*, doctoral dissertation, Princeton University, 1974, esp. ch. 1, "The localization of sensibility and contractility." A useful published distillation is idem, "The lessened locus of feelings: a transformation in French physiology in the early nineteenth century," *Journal of the History of Biology* (1979), *12:* 231–271. An older literature, still of some use in approaching this subject, includes: Pedro Lain-Entralgo, "Sensualism and vitalism in Bichat's *Anatomie générale*," *Journal of the History of Medicine*, (1948), *3:* 47–64; E. Gley, "Xavier Bichat et son oeuvre biologique," *Bulletin de la Société Française d'Histoire de la médecine* (1902, repr. 1967), *1:* 285–82; A. Arène, "Essai sur la philosophie de Xavier Bichat," *Archives d'anthropologie criminelle* (1911) *26:*753–825; Joseph Schiller, "Henri Dutrochet et la terminologie scientifique," *97ème Congrès de la Société des Savants* (1972); Adriana Amerio, " 'Sensibilita' ed 'Irritabilita' Nella Dottrina Vitalistica di Anthelme Richerand," *Medicina Nei Secoli* (1972), *9:*23–28; F. Fearing, *Reflex Action* (Baltimore: Williams & Wilkins, 1930), pp. 74–107; and T. S. Hall, *Ideas of Life and Matter*, 2 vols. (Chicago: University of Chicago Press, 1969), II, 121–132, 171–178.

56 Xavier Bichat, *Traité des membranes en général et de diverses membranes en particulier* (Paris: Richard, Caille et Ravier, an VIII [1799]), pp. 64–69.

57 Ibid., pp. 115–117.
58 Xavier Bichat, *Anatomie pathologique, cours fini le 23 Floréal an X*. Bibliothèque de l'Ecole de médecine, Université de Grenoble, pp. 1, 9v° – 13r°, 24r°, 35v° – 37r°, 38r°.
59 This has been pointed out most recently by Lesch (n. 16), pp. 78–79. See also T. S. Hall, "On biological analogs of Newtonian paradigms," *Philosophy of Science* (1968), *35*: 6–27.
60 This is implied by Genty, "Xavier Bichat" (n. 48), p. 293.

CHAPTER 2

1 MS Collections, Archives Nationales, Paris (abbreviated below AN), F¹⁷ 2165. Fragonard was the cousin of the illustrious painter.
2 For some detail on this episode see Maurice Genty, "Xavier Bichat," in P. Huard, ed., *Biographies médicales et scientifiques* (Paris: Dacosta, 1972), pp. 244–45.
3 M.-J. Imbault-Huart, *L'Ecole pratique de dissection de Paris de 1750 à 1822, ou l'influence du concept de médecine pratique et de médecine d'observation dans l'enseignement médico-chirurgical au XVIIIème siècle et au début du XIXème siècle*. Doctoral thesis, Université de Paris I, 1973 (Lille: Service de Reproduction des Thèses, 1975), pp. 36–56. Imbault-Huart's study is, like those of Erwin Ackerknecht and Jacques Léonard, an exceptionally useful synthetic work. She also provides useful chronology for the earlier eighteenth-century history of the *Ecole pratique*, and makes sensitive use of archival documents in her analysis of certain developments, especially those surrounding attempts to bring the *Ecole pratique* "into the bosom" of the Paris faculty. See also Toby Gelfand, *Professionalizing Modern Medicine* (Westport, Conn.: Greenwood Press, 1980), pp. 90–92.
4 Ibid., pp. 62–78.
5 Instead of tracing the strands of Bichat's work into that of each of these successors and students, I have chosen to focus on one of them, Théophile Laennec of Brittany. Laennec provided the crucial intellectual link between morbid anatomy and physical diagnosis, as well as the crucial cultural link between French and British pathology; see Chapter 4. Of note, however, is Pierre Huard's and M.-J. Imbault-Huart's recent discussion of Bayle as the critical transitional figure between "pure" pathological anatomy, typified by Bichat, and the "anatomico-clinical method" that would reach its apotheosis in Laennec. See "La clinique Parisienne avant et après 1802," *Clio medica* (1975), *10*: 173–82.
6 Starting points for this material are E. H. Ackerknecht, *Medicine at the Paris Hospital* (Baltimore: Johns Hopkins, 1967), ch. 4; and, on Fourcroy in particular, C. C. Gillispie, *Science and Polity in France at the End of the Old Regime* (Princeton, N.J.: Princeton University Press, 1980), pp. 178–82.
7 In all probability Chaussier was intimately involved in the School's genesis as well, with an important role in framing the early programmatic documents: for discussion of the point see Toby Gelfand, *Professionalizing Modern Medicine* (n. 3), p. 166.
8 Antoine Fourcroy, *Rapport et projet de décret sur l'établissement d'une Ecole centrale de Santé à Paris, fait à la Convention nationale au nom des comités de salut public et d'instruction publique* (Paris: Imprimerie nationale, an III), pp. 3–9. This document may be found in printed form in AN, AD VIII 30, and in MS form in the *Recueil* of the Faculté de médecine, in AJ¹⁶ 6306.
9 Ibid., pp. 11–12. The similarity of this language to that of the 1790 "New Plan" of the Society of Medicine was almost assuredly no accident. The latter was probably penned by Fourcroy's protector, Felix Vicq d'Azyr: compare, e.g., Gelfand, *Professionalizing Modern Medicine* (n. 3), pp. 157–58.
10 "L'état de l'indemnité pour les membres, employés, artistes, et entretenus divers de l'école de santé de Paris, conformément à la loi du premier Messidor an 4ème": AN, F¹⁷ 2289; and Antoine Fourcroy *et al.*, *Plan générale de l'enseignement dans l'école de santé de Paris* (Paris: Ballard fils, an III): AN, AD VIII 30.

11   The full list of early chair holders is in Ackerknecht, *Paris Hospital* (n. 6), p 35, and *Plan générale* . . . (ii. 10), pp. 3–4.
12   "Etat des employés, artistes, prosecteurs et attachés à l'école de Santé de Paris," AN F^{17} 2289. On financial arrangements in this period at the *Ecole pratique* see Imbault-Huart, *L'Ecole pratique* . . . (n. 3), pp. 47–49, 58–61, and passim.
13   "Extrait du registre du comité des finances de la Convention Nationale," AN, AJ^{16} 6307, pp. 71–72.
14   Cf. Chapter I for a brief survey of some of these ideas.
15   "Plan générale," pp. 26–28.
16   Ibid., pp. 28–32.
17   On the coexistence of alternative mentalities in medicine, even in a situation where the communities harboring those mentalities are confronting a common biological reality, see the important and only recently rediscovered early monograph by Ludvik Fleck, *Genesis and Development of a Scientific Fact* (Basel, 1935; Chicago: University of Chicago Press, 1979). By the term *Denkkollectiv* Fleck denotes a community – the "thought collective"—whose mentality reflects a set of coherent cultural habits.
18   [Michel Thouret], *De l'état actuel de l'Ecole de Santé de Paris* (Paris: Didot Jeune, an VI – 1798).
19   Ibid.
20   Louis Liard, *L'enseignement supérieur en France, 1789–1889* (Paris: Armand Colin, 1888), I, pp. 166–67.
21   The point is amplified in the useful introductory essay by Robert Fox and George Weisz, "The institutional basis of French science in the nineteenth century," pp. 1–28 in their edited volume, *The organization of science and technology in France, 1808–1914* (Cambridge and Paris: Cambridge University Press, 1980).
22   Rapport . . . au ministre de l'intérieur, 14 Messidor an V [1 July 1797]; and [Réponse du] ministre &c au cit. Thouret & aux membres composant le Bureau central du canton de Paris, 19 Messidor an V [7 July 1797]; both in AN F^{17} 2287.
23   Projet de loi sur l'organisation des écoles de médecine, le 1 Frimaire an VII [21 November 1798], cited at length in De Mercy, *Plan d'organisation de l'art médical* [Paris, 1815], pp. 92–97.
24   M.-J. Imbault-Huart, *L'Ecole pratique* (n. 3) pp. 241–45.
25   See, e.g., Le ministre [de l'intérieur] au citoyen Thouret, D^r de l'Ecole de médecine de Paris, 26 Floreal an XII [15 May 1803], AN F^{17} 2108; and Le Directeur de l'Ecole de Médecine
26   On Chaussier's role in the juries, see Chapter 4.
27   On Dupuytren and his controversy with Laennec, see also Chapter 3.
28   *L'ami des lois* no. 728, 1 Brumaire an VI [Oct. 1797], AN F^{17} 2287.
29   On Thouret's role see the following biographical writings: J. J. LeRoux and P. Süe, *Séance publique de la Faculté de Médecine de Paris, tenue le 14 novembre 1810, pour la rentrée des écoles, et discours prononcés par M. J. J. LeRoux et par M. Süe* (Paris: Didot jeune, 1810), AN AJ^{16} 6308; J. J. LeRoux, *Discours prononcé le 23 juin 1810 sur la tombe de Monsieur Thouret. . .* , AN AJ^{16} 6551; and the useful article in A. L. Bayle and A. Thillaye, *Biographie médicale par ordre chronologique*, (2 vols.), (Paris: Delahays, 1855), vol. II, pp. 720–25.
30   Thouret to Minister of Interior, 7 Vendémiaire an VI [28 Sept. 1797], AN F^{17} 2287.
31   *L'ami des lois* (n. 28).
32   Exchange of letters between Thouret and Minister of Interior, 13–17 March 1798; *Rapport présenté au Ministre de l'Intérieur . . . le 6 Germinal an VI* [26 Mar. 1798]; AN F^{17} 2287.
33   *Rapport presenté au Ministre de l'Intérieur*, 7 Brumaire an VI [28 Oct. 1797], AN F^{17} 2287. Thouret again pointed to the increase in enrollments from 300 to 1,000 and noted that besides anatomical dissection other subjects, which included surgical operations, chemical and pharmaceutical manipulations, the application of bandages and orthopedic appliances, and obstetrical *accouchement* were now taught.

On the subdivision of personnel in 1798 see, in the faculty *registre*, "Rapport sur le mode de composition de l'école pratique pour l'an 7," AN AJ¹⁶ 6307.

34 On this episode and for the most recent and exhaustive guide to Pinel's biography and bibliography, see the "Introductory essay" in Weiner's monograph: Dora Weiner, ed., *The Clinical Training of Doctors: An Essay of 1793, by Philippe Pinel* (Baltimore: Johns Hopkins University Press, 1980), pp. 1–22.

35 Ibid.

36 "Rapport sur le plan gᵃˡ. de l'enseignement vous nous avez chargés de revoir *le plan générale* [qui] fut adopté lors de la formation de l'Ecole. . . ," 29 Fructidor an VI [15 September 1798], *Rapports faits dans les differentes séances de l'Ecole de Santé de Paris, ans III–VIII (1794–1800)* (Manuscript register), AN AJ¹⁶, entry no. 143. [Emphasis added.]

37 Rapport présenté au Ministre de l'Intérieur, Germinal [March – April] an VII [1799], AN F¹⁷ 2165.

38 Minister of Interior to Minister of War, 15 Germinal an VII [4 April 1799], AN F¹⁷ 2165.

39 Rapport sur les moyens de prouver l'identité des candidats qui se présenteront à la place du Cit. Fragonard[,] chef des Travaux anatomiques, 9 Floréal an VII [28 April 1799]; AN AJ¹⁶ 6307 [MS register], no. 93.

40 Ibid., 8 Thermidor [26 July], no. 102.

41 Rapport présenté au Ministre de l'Intérieur, 20 Prairial l'an VII [8 June 1799], AN F¹⁷ 2165. Doubtless it was no accident that another internal report, devised, like the other internal documents mentioned here, at the level of the ministry's Bureau of Instruction [*Bureau d'enseignement*], found its way to the Minister at precisely that same moment. It detailed Thouret's desire further to expand the examination and instruction of surgeons in the *Ecole pratique*, "to the extent that the war proceeds more briskly [*prend une nouvelle activité*]." The report indicates the Minister's probable approval of such an authorization: Rapport presente au Min. de l'Int. ["autorisation de multiplier . . . les examens rélatifs aux opérations et d'admettre . . . un nombre double d'élèves"].

42 Rapport . . . No. 102 (n. 40).

43 Rapport presenté au Ministre de l'Intérieur, 20 Thermidor an VII [7 August 1799]. AN F¹⁷ 2165.

44 This was a faculty-level, though, it must be remembered, not officially professorial post in the school.

45 *Mutation* has been discussed somewhat invidiously by Ackerknecht: see *Medicine at the Paris Hospital*, p. 33.

46 On Cuvier's administrative career see Erik Nordenskiöld, *The History of Biology: A Survey* (New York: Tudor, 1949), pp. 331–33; William Coleman, *Georges Cuvier: Zoologist* (Cambridge, Mass.: Harvard University Press, 1964) esp. pp. 6–11; and Georgette Legée, "La participation de Georges et de Frederic Cuvier à l'organisation de l'instruction publique (1802–38)," *Histoire et Nature* No. 4 (n.s.) fasc. 2 (1974) 47–72.

47 Cuvier to Minister of Interior, 23 February 1801, AN F¹⁷ 2165.

48 Ibid.; Legée ("La participation," n. 46) points out that three years later Cuvier consigned to Duméril the task of producing an elementary treatise on natural history for the nation's lycées, based on the work both had conducted in comparative anatomy at the Muséum.

49 [Arrête de] Bonaparte sur le rapport du Ministre de l'intérieur. . . , 29 Ventôse an IX [20 March 1801]. AN F¹⁷ 2165.

50 "Procès-verbal d'exhumation des restes de Bichat," *Journal des connaissances médicales pratiques et de pharmacologie* (1845), *13:* 119–20.

CHAPTER 3

1 To assess the full extent and amplitude of this movement would represent a daunting prospect. One might, for example, find shifts in student acceptance of

the Bichatian schema by analyzing the shifts in emphasis in their M.D. theses. That, however, is not where I wish to place most of my emphasis. The very hagiography that grew up around Bichat is evidence of his having become a talisman. His image came to assume totemic stature for French medical men, a process that reached its ritual conclusion in the 1840s (see Introduction).

2 Emblematic of this continued conservative emphasis in the central faculty was the appointment of Dupuytren over Bichat to the position of *chef*, discussed in Chapter 2.

3 The assertion that this course and the material covered in it had grown into a state of relative disuse is not intended as a breezy aside, but is borne out by the documentary evidence. An extraordinarily intriguing statement appears, for example, in Thouret's successor as Dean, J. J. Leroux's (1749–1832) letter to MM. la Commission de l'instruction publique, 21 IX 1815, an accounting of courses for 1814–1815 (AN F^{17} 2168). Leroux remarks (f. 2), about this course, that "la pathologie interne n'a été professée que par M. Pinel. Ce cours fait par un tel professeur ne peut enseigner d'être très suivi."

4 There is now a bewildering array of historical analyses of this search for signs of disease through physical diagnosis and clinicopathological correlation. Many, such as Paul Delaunay (*L'évolution des théories et de la pratique médicales* [Paris: Hippocrate, 1949]), conflate the two pathologies. Two treatments representing radically disparate methods and conceptions but both useful points of departure are: Michel Foucault, *Naissance de la clinique* [Paris: Presses Universitaires de France, 1963], and M.-J. Imbault Huart, *L'école pratique de dissection de Paris de 1750 à 1822*, thèse présentée devant l'Université de Paris I, 1973 [Lille: Service de Reproduction des Thèses, 1975], which, belying its title, is an eminently serviceable synopsis of many aspects of Paris medicine during the period stated; see esp. pp. 140–147, 164–169.

5 The former post placed Corvisart at the nerve center of internal medicine, since its location, the *Charité*, was both a critical teaching site and the faculty-identified center of research or *perfectionnement*. I thank Prof. Dale Smith for useful discussion of Corvisart's pivotal role.

6 At the same time, Antoine Fourcroy further consolidated his power through his appointment to the *conseil d'état*. Useful chronology of these events may be found in: Antoine Bayle et al., *Encyclopédie des science médicales*, II, *Biographie médicale* (Paris: Bureaux de l'Encyclopédie, 1841), and Henri Mondor, "Laennec," *Histoire de la médecine* (1958) 8: 7–17.

7 I discuss some of the more important societies later in this chapter.

8 The *Journal de médecine* was founded in 1754, had gone through various editors in the eighteenth century, and had finally ceased publication in year 2 (i.e., the twelve months beginning September 1793) of the Revolution.

9 *Journal de médecine, chirurgie, pharmacie, etc.* [henceforth abbreviated *Journal de Médecine* (an IX [1801]), I: 7–18, at pp. 7–8.

10 Ibid., 14–15; emphasis in original.

11 Mondor, "Laennec," n. 6 above; also P. Huard and M. J. Imbault-Huart, "La clinique Parisienne avant et après 1802," *Clio medica* (1975), 10: 173–182.

12 See Ackerknect, *Paris Hospital*, ch. 9, "Medical societies and journals," pp. 115–119, for a brief overview. Among the others not treated here but mentioned by Ackerknecht, are: the Société de Médecine de Paris (1796); the Société de Médecine Pratique (1802, sponsored by François Chaussier); the Société Medicopratique (1805); the Société Médicophilanthropique (1805); and the Athenée Médicale (1808, sponsored by Laennec). The first of these, and probably the most important, was steered by its secretary-general, the conservative surgeon R. B. Sabatier (1732–1811). A useful and well-contextualized look at that society and its junior counterpart, the Société Médicale d'Emulation (1796) is Terence D. Murphy's, "The French medical profession's perception of its social function between 1776 and 1830," *Medical History* (1979), 23:259–78.

13 C^{en} [Henri-Marie] Husson, "Premier mémoire historique sur l'Ecole de médecine

de Paris," *Journal de Médecine* (1800–1801), *1:* 65–73; see also N.A., "[Mémoire sur] Société de l'Ecole de médecine de Paris," ibid., 153–169.

14 Ibid.

15 This last no doubt provided for the inclusion, at least in theory, of influentials like the chemist Fourcroy and the biologist Cuvier.

16 The expenses of this society were to be borne by the faculty of the Ecole de médecine. See Husson, "Societe de l'Ecole," n. 13.

17 Ibid.

18 See, e.g., J. J. Leroux, Bayle, Fizeaux et Laennec, "Constitution medicale observée à Paris, depuis le mois de Novembre 1805, jusqu'au mois de Juin 1806, inclusivement," *Journal de Médecine* (1806), *12:* 30–39; and in most succeeding volumes of what was by now generally known as "Corvisart's journal." Later contributions were joined by A.-C. Savary (1776–1814), F. Chomel (1788–1856), and others; only after 1816, roughly speaking, did Bayle and Laennec drop out of this mammoth undertaking.

19 [R. T. H. Laennec?], Discours pour la Rentrée de la *Société d'anatomie* 1808, FMP MS 2186 (II); the qualification is necessary because these lecture notes, though attributed to Laennec and part of the Laennec archive, are not in his hand, yet seem clearly written for delivery verbatim. With this caveat in mind I will nonetheless follow the received assumption that Laennec was the lecturer at this opening ceremony. Some years later Cruveilhier revived the *Société d'anatomie.*

20 Ibid., f. 1ᵛ–2ʳ

21 The course at the faculty had been given, since 1801, by André Duméril (1774–1860), Bichat's and Dupuytren's competitor during the turn of the century *concours* for *chef des travaux anatomiques* discussed in Chapter 2; by 1808 François Chaussier may also have had a hand in it. See J. J. Leroux, Compte rendu MM. la Commission de l'instruction publique, 21 Sept. 1815, AN F¹⁷ 2170.

22 Laennec, Discours pour la Rentrée, ff. 2ᵛ, 4ʳ. Caroline Hannaway is preparing a study of French comparative anatomy and medicine during the period treated here. She demonstrates convincingly that veterinary medicine and animal dissection played a modest but significant role in the development of human medicine and pathological anatomy.

23 Ibid., f. 4ᵛ–5ʳ.

24 Bayle, *Encyclopédie,* n. 6, and Jean Cruveilhier, *Vie de Dupuytren* (Paris: Bechet Jeune et Labé, 1841).

25 [René Dupuytren], Extrait d'un Mémoire sur l'Anatomie pathologique, lu à l'Ecole de Médecine de Paris, par le citoyen Dupuytren," *Journal de Médecine* (1802), *4:* 575–83.

26 Jean Cruveilhier, *Vie de Dupuytren* (Paris: Bechet Jeune et Labe, 1841), pp. 20–25.

27 Ibid., p. 42.

28 R. T. H. Laennec, "D'inflammation du péritoine, recueillies à la clinique interne de l'école de médecine de Paris, sous les yeux des professeurs Corvisart et J. J. Leroux," *Journal de Médecine* (1802), *4:* 499–547.

29 See also "Sur des tuniques qui enveloppent certains viscères, et fournissent des gaines membraneuses à leurs vaisseaux," Ibid. (1802–1803), *5:* 539–75.

30 R. T. H. Laennec, "Note sur l'anatomie pathologique," *Journal de Médecine* (1804), *9:*360–78.

31 Ibid., pp. 362–63.

32 Ibid., pp. 366–67. Also of note in Laennec's hierarchy of pathological alterations, inflammatory changes were well separated from those causing either malignant or tuberculous affections. On the tendency in this period to conflate malignant and other, for example, inflammatory, tumors under various classificatory schemes see L. J. Rather, *The Genesis of Cancer* (Baltimore: Johns Hopkins University Press, 1978).

33 G. Dupuytren, "Observations sur la note relative aux altérations organiques, publiée par M. Laennec dans le dernier numéro du Journal de Médecine," *Journal*

de Médecine (1804), *9:* 441–46. Dupuytren's *Treatise* was never completed. Explaining the lapse, Cruveilhier (*Vie due Dupuytren,* n. 26 above, pp. 20–24, 35) would write that Dupuytren soon became the "slave of his professional duties" and that, absorbed by an immense surgical practice, he never had time to read to assimilate others' ideas.

34 Dupuytren, ibid.; Cruveilhier wrote (*Vie de Dupuytren,* n. 26, p. 35): "His enemies! *Voilà* the secret of his miserable life. . . . He saw them everywhere forming coalitions against him, taking away his favorite students; he saw them spying, penetrating his amphitheater . . . poisoning his success, exaggerating his faults and reverses," ending in an utter sense of isolation. In a useful article, Huard and Imbault-Huart allude to the debate with Laennec and to Dupuytren's "polemic," noting that it led to the dissolution of the *Société d'anatomie* in 1809 as well as to the cessation of Dupuytren's teaching in pathological anatomy: "La formation de l'oeuvre scientifique de Dupuytren (1777–1835)," *Histoire des sciences médicales* (1978), *12:* 217–31.

35 R. T. H. Laennec, "Réponse aux observations, etc., de M. Dupuytren," *Journal de Médecine* (1804), *10:* 89–95.

36 G. Dupuytren, "Nouvelles observations de M. Dupuytren sur la Note de M. Laennec," *Journal de Médecine* (1804), *10:* 96–102.

37 Mirko D. Grmek, "L'invention de l'auscultation médiate, retouchés à un cliché historique," in A. J. Rose, ed., *Commemoration du Bicentenaire de la Naissance de Laennec, 1781–1826: Colloque Organisé au Collège de France les 18 et 19 février 1981, Revue de Palais de la Découverte,* N° spécial 22, 1981, pp. 107–116. See also, in the same volume, M.-J. Imbault-Huart, "Bayle, Laennec, et le méthode anatomo-clinique." Ibid., pp. 79–90.

38 R. T. H. Laennec, "Anatomie pathologique," Adelon et al., eds., *Dictionnaire des Sciences Médicales* (Paris: Panckoucke, 1812–1822), vol. *II,* pp. 46–61.

39 G. L. Bayle, *Recherches sur la Phthisie Pulmonaire* (Paris: Gabon, 1810).

40 Ibid., p. 335. On Bayle's position vis-à-vis Laennec and Dupuytren, see Alfred Rouxeau, *Laennec après 1806* (Paris: Baillière, 1920), p. 74.

41 Ibid., pp. 336–41.

42 G. L. Bayle, "Considerations générales sur les secours que l'anatomie pathologique peut fournir à la médecine," in Adelon et al., *Dictionnaire* (n. 38), pp. 61–79.

43 Ibid, pp. 65–66.

44 Ibid, p. 69. Bayle's "physical symptoms" are related to, if not coextensive with, the elicited physical *sign* of which historians of this period have made much: see Imbault-Huart, "Bayle, Laennec, et le méthode anatomo-clinique," n. 37; and P. Huard, "La clinique Parisienne avant et après 1802," (n. 11). In these articles. Imbault-Huart engages in a nice dispute with Michel Foucault (*Naissance de la Clinique* [Paris: Presses Universitaires de France, 1963]) over whether to credit Bichat or Bayle with this notion. Even if I were certain whether Bayle meant the modern "sign" when he spoke of the "physical symptom," which I am not, I would be agnostic about the issue. Certainly Bayle was more concerned, and more concerned over a much longer period of years, about the symmetry and reciprocal relations between antemortem and postmortem findings.

45 Bayle, ibid., pp. 74–76.

CHAPTER 4

1 On the faculty's suppression in 1822 see Chapter 6, "Channel Crossing."

2 M. Leveille, *Mémoire sur l'état actuel de l'enseignement de la médecine et la chirurgie en France, et sur les modifications dont il est susceptible* (Paris: Dentu, 1816), p. 16. For a related argument see also A.-A. Royer-Collard, "L'institut de médecine de Paris," (Paris, 1810), in F[17] 2167.

3 De Grosbois, *Rapport de la Commission nommée par l'Ordonnance du Roi du 9 Novembre 1815, à l'effet de Lui rendre compte de l'Etat Actuel de l'Enseignement de la Médecine et de la Chirurgie en France* (Paris: Croullebois, 1816), pp. 5, 12–13, 16.

4 See, e.g., De Mercy, "Plan d'organisation de l'art médicale," Paris, 1815, pp. 61–85.

5 More detail is provided in the authoritative article by George Weisz, "Constructing the medical elite in France: the creation of the Royal Academy of Medicine, 1814–1820," *Medical History* (1986), *30:* 419–43; see esp. part 2, "The campaign to separate surgery from medicine."

6 See, e.g. De Montaigu, "Obervations des médecins de l'Hôtel-Dieu de Paris sur une réclamation," Paris, Egron, 1818, pp. 1–17, for a bald statement of this discontent.

7 Even at this level the gender denomination is appropriate. Virtually all *officiers de santé* were male, while the category of *sages-femmes*, also subjected to rigid scrutiny by the newly founded medical juries, was occupied by female practitioners.

8 There is no focussed study of this intriguing problem; but of considerable help is Dora B. Weiner, "French doctors face war, 1792–1815," in C. K. Warner, ed., *From the Ancien Régime to the Popular Front: Essays in the History of Modern France in Honor of Shepard B. Clough* (New York: Columbia University Press, 1969), pp. 151–73. A good overview of the *officiers de santé* cadre, their origins, regulation, and fate, to which I adhere for the most part in this section, is Robert Heller, "*Officiers de santé:* the second-class doctors of nineteenth-century France," *Medical History* (1978), *22:*25–43. Heller's account usefully appends a full translation of the 1803 law.

9 Heller, ibid., passim. That data on the makeup of the juries is sparse is partly because most of the demographic data were turned back to the individual départements, whose archives therefore now house most of the juries' records. See, e.g., Département de la Seine Inférieure, "Tableau des Docteurs en Médecine et des chirurgiens de ce Département qui on été reçus dans les collèges et qui sont presentés par le Préfet pour la formation du Jury de Médecine," Archives départementales de Seine Maritime 5MP 2696 (an XI [1803]). For Paris see [Bonaparte], "Arrête qui nomme les commissaires pour présider [sur] les Jurys de médecine dans les arrondissemens des Ecoles de Paris, de Montpellier, de Strasbourg, et les membres des Jurys dans plusieurs départmens," AN AD VIII 30 (October 1803). For Isère and other departements, see Décrets et Arrête sur la création, le renouvellement ou le maintien des Jurys . . . dans les Départements de l'Empire: Archives départementales d'Isère, 2 T 9.

10 Rapport de la commission d'instruction publique et project de résolution sur les examens des officiers de santé (24 November 1798), AN AD VIII 30.

11 Most of these appeals and some of Thouret's responses are collated in AN F^{17} 2287.

12 Michel Thouret, Rapport fait an nom de la Section de l'Intérieur, sur le projet de loi rélatif à l'éxercise de la médecine, 16 Ventôse an 11. AN AD VIII 33. For a list of the commissioners chosen, see Minister of Interior to Bonaparte, arrête de 29 Brumaire an XII (20 Nov. 1803), F^{17} 2386.

13 Ibid.

14 Ministère de l'Intérieur, Convocation des Jurys de Médecine pour l'an 13 (29 Prairial an XIII [17 June 1805]); AN AD VIII 30.

15 Procès-verbal des Operations du Jury Medical du Département de l'Isère du 3 Brumaire au 14 et jours suivants, an XIV. Archives départementales de l'Isère 2 T 9.

16 Procès-verbaux des séances [du Jury medical] du département de la Gironde pendant cette session [1816]; Archives départementales de Gironde, 5 M 2.

17 Procès-verbaux des opérations du Jury médical de Département de l'Isère, Session de 1821. Archives départementales d'Isère, 2 T 9.

18 *Traité d'Anatomie pathologique ou Exposition des altérations visibles qu'éprouve le corps humain dans l'aaetat de maladie,* MS FMP 2186 (III a); a nineteenth-century edition of this MS was published by V. Cornil as *Traite inédit sur l'anatomie pathologique . . .* (Paris: Felix Alcan, 1884).

19 Ibid, pp. 14ʳ–14ᵛ. Nonetheless, Laennec averred, Germany was not without its zealous pathological anatomists, mentioning in particular Conrad (*Handbuch der pathologischen anatomie*, 1796) and Vetter (*Aphorismen aus der pathologischen anatomie*, 1803).

20 Ibid., pp. 15ʳ–15ᵛ.

21 The postmortem reports, coming mainly from the Hôtel-Dieu, the Hôpital Necker and the Hôpital de la Charité, are preserved primarily at the Bibliothèque Universitaire de Nantes, whose permission to examine them I gratefully acknowledge. Most are housed in Classeurs I, II, and III, as well as in a few of the consultation reports in Classeur 1, in the Musée Laennec of that institution. A full and most helpful description is in Lydie Boulle, Mirko D. Grmek, and Janine Samion-Contet, eds., *Laennec: Catalogue des Manuscrits Scientifiques* (Paris: Masson, 1982), pp. 11–87.

22 Nantes MS Cl. 1, lot f [VI], feuillets 186ʳ–189ᵛ.

23 *A Medical Bibliography* of Fielding Garrison and Leslie Morton (4th ed. [London: Gower, 1983], p. 358), for example, locates the work squarely among exclusively *diagnostic* texts from Sir John Floyer on the pulse-watch to Ian Donald on ultrasonographic diagnosis of abdominal masses.

24 *Traite d'Auscultation Médiate, ou Traité du Diagnostic des Maladies des Poumons et du Coeur* (2 vols., Paris: Brosson & Chaude, 1819), ii:128–43.

25 Andre Hahn, "Laennec à la Faculté de Médecine," *Histoire de la médecine* (1958), 8: 17–31.

26 Laenneck [sic], "Régistre des délibérations prises aux Assemblés des Lecteurs et Professeurs du Roi au Collège de France depuis le 9 Janvier 1780," Archives du Collège de France G.II.3, pp. 185–87. I thank M.-C. Delangle, archivist of the Collège, for allowing me to examine these materials. I know of no adequate treatment of this episode. But see Yves Laporte, "Allocution d'ouverture," in *Laennec, 1781–1826: Colloque organisé au Collège de France les 181 et 19 février 1981*, Revue du Palais de la Découverte, N° spécial 22, Août 1981, pp. 12–21; and J. Jolly, "Les sciences biologiques au Collège de France," ch. VIII, pp. 133–45 in A. Lefranc et al., *Le Collège de France (1530–1930)* (Paris: P.U.F., 1932).

27 Ibid.

28 Yves Laporte, "Allocution d'ouverture," n. 26 above pp. 20—21.

29 I comment further in my review of the catalog of Grmek et al. (n. 21): Compare *Isis* (1984), 75: 442. On the lecture notes a useful point of departure is Erwin H. Ackerknecht, "Laennec und sein Vorlesungsmanuskript von 1822," *Gesnerus* (1964), 21: 142–54.

30 Nantes MSS, Musée Laennec, Cl. 2, Lot a[B]. Unpaginated.

31 Ibid., 27th lecture.

32 Ibid., lecture 45.

33 For the intimate biographical details see the standard work by the author who provided the basic classification for the Laennec archives: Alfred Rouxeau, *Laennec après 1806: 1806–1826, d'après des Documents Inédits* (Paris: Baillière, 1920); see especially pp. 385–98.

CHAPTER 5

1 The role of the surgeon–apothecary is the usual choice for historians wishing to identify the "precursor" of the general practitioner in England. Among the best accounts that adopt this approach are: Irvine S. L. Loudon and Rosemary Stevens, "Primary Care and the Hospital," in John Fry, ed., *Primary Care* (London: Heinemann, 1980), pp. 139–75; M. Jeanne Peterson, *The Medical Profession in Mid-Victorian London* (Berkeley: University of California Press, 1978) and what is probably the most detailed account: Rachel E. Franklin, "Medical Education and the Rise of the General practitioner, 1760 to 1860," unpublished doctoral dissertation, Faculty of Medicine, University of Birmingham (England), 1950.

2 Adroitly making this point is Othmar Keel in his useful recent essay, "The politics of health and the institutionalisation of clinical practices in Europe in the second

half of the eighteenth century," pp. 207–56 in W. F. Bynum and Roy Porter, eds, *William Hunter and the Eighteenth Century Medical World* (Cambridge, England: Cambridge University Press, 1985); compare esp. pp. 233–34.

3 See Peterson (n. 1), p. 21; An analogous position may be perceived in the discipline of chemistry in the same period: compare Robert F. Bud, "The Discipline of Chemistry: The Origins and Early Years of the Chemical Society of London," (unpublished doctoral dissertation, University of Pennsylvania, 1980).

4 James D. Bailey, "The Medical Societies of London," *British Medical Journal,* (1895), 2:25. See also D'Arcy Power, ed., *British Medical Societies* (London: The Medical Press and Circular, 1939).

5 Norman Moore and Stephen Paget, *The Royal Medical and Chirurgical Society of London Centenary, 1805 to 1905* (Aberdeen: Aberdeen University Press, 1905), esp. pp. 2–3. The careful balance between physicians and surgeons with respect to numbers within the membership was no mere accident: there were thirteen surgeons and thirteen physicians as ordinary members; of these, six surgeons and eleven physicians were committee members such that the physicians dominated the inner circle.

6 For an example of this style and its transitional form after 1810, see pp. 123, 176–197.

7 Moore and Paget, *The Royal Medical and Chirurgical Society* (n. 5), p. 29.

8 Ibid., p. 75 and passim.

9 Ibid., pp. 88–89.

10 Christopher Lawrence, "Ornate physicians and learned artisans: Edinburgh medical men, 1726–1776," pp. 153–76, in W. F. Bynum and Roy Porter, eds., *William Hunter and the Eighteenth Century Medical World* (Cambridge, England: Cambridge University Press, 1985). Lawrence discerns in the Munros an interest in crucial problems like edema and hydrothorax, problems that will by now be readily recognized to be resonant with the concerns of the nascent Bichatian school in France.

11 Guenter Risse, *Hospital Life in Enlightenment Scotland* (Cambridge: Cambridge University Press, 1986), pp. 287–95.

12 See Chapter 6.

13 Lawrence, "Ornate physicians," n. 10, 163; the quotation is from p. 161.

14 Risse, *Hospital Life,* (n. 11), 261–66.

15 L. S. Jacyna, "Images of John Hunter in the nineteenth century," *History of Science* (1983), *21:* 85–108.

16 Ibid.

17 John Hunter, *The Works of John Hunter, F.R.S., with Notes,* ed. James F. Palmer (London: Longman, Rees, 1837). 4 vols.; vol. III, pp. 349–50, and (on the "Animal Oeconomy," first published 1786, 2nd ed. 1792) vol. IV in toto. Instructive with respect to Hunter as comparative anatomist is Richard Owen's 1837 "Preface" (pp. i-xl) lamenting the lack of attention, especially from Cuvier and the continental school of comparative anatomy, to Hunter's work on this field, "meting out but scanty justice to the author of the Treatise on the Blood and of the Observations on the Animal Oeconomy, which abound with so many general propositions in comparative anatomy and physiology" (v). With this new edition of Hunter's fully collected works, claimed Owen, the oversight became "unpardonable."

18 Hunter, *Works* (n. 17), vol. III.

19 Ibid., vol. III, p. 363.

20 Cf. chs. I and II.

21 Jacyna, "Images of John Hunter" (n. 15).

22 Susan Lawrence, *Science and medicine at the London Hospitals: the Development of Teaching and Research, 1750–1815* (doctoral dissertation, University of Toronto, 1985); cf. esp. ch. 9. Only Keel ("The politics of health," n. 2) makes an unqualified claim for the importance of the Hunterian *problématique,* "one of whose leading characteristics [was] *the interpenetration of medicine and surgery.*" This claim, to reiterate, though it seems reasonable for the Hunters and their earliest followers,

must be carefully hedged by recalling that medicine and surgery remained distinct in Britain and that theoretical pathological anatomy, though adumbrated by John Hunter, was not, in fact, enrooted by his later followers. Meanwhile, as S. Lawrence (ibid., ch. 12) shows, as far as practical pathological anatomy was concerned, London hospital physicians (with the notable exceptions of Matthew Baillie and John Yelloly) left postmortem dissection to the labors of their surgical colleagues; cf. esp. pp. 576–90.

23 I extend this point to London, but the quotation refers only to the Edinburgh scene in C. Lawrence's useful recent overview of that topic: "Ornate physicians," (n. 10), at p. 173.

24 This interpretation is possible both in traditional and revisionist views. The standard, older account most often cited is Charles Newman, *The Evolution of Medical Education in the Nineteenth Century* (London: Oxford University Press, 1957); a modern sociological view, while rehearsing the controversy about this interpretation, that maintains the essential evolutionary sequence is Noel and Jose Parry, *The Rise of the Medical Profession: A Study of Collective Social Mobility* (London: Croom Helm, 1976).

25 Newman, *Evolution of Medical Education*, n. 24, p. 75.

26 For other versions of this interpretation see S. W. F. Holloway, "The Apothecaries Act, 1815: A reinterpretation," *Medical History* (1966) *10*:107–29, 221–36.

27 Such accounts, typified by Holloway, "The Apothecaries Act," n. 26, are more valuable particularly with respect to the apothecaries' role in stimulating the growth of new institutions.

28 Holloway, "The Apothecaries Act." The quotation is to be found on p. 129.

29 Ibid., p. 128.

30 M. J. Peterson (n. 1) provides the one recent account that does seem to note, if only in passing, the significance of this state of affairs; see pp. 17–22.

31 Robert Masters Kerrison, "Observations and Reflections on the Bill Now in Progress through the House of Commons, for 'Better Regulating the Medical Profession as Far as Regards Apothecaries,' " (London, 1815) p. 326.

32 Peterson, *The Medical Profession* (n. 1) pp. 20–21.

33 Kerrison, "Observations and Reflections," (n. 31), p. 315.

34 Ibid.

35 Holloway, "The Apothecaries Act," (n. 26), p. 128.

36 Ibid., p. 119.

37 Kerrison, "Observations and Reflections," p. 322.

38 See *Transactions of the Associated Apothecaries and Surgeon – Apothecaries of England and Wales* (London: Burgess and Hill, 1823), p. xci for the group's composition, bearing out this notion in 1822/23.

39 Ibid., p. viii.

40 See Kerrison (n. 31), p. 81.

41 *Transactions* (n. 38), p. xli.

42 Ibid.

43 Ibid., pp. lvi, lxiv.

44 See Chapter 7.

45 David Allen, *The Naturalist in Britain* (London: Allen Lane, 1976).

46 Ibid., p. 107.

47 See Great Britain, Parliament, House of Commons, Report from the Select Committee on Medical Education (London: 1834), Appendix 24.

48 See Great Britain, Parliament, House of Commons, Report from the Select Committee on the Matter of Obtaining Subjects for Dissection in the Schools of Anatomy, and into the Laws Affecting Persons Employed in Obtaining or Dissecting Bodies (Session 1828, 568. Volume 7, pp. 1–550); hereafter I shall refer to this document as *SCA* (1828), and the former report as *SCME* (1834).

49 Newman, (n. 24), p. 107; *SCME* (1834) III, Appendix 24, pp. 120–24.

50 Testimony of J. Rideout in Newman (n. 49), p. 41.

51 Incentives that gave rise to this demand form the subject of the first part of Chapter 6.

52 The College of Surgeons, of course, and only that body, did require dissection; but see Newman, *Evolution of Medical Education*, n. 24, p. 106, and *SCA* (1828), passim., regarding its inadequacy. The effects of changing regulations at the Royal College of Surgeons in the 1820s are also discussed in Chapter 7.

53 *Allison v. Haydon*, 1828, quoted in Holloway, "The Apothecaries Act," (n. 26) p. 129.

54 Kerrison, *Inquiry*, pp. 90–91.

55 [Charles Haden], "Introductory essay," *Transactions of the Associated Apothecaries and Apothecary–Surgeons* (n. 38), pp. i–cxl; and Thomas Alcock, "An Essay on the Education and Duties of the General Practitioner in Medicine and Surgery," ibid., pp. 57–133.

56 Haden, "Introductory essay" (n. 55), p. xciii.

57 Alcock, "Essay on the education and duties," (n. 55) p. 128.

58 For a list of the various modes of certification, see Peterson, *The Medical Profession* (n. 1), pp. 289–90.

59 A related example is that provided by John Saunders, discussed in Chapter 8.

60 *Medico-Chirurgical Review*, 1824, 1:iii; the passage was probably written by James Johnson (1777–1845), discussed below.

61 On this point see Allen, *The Naturalist in Britain* (n. 45).

62 Philip Gaskell, *A New Introduction to Bibliography* (New York: Oxford University Press, 1972), p. 298; see also pages 251–58, 297–300.

63 Long-range survival of journals was another matter. Many of them did, in fact, become absorbed or defunct after a very few years.

64 See, e.g., "Preface, Advertisement, Address and a Rare Wack at the Voracious Bats, Not Forgetting a Few Useful Hints to Our Beloved but Cruelly-Plundered Friends, the British Students of Medicine," *Lancet*, 1831–32, i, pp. 1–16.

65 J. F. Clark, *Autobiographical Recollections of the Medical Profession* (London: Churchill, 1874, 1874); see pp. 34–35 regarding Cooper v. Wakley.

66 Also included were John Bostock of Liverpool, John Richard Farre from the London Dispensary (Chapter 8), Edward Jenner from Cheltenham, and a number of other key figures; see *Medico – Chirurgical Transactions* (1805–1809, 1:ix–xiii; the membership list is on pp. xiv–xvii.

67 In this forum one sees the process of chemistry being grafted aggressively onto physicians' humoralist suite of ideas. Such a process is evident for example in the work of John Bostock; see also, e.g., Alexander Marcet, "A Chemical Account of Various Dropsical Fluids," ibid., pp. 340–81.

68 Ibid., p. 236.

69 Ibid., p. 240.

70 Ibid., p. 241.

71 Ibid.

72 Ibid., p. 237.

73 Ibid., p. 258.

74 Young cited (p. 262) a similar case of which he had been made aware, noting it had been published "a few years since" in the *Bulletin de l'Ecole de médecine de Paris*.

CHAPTER 6

1 An important recent example is Othmar Keel, *La Généalogie de l'Histopathologie: Une révision déchirante Philippe Pinel, lecteur discret de J.-C. Smyth* (Paris: Vrin, 1979). Keel's monograph is instructive in two respects. It deals specifically with the origins of tissue pathology, an intellectual tradition that served, in fact, as the medium of discourse for the Anglo-French medical relations during the period under discussion. Keel's thesis is also instructive with respect to the limitations of the "hierarchy-of-texts" approach to medical history. His contention seems to be that, having traced the notion of tissue specificity to James C. Smyth (1741–1821), a London-based Scot, he thereby upends previous historiographic notions. If, however, innovation involves elements of the amplification and dissemination

of ideas, not just their isolated proposition, then Keel's claims for the British origins of histopathology are probably not quite as "déchirante" as he suggests.

2 I have discussed the impact of these techniques in two articles: "Rudolf Virchow, Julius Cohnheim, and the program of pathology," *Bulletin of the History of Medicine* (1978), 52:162–82; and "Pathology," in Ronald L. Numbers, ed., *The Education of American Physicians* (Berkeley: University of California Press, 1980), pp. 122–42.

3 [Review of] John Forbes, *Original Cases Illustrating the Use of the Stethoscope and Percussion in the Diagnosis of Disease of the Chest* (London: Underwood, 1824), *Anderson's Quarterly Journal of Medical Sciences* (1824), 1:625.

4 There is no reliably exhaustive guide to translations published in Britain. Useful, however, is Eric Gaskell, "Early American English translations of European medical works," *Medical History*, (1970), 14:300–307.

5 On Laennec's students, see Pierre Huard and Mirko D. Grmek, "Les élèves étrangers de Laennec," *Revue d'histoire des sciences*, 1973, 26: 315–37. The standard work on the Paris experience in this period remains E. H. Ackerknecht, *Medicine at the Paris Hospital, 1794–1848* (Baltimore: The Johns Hopkins University Press, 1970). See esp. ch. 16, "Foreign Students and Doctors," pp. 191–94.

6 R. T. H. Laennec, *De l'auscultation médiate, ou traité du diagnostic des maladies des poumons et du coeur* (Paris: Brosson et Chaude, 1819).

7 Archives Nationales, Paris, AJ¹⁶6313.

8 This was, of course, precisely the circumstance in which Bichat and his students in pathological anatomy found themselves at the turn of the century when he failed to obtain the post of *Chef des travaux anatomiques* at the Paris Faculty.

9 Archives Nationales, Paris, AJ¹⁶21.

10 The closely observed balance and symmetry between these two entities was part of the carefully nurtured *rapprochement* between medicine and surgery at the Paris Faculty.

11 Both by death, and by the practice of *mutation*, the faculty roster did slowly change, of course, over time. I give here that for the winter of 1821–22 (AN, AJ¹⁶21, dossier 4).

12 Jean Cruveilhier, *Médecine éclairée par l'anatomie et la phisiologie pathologique* (Paris, 1821); in the same place, *Anatomie pathologique du corps humain* (Paris, 1830–42).

13 Throughout the period under discussion, the chair at the Collège de France remained the sole medical post at that institution.

14 The implied contention should be made explicit: the microscope was instrumental in this process. See Maulitz, "Rudolph Virchow, Julius Cohnheim, and the program of pathology," 162–82; and *idem*, "Pathology," in *The Education of American Physicians*.

15 On the epistemological basis of the new methods, see: Michel Foucault, *Naissance de la clinique* (Paris: Presses Universitaires de France, 1963), and Georges Canguilhem, *On the Normal and the Pathological* (Dordrecht: Reidel, 1978). On the institutional basis, see Marie-José Imbault-Huart, "L'Ecole Pratique de dissection de 1750 à 1822," (Thesis, Université de Paris, 1973) and Toby Gelfand, *Professionalizing Modern Medicine* (Westport, Conn.: Greenwood Press, 1980).

16 Henri Meding, *Paris Médical: Vade-Mecum des médecins étrangers* (Paris, Baillière, 1853), p. 323.

17 See M. J. Durey, "Body-snatchers and Benthamites: the implications of the dead body bill for the London schools of anatomy, 1820–42," *London Journal* (1970, 2:200–225; see also Great Britain, Parliament, House of Commons, *Report from the Select Committee on the manner of obtaining subjects for dissection in the schools of anatomy, and into the laws affecting persons employed in obtaining or dissecting bodies* (Session 1829, 568. Vol. 7, pp. 1–550); see especially pp. 26ff. Benjamin Brodie, testifying before the Select Committee, claimed that the resistance in England to postmortem examinations *per se* decreased as the 1820s wore on. Hereafter I refer to this work as *SCR, Anatomy*.

18 More information about this phenomenon can be found in two additional articles:

Lester S. King and Marjorie C. Meehan, "The history of the autopsy," *American Journal of Pathology* (1973), *73*:514–44; and Alan F. Guttmacher, "Bootlegging bodies: a history of body snatching," *Bulletin of the Society of Medical History (Chicago)*, (1935), *4*:353–402.

19 Even before hostilities ended between England and France, it was theoretically possible, if only rarely undertaken, for students from English-speaking countries to take the diploma of the Paris Faculty. This was an unusual circumstance, however, requiring four years of time and an expenditure of substantial funds, and it remained unusual throughout the period here under discussion. It is therefore entirely true, as R. M. Jones has pointed out for the case of American students in the 1830s, that the surviving inscription registers afford no clear-cut determination of the absolute number of students from any given country studying in Paris. But a rough idea of this number is available by other means; see note 20. Jones's analysis is to be found in his "Introduction" to the *Parisian Education of an American Surgeon* (Philadelphia: American Philosophical Society, 1978), pp. 1–70, especially pp. 1–5. Since Professor Jones's important work, Catherine Moureaux, Archiviste de l'Université, has compiled a partially rectified list of foreign students in the Paris registers; I wish to thank her for providing access to these documents during research for this book.

20 Manipulating the data derived from these registers is most instructive if one assumes that the ratio of those inscribing to those not doing so remained roughly constant. The latter group consisted of those enrolled only in private courses (of which no systematic records survive), or merely taking advantage of the forbearance of the French authorities in regard to free attendance at official lectures and clinics. The problem is that of an indeterminate denominator in a ratio that one might wish to see held constant. What therefore remains to be seen is the extent to which the change in the number of Paris Faculty registrants is in fact an adequate indicator of the actual rate of increase in the overall number of English medical students streaming to Paris. The evidence for this contention is circumstantial but persuasive. That the graph of Paris faculty registrants responds precisely to the sort of social and institutional pressures, and at precisely the "right" moments, that one would expect the missing graph of overall students to reflect, must be discounted as both a historically and statistically improper inference. But the information available suggests that there were no intervening factors in the 1820s that would have made a student more likely to inscribe for the diploma, thus skewing the curve and imposing on it a speciously increased slope. If anything, the reverse was true: not only were there progressively more options for a reasonably promising level of certification on one's return to England in the course of the period between 1816 and 1830, but it became progressively easier, at least during the first half of that period, for those desiring lecture tickets at the faculty to obtain forgeries from black marketeers, for the nominal outlay of a *douceur* to the forger. The forgery problem was said to have had a part in precipitating the notorious *affaire Bertin* that closed down the Faculty in the winter of 1822–23.

21 That is, the conditions stated (n. 20) are a reasonable account of those that obtained.

22 It is difficult to determine the number of private courses, which varied widely from year to year, but see AN, AJ[16]21, which provides a list of *cours particuliers* for 1822. Thirty-six private courses are listed, including offerings from the likes of Magendie, Breschet, Lisfranc, Dupuytren, Rayer, and Spurzheim.

23 The notion of *terminaison* (roughly, termination) was an important one that represented a holdover or bridging idea between the current Bichatian system of tissue pathology and an older medical pathology that relied on natural history concepts. *Terminaison*, which implied both the final appearance of the lesion and the point at which the patient's illness reached a plateau, was an especially commodious concept.

24 Jones, *Parisian Education* (note 19), pp. 22–25; also R. C. Maulitz, "A Treatise on Membranes: Concepts of Tissue Structure, Function, and Dysfunction from

Xavier Bichat to Julius Cohnheim," (doctoral dissertation, Duke University, 1973) for discussion of Bichat and tissue pathology.

25   On the Edinburgh picture generally, see Anand Chitnis, "Medical Education in Edinburgh, 1790–1826, and Some Victorian Social Consequences," *Medical History* (1973), *17*:173–85. On Edinburgh–London rivalry in medical education, see Noel and Jose Parry, *The Rise of the Medical Profession: A Study of Collective Social Mobility* (London: Croom Helm, 1976), pp. 105–107.

26   To identify this receptivity with "French ideas and techniques" would be to oversimplify the position. In the first place, the now-dominant Bichatian mode of tissue pathology was not, strictly speaking, a French innovation at all. It could have sprung equally well from the English Hunter–Baillie tradition, had English medicine and surgery been in a position to foster it. But it was the French who seized on the pathology of tissues and textures that had been generated in both countries in the 1790s and it was elaborated most completely by Xavier Bichat in 1799–1801; and it was the French who put this knowledge to work in the clinic. On the availability of the tissue model in both medical cultures, see Keel, *La Généalogie* (note 1). The Scottish knew all this. What they did not know at all well in the period 1816–20 were the French techniques of percussion and auscultation. Physical diagnosis did not, therefore, loom large in this earliest expression of a British (and mainly Scottish) inclination toward Paris.

27   W. H. McMenemey, *The Life and Times of Charles Hastings* (Edinburgh and London: Livingstone, 1959), pp. 19–34; cf. p. 19. See also *The Scottish Nation*, vol. II, pp. 89–90.

28   Andrew Duncan, Jr., to Andrew Duncan, Sr., 13 January 1795; Andrew Duncan Correspondence, Edinburgh University Library, MS Dc.1.90 (Letters and Papers, 1818–22). John Forbes, in his "Translator's Preface" to the first English edition of Laennec's *Médiate Auscultation* (London: Underwood, 1821), pp. vii–xxviii, expatiated at some length on Duncan's role. Forbes identified Duncan, along with James Clark in Rome, as prime movers in gaining adherents for Laennec's method; see especially pp. xx–xxi.

29   James Clark to Théophile Laennec, 12 May 1823. Musée Laennec, Nantes.

30   *Transactions of the Medico-Chirurgical Society (Edinburgh)*, (1824), I:470–650. According to Keel, *Généalogie*, Smyth was the "missing link" in the tissue pathology tradition. But see Edwin Ackerknecht's percipient review of this book and its central tenet re Smyth's role in *Gesnerus* (1980), *37*:147–48. Ackerknecht correctly points to the intellectualist fallacy involved in this argument. He notes that there is more to intellectual history than the antecedents of a given idea without careful attention to context – such that establishing anteriority becomes somewhat pointless in the history of ideas.

31   It was at Duncan's behest that a young Englishman, Charles Locock, published an early (1821) Edinburgh M.D. thesis on auscultation. See Saul Jarcho, "An early mention of the stethoscope (Locock 1821)," *Bulletin of the New York Academy of Medicine* (1965), *41*:374–77; and R. C. Maulitz, "Metropolitan medicine and the man–midwife: the early life and letters of Charles Locock," *Medical History* (1982), *26*.

32   John Thomson, *Lectures on Inflammation, Exhibiting a View of the General Doctrines, Pathological and Practical, of Medical Surgery* (Edinburgh: Blackwood, 1818).

33   "Notice of some of the leading Events of the life of the late Dr. John Thomson. . . ," *Edinburgh Medical–Surgical Journal* (1847), *67*:131–93; pp. 81–82.

34   Ibid., p. 188.

35   Ibid., pp. 188–90.

36   J. D. Comrie, *History of Scottish Medicine to 1860*, 2nd ed. (London: Wellcome Research Institution, 1932), p. 506.

37   Carswell's paintings and drawings are currently housed in the University College, Medical School Library, London; many of them became the basis for the important atlas, *Pathological Anatomy* (London, 1838), which reflected unequivocally the French influence.

38 C. J. B. Williams, *Memoirs of Life and Work* (London: Smith, Elder, 1884), pp. 10–19; the quotation is found on p. 11.

39 See, e.g., S. J. Reiser, "Aspects of the role of the stethoscope in the introduction of auscultation to Great Britain and the United States," *Proceedings 23rd International Congress of the History of Medicine,* [London, 1972] (London, 1974), 1:832–40; S. J. Reiser, *Medicine and the Reign of Technology* (Cambridge: Cambridge University Press, 1978), ch. 2, "The Stethoscope and the Detection of Pathology by Sound," pp. 23–44; George Rosen, "A note on the reception of the stethoscope in England," *Bulletin of the History of Medicine* (1939), 7:93–94; and Saul Jarcho, "Early mention of the stethoscope."

40 [Review of] Charles Scudamore, *Observations on M. Laennec's Method of Forming a Diagnosis of Diseases of the Chest, by means of the Stethoscope, and Percussion; and upon some Points of the French Practice of Medicine* (London, 1826), *Anderson's Quarterly Journal of Medicine and Surgery* (1826), 3:525.

41 These developments must be seen against the wider background of the general decline of science controversy that engaged elite English academics and professional men during the second quarter of the nineteenth century.

42 The dramatic increase in numbers through the mid-1820s no doubt served to heighten the alarm mounting at home among educators and parliamentarians: thus, the timing of the Select Committee's deliberations, beginning in 1828, was far from coincidental.

43 On early skepticism about the interposition of instrumentation between patient and medical man, see Reiser, *Medicine and the Reign of Technology.*

44 A plot of the cumulative number of journal "starts" over this period reveals, in fact, an almost perfect exponential growth curve; see W. R. Lefanu, "British periodicals of medicine: A chronological list," *Bulletin of the History of Medicine,* 1937, 5: 735–61.

45 This was the dictum of a detractor, in a review of Bouillaud's treatise on encephalitis, in *Anderson's Quarterly Journal of Medicine and Surgery* (1826), 3:48.

46 One of the excuses made, as noted earlier, was the difficulty of managing the problem of students gaining admission with false entrance cards (AN, AJ[16]21, dossier 4).

47 Though the actual period of closure was relatively brief, the "ripple effect" of the *désordres* was real enough, and was reflected in English enrollments (Fig. 6.1).

48 There seems, in other words, to have been a suppressive or retardant effect followed by a release effect generated by the Faculty's 1823 troubles. The extent to which these effects were mirrored in overall foreign enrollments and studies in Paris by Britons is difficult to gauge. It is equally plausible, for example, to argue that the upswing in the number of English students seen in the table for 1824 was a local phenomenon confined to the Faculty itself, a result perhaps of the release phenomenon made possible by the reestablishment of a stable regime within that body. But see Ackerknecht, (n. 5), *Medicine at the Paris Hospital*, pp. 39–41.

49 SCR, *Anatomy*, (17), testimony of Thomas Wakley; in the recent secondary literature, the best chronicle of these events is M. J. Durey, "Bodysnatchers and Benthamites" (n. 17).

50 SCR, *Anatomy*, testimony of Wakley.

51 Ibid., p. 4. There is little to indicate that Paris was often "recommended by the medical establishment," but there was much to recommend it otherwise, especially for those English provincials whose local surgical academies were newly disenfranchised.

52 Ibid., pp. 51–56, 61–62, testimony of J. R. Bennett.

53 Letter from Robert Carswell to J. R. Bennett, 1 May 1828, quoted in SCR, *Anatomy*, pp. 55–56.

54 Ibid.; since Carswell estimated this number to break down into roughly half (about one hundred) the students taking out Faculty inscription tickets and the balance omitting to do so, it bears noting that the figures in his letter tally, roughly speaking, with the appropriate point on the curve in Figure 6.1.

55 Sometimes also referred to as John Richard Bennett. Bennett was an Irishman who later became part-proprietor of the private anatomy school in Little Dean Street, Soho, and still later, the first Professor of Practical Anatomy at University College, London.

56 Ibid., p. 53.

57 Ibid., pp. 53–54.

58 AN, F^{17}2182.

59 Ibid.

60 Ibid.

61 *Lancet* (1830–31), 2:401–406, 437.

62 Ibid., p. 404. I have not found corroboration elsewhere of Armstrong's reckoning of a 7:1 distribution of physicians and surgeons. It is, however, at least plausible: whereas surgeons continued to seek instruction in practical and pathological anatomy as a means of honing their therapeutic skills, the physicians were even more strongly drawn to the Bichat–Laennec system as a means of refining their diagnostic ability.

63 Williams, *Memoirs* (n. 38), pp. 29–32, 42–47. W. F. Edwards is a particularly intriguing and overlooked figure in any account of international medical and scientific relations during this period. Little is written about this Englishman who was naturalized as a French citizen, and who would be a central figure in this account if medical chemistry rather than pathological anatomy were the chosen leitmotif. His work on chemical and physical effects of the environment on living organisms, *De l'influence des agens physiques sur la vie* (Paris: Crochard, 1824) was owned (via a presentation copy) by Laennec and translated by Hodgkin into English (London: S. Highley, 1832).

64 Williams, *Memoirs* (n. 38), pp. 29–32.

65 Ibid., pp. 40–42.

66 Ibid., pp. 41–49.

CHAPTER 7

1 It was introduced initially as the *London Medical, Surgical, and Pharmaceutical Repository.*

2 A. B. Granville, *Autobiography of A. B. Granville, M.D., F.R.S., – Being Eighty-eight Years of the Life of a Physician,* II (London: Henry S. King, 1874), pp. 76–77.

3 By "passive" I mean, simply, the nonexperiential nature of this exposure to pathological anatomy. For an appraisal of the active step taken by those who traveled abroad for the *tour de main,* see Chapter 6.

4 While I have not yet located circulation figures, there is no question that the competition was fierce: see Granville, *Autobiography,* (n. 2).

5 The *Journal* actually began its existence as the *Medico-Chirurgical Journal and Review;* it changed its name approximately every two years, moving to London in 1818.

6 This account is based on standard sources including Munk's *Roll of the Royal College of Physicians,* III, pp. 238–41; *Dictionary of National Biography,* XXX, pp. 16–17; and *SCME,* 1834, pp. 235–38.

7 Charles J. B. Williams, *Memoirs of Life and Work* (London: Smith, Elder: 1884), p. 121.

8 *SCME,* 1834, p. 237.

9 In 1818 yet another review journal, *The Quarterly Journal of Foreign Medicine and Surgery,* was established. I find few data on its origins and early personnel. The *Medical Intelligencer* was unique in one key respect: It was primarily a review of reviews.

10 Granville, *Autobiography* (n. 2), pp. 174–75; Granville refused, of course, to remain an outsider for long. Like Johnson, he settled in London and became part of the new scientific establishment of moderate reformers.

11 Ibid., p. 175.

12   Charles T. Haden, *Practical Observations on the Management and Diseases of Children* (London: Burgess and Hill, 1827), pp. v–xii; Zachary Cope, "Dr. Charles T. Haden (1786–1824), a Friend of Jane Austen," *British Medical Journal*, i, 9 April 1966, p. 974.

13   Without doubt the most Francophilic of the editors, Haden was involved in the *Medical Intelligencer*, the *Journal of Popular Medicine*, and the *Transactions of the Associated Apothecaries and Apothecary–Surgeons*.

14   The publication of this work marked the intersection of the Bichatian tradition of membrane pathology and the new chemical medicine, particularly with respect to the study of chemical poisons that was coming to serve as the basis of experimental physiology: cf. John E. Lesch, *Science and Medicine in France: the Emergence of Experimental Physiology, 1790–1855* (Cambridge, Mass.: Harvard University Press, 1984). Before his early death, Haden continued to press his interest in chemical medicine, including the American edition (Philadelphia, 1824) of the Magendie *Formulary*, and a monograph of his own authorship on colchicine (London, 1820).

15   *Medical Intelligencer* (1820), 1:7, 15; John Forbes's translation superseded Haden's, and the latter's was never published.

16   Ibid., pp. 311–32.

17   Ibid., pp. 151–57, 196–202.

18   Ibid., pp. 152–53.

19   See "Researches on the Pathology of the Intestinal Canal," *Edinburgh Medical and Surgical Journal* (1820), 44:321–48.

20   Joseph Houlton, trans., Xavier Bichat, *A Treatise on the Anatomy and Physiology of the Mucous membranes, with Illustrative Pathological Observations* (London, 1821).

21   See Chapter 8.

22   Though later president of the Pathological Society, he "did not obtain the respect" of his peers in the community of morbid anatomists according to one biographer (*Dictionary of National Biography*, XII, pp. 171–72).

23   [Probably James Copeland], *London Medical Repository* (1821), XVI:462.

24   [Charles T. Haden], *Medical Intelligencer* (1822), III:119.

25   Ibid., pp. 68–69.

26   Charles T. Haden to R. T. Laennec, 13 September 1822, Musée Laennec, Nantes.

27   Charles T. Haden to Thomas Alcock, quoted by Alcock in the "Biographical Notice" in his edition of Haden's *Practical Observations* (n. 12), p. ix.

28   *Medical Intelligencer* III:iii–xix, at pp. vi–vii.

29   Alcock, "Biographical Notice", n. 27.

30   *Medical Intelligencer* (1822), 3:69.

31   *London Medical and Physical Journal* (1822), 47:140–46; *Medical Intelligencer* (1822), 3:69.

32   The second "deviation" was the considerable abridgement of Laennec's work, a step that was predictably deprecated by many critics but doubtless effective at widening the book's audience.

33   *London Medical and Physical Journal*, n. 31, p. 142.

34   John Forbes, trans., R. T. H. Laennec, *Treatise on Diseases of the Chest* (London, 1821), p. x.

35   Ibid., pp. ix–x.

36   Ibid., p. xix.

37   For example see *London Medical and Physical Journal*, (n. 33).

38   *Medical Intelligencer*, n. 31, p. 69. The immediate effect was, of course, much the same as it would have been had Forbes, in fact, expected to capitalize quickly on the stethoscope: the "skimming" of auscultation away from the pathological anatomy that, for Laennec, undergirded it.

39   See Chapter 6.

40   Robert Kerrison was listed as an active member and former committeeman. Several individuals with the surname Johnson were listed only as active members.

41   *Transactions of the Associated Apothecaries and Apothecary–Surgeons* (1823), 1:li–cxxxvii.

42 Ibid., pp. 57–133; at p. 57.
43 See Alcock's "Biographical Notice" of Haden in his posthumous edition of the latter's *Practical Observations* (n. 12).
44 *Transactions of the Associated Apothecaries and Apothecary–Surgeons*, ibid., p. xciii.
45 Ibid., p. xcix.
46 Ibid., pp. ci–cii.
47 Ibid., pp. cvi–cix.
48 Ibid., pp. cxiii–cxiv.
49 Ibid., pp. cxxii–cxxix; emphasis added.
50 Ibid., pp. cxxxi–cxxxii; he cites Béclard's additions to Bichat's *Anatomie Générale* and J. F. Meckel in Germany.
51 On the role of elites, such as that operating at the intersection of the journalistic and surgeon–apothecaries' leaderships, see Michael Mulkay, "The Mediating Role of the Scientific Elite," *Social Studies of Science*, (1976), 6:445–70.
52 *Transactions of the Associated Apothecaries and Apothecary – Surgeons*, p. cxli.
53 *Anderson's Quarterly Journal of the Medical Sciences* (1824), 1:118; around 1824 this journal had taken a new title, formerly having been known as the *Quarterly Journal of Foreign Medicine and Surgery*.
54 Ibid.
55 Ibid., p. 139.
56 Ibid., p. 180.
57 *Anderson's Quarterly Journal of the Medical Sciences* (1824), 2:90.

CHAPTER 8

1 Adolph Muehry, *Observations on the Comparative State of Medicine in France, England, and Germany, during a Journey into these Countries in the Year 1835* (Philadelphia, 1838), pp. 65–66.
2 John Richard Farre, *An Apology for British Anatomy, and an Incitement to the Study of Morbid Anatomy* (London, 1827), p. 5. See also, "Introductory and leading article," *Journal of Morbid Anatomy* (1828), 1:x. In my research on the work of Farre and his associates I received invaluable assistance from Dr. Bonnie Blustein; I wish to acknowledge that debt with gratitude.
3 Although there is no adequate historical treatment of this point, see Humphrey Rolleston, "The early history of the teaching of I. Human Anatomy in London. II. Morbid anatomy and pathology in Great Britain," *Annals of Medical History*, 1939, 1:203–38.
4 On the latter group see Chapters 1–4, 6.
5 The French use of this imagery is discussed in preceding chapters.
6 On tissue theory see my "A treatise on membranes: concepts of tissue structure, function, and dysfunction from Bichat to Cohnheim," unpublished doctoral dissertation, Duke University, 1973, and Othmar Keel, *La généalogie de l'histopathologie* (Paris, 1979).
7 Cf. Chapters 2–4.
8 Cf. Chapter 6.
9 Ibid. On the periodical literature also see M. J. Peterson, "Specialist journals and professional rivalries in Victorian medicine," *Victorian Periodicals Review* (1979), 12:25–33.
10 John Richard Farre, *An Apology for British Anatomy* (n. 2), p. 5 and passim.
11 See Great Britain, Parliament, House of Commons, *Report from the Select Committee on Anatomy* (Sessional Papers, VII, 1828), p. 138, for a list of the private schools ca. 1826. Four hospital and eight strictly private schools provided returns to the Select Committee's questions, supplying information as to numbers of students *in toto*, number per dissecting room, number who actually dissected, and number of bodies dissected.
12 Farre, *Apology*, p. 8.
13 Keel, (n. 6), and see also, "La pathologie tissulaire de John Hunter," *Gesnerus* (1980), 37:4761, by the same author.

14 John Hunter, *A treatise on the Blood, Inflammation, and GunShot Wounds* (London, 1794), pp. 240–243.

15 John Cunningham Saunders, *A Treatise on Some Practical Points Relating to Diseases of the Eye . . . to Which are Added, a Short Account of the Author's Life, and His Method of Curing the congenital Cataract, by J. R. Farre.* New [2nd] ed. (London, 1816), p. 4.

16 J. R. Farre, *Pathological Researches. Essay 1. On Malformations of the Human Heart: Illustrated by Numerous cases, and Five Plates . . . and Preceded by Some Observations on the Method of Improving the Diagnostic Part of Medicine* (London, 1814).

17 Saunders, *Treatise on . . . the Eye* (n. 15), p. xix.

18 See Maulitz, "Treatise on membranes" (n. 6), pp. 93–97. I have not, however, been able to find an explicit statement of the microcosm concept in Farre's own writings.

19 Saunders, *Treatise on . . . the Eye*, p. xlii.

20 Farre, *Apology*, p. 8; one younger colleague who emulated this model to Farre's evident satisfaction was John Dalrymple, whose paper on "The muscularity of the iris" he published, lauding it as having met "a principal object for which the academy was instituted, and the inquiry having been physiologically conducted and pathologically directed, assumes the very spirit which the Editor is most desirous of encouraging amongst the rising British candidates for anatomical character." *Journal of Morbid Anatomy* (1828), *1*:59–64.

21 Anatomical illustration in this period awaits a historian's careful survey and analysis. Steven Peitzman has provided some useful comments in "Bright's disease and Bright's generation: Toward exact medicine at Guy's Hospital," *Bulletin of the History of Medicine* (1981), *55*:307–321; this paper advances a persuasive argument about the exactitude of description afforded by the new techniques of illustration. On the rapidly changing social, intellectual, and economic picture of publishing book illustration more generally during this period, see: David E. Allen, *The Naturalist in Britain* (London, 1976), esp. pp. 96–99; M. J. Rudwick, "The emergence of a visual language for geological science 1760–1840," *History of Science* (1976), *14*:149–195; William M. Ivins, Jr., *Prints and Visual Communications* (London, 1953); Celina Fox, "The engravers' battle for professional recognition in early nineteenth century London," *London Journal* (1976), *2*:3–25.

22 John Dalrymple, *Pathology of the Eye* (London, 1852)). On the cost of this volume see Treacher Collins, *The History and Traditions of the Moorfields Eye Hospital* (London, 1929), p. 77.

23 On this point see Great Britain, Parliament, House of Commons, *Report of the Select Committee on Medical Education* (London, 1834), p. 300, testimony of John Yelloly. This volume is cited hereafter as *SCR, Medical Education.*

24 Other formats included quizcompends and manuals, the published transactions of the Medico-Chirurgical Society, and the published lectures delivered at the College of Physicians.

25 Farre, *Apology*, p. 79.

26 Ibid., p. 7.

27 Farre, *Pathological Researches* (n. 16), p. xiv.

28 Ibid., pp. ix, vi.

29 Farre, *The Morbid Anatomy of the Liver* (London: Longman, Hurst, Rees, Orne, and Brown, 1812), pp. 23.

30 Farre, *Apology*, p. 910.

31 On Forbes see Ch. 7.

32 Collins, *History of Moorfields* (n. 22), gives a reasonable account of this institution, which was successively called the London Dispensary for Curing Diseases of the Eye and Ear (1804–1807), the London Infirmary for Curing Diseases of the Eye (1808–1821), the London Ophthalmic Infirmary (1821–1837), and the Royal London Ophthalmic Hospital (from 1837). After 1821 it was commonly known as the Moorfields Eye Hospital. In 1872 it merged with the competing Royal Infirmary for Diseases of the Eye, also founded in 1805. A third institution, the Royal Westminster Ophthalmic Hospital, was begun in 1816.

33 Standard accounts of Saunders's life are drawn mainly from Farre's preface to Saunders, *Treatise* (1st ed., London, 1811). I have used the second edition (1816), which reprinted the first unaltered save for the addition of substantially more prefatory material. See also passim in Collins, *History of Moorfields*.

34 M. J. Peterson, *The Medical Profession in Mid-Victorian London* (Berkeley, California, 1978) provides an excellent account of the system of nepotism and aristocratic patronage. See Chapter 4, "The formation of a professional elite," pp. 136–93; the quotation is from p. 148. Useful background regarding the critical tension during this period, in science more generally, between London and the provinces is in Ian Inkster and Jack Morrell, eds., *Metropolis and Province: Science in British Culture, 1780–1850* (Philadelphia: University of Pennsylvania Press, 1983). See esp. Chapter 9, Michael Durey, "Medical elites, the general practitioner and patient power in Britain during the cholera epidemic of 1831–32," pp. 257–78.

35 *SCR, Medical Education* (n. 23), p. 222 (testimony of J. R. Farre).

36 Ibid.

37 Collins makes this argument; there is little reason to question it: compare Fielding H. Garrison, *History of Medicine*, 2nd ed. (Philadelphia, 1917), pp. 511, 389–90.

38 Quoted in Collins, *History of Moorfields*, pp. 13–14.

39 *SCR, Medical Education*, p. 222; compare Collins, *History of Moorfields*, p. 11.

40 *SCR, Medical Education*, p. 222.

41 Collins, *History of Moorfields*, pp. 13–14.

42 Ibid., p. 3.

43 On Farre's life, see *SCR, Medical Education*, and the *Dictionary of National Biography*. Where these accounts differ, I have followed Farre's own testimony in the *SCR* of 1834. A sketchy and undocumented account is found in Simon Behrman, "John Farre (1775–1862) and other nineteenth century physicians at Moorfields," *Medical History*, 1962 6: 73–76. The irony of his sons' education may be sharp but is neither atypical of his generation, nor hard to fathom.

44 This account of Battley's life is summarized from the *Dictionary of National Biography*, which relied in turn, it appears, on an obituary in the *Gentleman's Magazine*, n.s., (?)1856, 45: 534–36.

45 Collins, *History of Moorfields*, passim.

46 On the changing role of the general practitioner see Rosemary Stevens and Irvine Loudon, "Primary care and the hospital," ch. 7 (pp. 139–75) in John Fry, ed., *Primary Care* (London, 1980).

47 Peterson, *The Medical Profession* (n. 34), pp. 11, 17, 21; see also S. W. F. Holloway, "The Apothecaries' Act of 1815: a reinterpretation," *Medical History* (1966), 10:107–129, 221–36. An indispensable primary source is the "Introductory essay," (cf. Ch. 5 above), pp. iii–cxxxviii in the single published volume of *The Transactions of the Associated Apothecaries and Surgeon–Apothecaries of England and Wales, 1* (London, 1823).

48 That is, posts such as that of the apothecary at the Ophthalmic Infirmary could now go in an institutionally sanctioned manner to a surgeon-apothecary. This change is also consistent with Holloway's view that the Apothecaries' Act was in many ways a blow as much as it was a boon to the apothecaries.

49 *Transactions of the Associated Apothecaries and Surgeon-Apothecaries* (n. 47), pp. cvi–cxiv.

50 Collins, *History of Moorfields*, p. 57.

51 Saunders, *Treatise*, pp. xvii ff.

52 Farre, "Introductory article," p. x.

53 Collins, *History of Moorfields*, p. 38.

54 *SCR, Anatomy* (n. 11); significantly, perhaps because he was not a surgeon and hence not involved in instruction in gross anatomy, Farre was not called as a witness in the 1828 inquiry. See also M. J. Durey, "Bodysnatchers and Benthamites: the implications of the dead body bill for the London schools of anatomy, 1820–42," *London Journal* (1976), 2:200–25.

55 Farre, *Apology*, p. 10.

56 SCR, *Medical Education*, pp. 222–23.
57 One such controversy, with William Adams, inspired a series of published po-
    lemics and, apparently, a parliamentary investigation. Another was conducted
    at least partly in the pages of the *Edinburgh Medical and Surgical Journal* and involved
    Benjamin Gibson and his biographer James Wardrop (who was also editor and
    biographer of Baillie). For Farre's defense of Saunders, see Saunders, *Treatise*,
    pp. vi–xvi.
58 Farre, *Pathological Researches*, p. v.
59 Saunders, *Treatise*, pp. xviii–xix.
60 See Farre, "Introductory article," pp. xxi–xxiii.
61 Collins, *History of Moorfields*, pp. 53–57, and William Lawrence, *Treatise on Diseases
    of the Eye* (London, 1833), p. 4.
62 Ibid.
63 Garrison, *History*, pp. 563, 643 ff.
64 Farre, "Dedication" and "Advertisement," *Journal of Morbid Anatomy* (1828), *1*;
    SCR, *Medical Education*, p. 222; Collins, *History of Moorfields*, p. 35.
65 Farre, *Apology*, p. 6; Collins, *History of Moorfields*, pp. 55–57.
66 On John Dalrymple see Collins, *History of Moorfields*, pp. 75 ff., and standard
    biographical sources. Obituary notices appeared in *Lancet* (1852), i, 452; *Medical
    Times* (8 May 1852), p. 471; the *Times* of London, 6 May 1852; and *Gentleman's
    Magazine* (1852), i, p. 626. His papers are enumerated in the *Royal Society Catalogue
    of Scientific Papers*.
67 Collins, *History of Moorfields*, pp. 58–61; Squire Sprigge, *Life and Times of Thomas
    Wakley* (London, 1897), pp. 102–126.
68 Farre's comment appeared in Saunders, *Treatise*, p. 26.
69 See Holloway, "The Apothecaries' Act," (n. 47) for the elaboration of this ar-
    gument.
70 Farre, *Journal of Morbid Anatomy*, p. ix.
71 Ibid., p. 11 and *passim*.
72 SCR, *Medical Education*, p. 222.
73 Farre, "Introductory article," p. x (emphasis in the original).
74 SCR, *Medical Education*, pp. 220–25. Other excerpts from Farre's testimony are
    cited above.
75 Ibid.

CHAPTER 9

1 With the awarding of the Royal Charter in 1800, the Company of Surgeons had
   become the Royal College of Surgeons; its Council remained, however, under
   the firm control of the London establishment – until 1842–43, only those residing
   within five miles of the City Centre could be Members of Council. See Zachary
   Cope, *The History of the Royal College of Surgeons of England* (London: Anthony
   Blond, 1959), p. 69.
2 A sophisticated analysis of this process is M. Jeanne Peterson, *The Medical Profession
   in Mid-Victorian London* (Berkeley: University of California Press, 1978), esp.
   Chapter IV, "The formation of a professional elite," pp. 136–93; on Hodgkin
   and Harrison, compare pp. 144–46.
3 There is no satisfactory full-scale biography of Thomas Hodgkin, although Edward H. and Amalie Kass of Boston are nearing completion of such a project.
   But see Samuel Wilks and G. T. Bettany, *A Biographical History of Guy's Hospital*
   (London: Ward, Lock, Bowden and Co., 1892), pp. 380–86; and *Dictionary of
   National Biography XXVII*, 63–64.
4 Samuel Wilks, "Cases of enlargement of the Lymphatic Glands and Spleen, or
   Hodgkin's Disease, with remarks," *Guy's Hospital Reports* (1877), *22* (ser. 3):
   259–74.
5 Gerald Geison, in his important book-length essay on the development of physiology in England, makes this point in relation to the slow beginnings of that

discipline and the obstacles posed to physiology by the entrenchment of normal anatomy: *Michael Foster and the Cambridge School of Physiology* (Princeton, N.J.: Princeton University Press, 1978), pp. 26–31.

6   In addition to the works cited above (n. 3) see, on Hodgkin, E. H. Kass, and A. H. Bartlett, "Thomas Hodgkin, M.D. (1798–1866): an annotated bibliography," *Bulletin of the History of Medicine* (1969), *43*:138–77; and the several essays by this author and others collectively titled "Thomas Hodgkin: the man and the work," *Guy's Hospital Reports* (1966), *115*:243–303. On Robert Carswell there is even less; but J. F. Payne's entry in *Dictionary of National Biography* (*IX*, 199) is quite serviceable and accurate.

7   Thomas Hodgkin, "On some morbid appearances of the absorbent glands and spleen," *Medico-Chirurgical Transactions*, (1832), *17*:68–114, at p. 89 (in this article Hodgkin described the affection that would later be assigned his name).

8   Charles J. B. Williams arrived between two and three years after Hodgkin. He described the experience in great detail in *Memoirs of Life and Work* (London: Smith, Elder, 1884), the fullest impressionistic account I have seen of what was by now (Chapter 6) an increasingly common experience.

9   Thomas Hodgkin to John Hodgkin, Jr., 15 October 1821. The entire Hodgkin correspondence has been microfilmed by Dr. E. H. Kass and deposited at the Countway Library in Boston as well as at the Wellcome Institute, London. It has been assigned microfilm locator numbers to which I conform in these notes; the first refers to reel number. Thus the locator for this letter is 3:262, 15 October 1821.

10 Hodgkin to a family member, 25 November 1821, 3:271.

11 Ibid.; in an undated letter he further noted that "Dr. Knox, one of my fellow students at Edinburgh and myself have formed ourselves into a little Physiological Society." (3:278:636).

12 Hodgkin to a family member, 5 January 1822, 3:282.

13 Hodgkin to Joseph A. Gillett, 3 March 1822. Friends Library, London, Temp. MSS 13/8.

14 The *régistres*, used to generate the curve above, Chapter 6, describing foreign student enrollments, bear Hodgkin's name in the appropriate sequence of terms, but do not provide the specific designations of courses that the students, native or foreign, actually took.

15 "Lists des élèves et de médecins étrangers qui ont suivi mes cours, et dont j'ai connu les noms, 1821–22/1823–24," Musée Laennec, Nantes.

16 Hodgkin to Gillett (n. 13).

17 Ibid.

18 On 29 August 1822 Thomas Hodgkin and his brother, John Hodgkin, Jr., wrote to their father (4:66:133–34) that "on 7th day evening we went to Cuvier's soirée. Thomas presented the baron with the *Calligraphia Graeca* from thee; with which appeared pleased. . . . We yesterday joined Thomas Forster, my fellow pupil Oxnam, and his fellow traveler Coleridge, the nephew of the poet, in going to the Veterinary College at Alfort; here we saw the junction of the Seine and the Marne. After examining the Museum at Alfort we proceeded to the lunatic asylum where Dr. Roche (the brother of the gentleman who lives in . . . Lincoln's Inn) is Physician. . . ."

19 Thomas Hodgkin, *Dissertatio physiologica inauguralis de absorbendi functione* (Edinburgh: J. Pillans and Son, 1823).

20 No later than 1827 Hodgkin began lecturing on the membrane at Guy's, publishing his emended lectures *in extenso* in two volumes a decade later: *Lectures on the Morbid Anatomy of the Serous and Mucous Membranes* (London: Sherwood, Gilbert, and Piper, 1836–40). His appointment to the curatorship in morbid anatomy may be dated to the 1825 founding of the Museum.

21 On the role of the Quakers, especially from the late 1830s on, see Elizabeth Isichei, *Victorian Quakers* (London: Oxford University Press, 1970); for the earlier nineteenth century, compare Ian Inkster, "Science and society in the metropolis:

a preliminary examination of the social and institutional context of the Askesian Society of London, 1796–1807," *Annals of Science*, (1977), *34*:1–32. This group, according to Inkster, was characterized by an aggressive mercantilism, political reformism, and an avidity for scientific culture.

22 The globularist notion of tissue structure, usually referred to as a "fallacy," revolved around a perception of the microscopic anatomy of plants and animals being composed of ultimate units that were homogeneous and globular in makeup. Perhaps related to halo artifacts in lenses with high spherical aberration, the globularist notion was popular in both France and England, especially among the followers of René Dutrochet.

23 At the third meeting of the fiftieth session, on 16 October, 1819, Mr. Hodgskin [sic] was proposed for membership in the Society (Minute Books, 1813–1820).

24 Wilks and Bettany, *Biographical History* (n. 3), pp. 87, 189; also J. R. Wall, "The Guy's Hospital Physical Society," *Guy's Hospital Reports* (1974), *123*:159–70.

25 J. M. H. Campbell, "The history of the Physical Society," *Guy's Hospital Gazette* (1925), pp. 107–119. Many of these individuals, e.g., John Lettsom, were focal points for the network of well-placed Quakers that included Lister and Hodgkin.

26 R. C. Maulitz, "Metropolitan medicine and the man–midwife: the early life and letters of Charles Locock," *Medical History* (1982), *26*:25–46.

27 See, e.g., Minute Books for 1838–39, Wills Library, Guy's Hospital, London. The Physical Society continued to flourish until midcentury. In the 1850s, fading, and supplanted in importance to the Guy's faculty by specialty groups such as the Pathological Society, it was superseded by a Pupils Physical Society, organized by the students of medicine.

28 Thomas Hodgkin, *An Essay on Medical Education, read before the Physical Society of Guy's Hospital, at the First Meeting of the Session 1827–28* (London: William Phillips, 1828), pp. 12–13.

29 Ibid., p. 13.

30 Thomas Hodgkin, Medical lecture notes, n.d. [?1830], 5:288:654–64.

31 Ibid.

32 Ibid., 5:289:664–70.

33 Kass and Bartlett, "Annotated bibliography," (n. 6), p. 151.

34 See n. 20; the second volume was delayed in publication for four years as a result both of illness and (perhaps more important) the difficulties that were soon to unfold in his career.

35 See, e.g., [Review of] Thomas Hodgkin, *Lectures on the Morbid Appearances of the Serous and Mucous Membranes, Edinburgh Medical and Surgical Journal* (1843), *59*:155–69.

36 Hodgkin, *Lectures* (n. 20), pp. vii–viii.

37 Ibid., pp. 4, 6.

38 Ibid., p. 12.

39 Ibid., p. 16.

40 Ibid.

41 Ibid., p. 25.

42 Ibid.

43 Ibid., pp. 24–65.

44 Hodgkin MSS (n. 9), 5:292:679—87.

45 Ibid.

46 Ibid.

47 Surprisingly, there is no full study of nineteenth-century humoralism. Some helpful clues may be found, however, in Robert Miciotto, "Carl Rokitansky: a reassessment of the hematohumoral theory of disease," *Bulletin of the History of Medicine* (1978), *52*:183–99.

48 R. C. Maulitz, "A treatise on membranes: concepts of tissue structure, function and dysfunction, from Xavier Bichat to Julius Cohnheim," doctoral dissertation, Duke University, 1973, pp. 10–17.

49 On paracentesis see Kurt Sprengel, *Histoire de la médecine*, tr. A. J. L. Jourdan

(Paris: Baillière, 1815–32), *9*, ch. 5, "De l'operation do l'empyème," pp. 1–90; Hugo Gierlich, "Zur Fruhgeschichte der Paracentesis pericardii," *Sudhoffs Archiv für Geschichte der Medizin und der Naturwissenschaften* (1956), *40*:119–55; Saul Jarcho, "The differentiation of the diagnosis of pericarditis (Bouillier, 1812)," *American Journal of Cardiology*, (1963), *12*:853–59; and "Henry I. Bowditch on pleuritic effusion and thoracentesis (1852)." Ibid., 1965, *15*:832–36.

50 Tuberculosis could and did cause a very large number, and probably the majority, of such cases.

51 See for example Hodgkin's warning about pathological events at remote sites (n. 37 above).

52 See, e.g., a case discussion (Charles Locock, et al.) of ovarian tumor resulting in fluid redistribution and probable shock at Guy's Hospital (Minute Books, Wills Library, 1838–39, entry for 17 November 1838); another interesting case of paracentesis in a patient with ascites is related in a letter from John Howship to John Thomson, ca. 21 August 1821: Edinburgh University Library MSS. Gen. 591 (II)–91.

53 Hodgkin, for example, used the economic metaphor on repeated occasions in his own work.

54 Here one recalls Hodgkin's role as Edwards's translator (see Chapter 6).

55 Edward H. Kass, Anne B. Carey, and Amalie M. Kass, "Thomas Hodgkin and Benjamin Harrison: Crisis and promotion in academia," *Medical History* (1980), *24*:197–208. Enunciating the more traditional, conservative view of this affair, H. C. Cameron, in *Mr. Guy's Hospital* (London: Longmans, Green, 1954) attributed Harrison's action to Hodgkin's "unpredictable" and "perhaps not reliable" conduct (p. 132).

56 Benjamin Babington was the son of the highly influential Quaker physician William Babington, who was Physician to Guy's until his death in 1811.

57 Cameron, *Mr. Guy's Hospital* (n. 55), pp. 281–82.

58 Wilks and Bettany, *Biographical History* (n. 3), p. 384.

59 A personal animus could, of course, have underlain Harrison's particular actions in some more general sense, with the Hudson's Bay episode serving as a trigger in the 1837 promotion crisis.

60 Kass, Carey, and Kass (n. 55).

61 John Herschel Correspondence, Royal Society, London, MSS for 1834–36, pp. 408–410.

62 Thomas Hodgkin, *Lectures on the Means of Promoting Health, delivered at the Mechanics' Institute, Spitalfields, 12mo 1835* (London: Arch, 1835, reprinted London: Simkin, Marshall, 1841).

63 On the Mechanics' Institutes phenomenon in general, see Steven Shapin and Barry Barnes, "Science, nature and control: interpreting the mechanics' institutes," *Social Studies of Science* (1977), *7*:31–74.

64 See, e.g., Michael Durey, "Medical elites, the general practitioner and patient power in Britain during the cholera epidemic of 1831–2," pp. 257–78 in Ian Inkster and Jack Morrell, eds., *Metropolis and Province: Science in British Culture, 1780–1850* (Philadelphia: University of Pennsylvania Press, 1983).

65 H. Hale Bellot, *University College London: 1828–1926* (London: University of London Press, 1929).

66 W. R. Merrington, *University College Hospital and its Medical School: a History* (London: Heinemann, 1976), p. 5; see also University of London Council Minutes, *I* (1825–29), p. 98.

67 Minutes (n. 65), *I*, 130, Charles J. B. Williams, in his *Memoirs* (n. 8) recalled that Thomson had sent Carswell to Paris for this express purpose; compare p. 17.

68 J. F. Clarke, *Autobiographical Recollections of the Medical Profession* (London: Churchill, 1874), p. 321.

69 University of Edinburgh MS Collections Gen. 590–91, Notes of Medical Cases made in France with a few letters and other papers [Robert Carswell], ca. 1822–

25; Carswell gleaned his cases of dissection not only from London and Paris but also Chatham, Lyons, and Rome.

70 The representations have been preserved in the Library of the School of Medicine, University College, London.

71 In his case descriptions Carswell described the following patient, for example, from the *Enfants Malades* dated 22 November 1822 (p. 158): "Pericarditis terminating in general Dropsy in a Girl about 12 years of age – External appearance of the body – Inferior extremities oedematous to a high degree – abdomen distended – Breast, neck, and face particularly under the ear and margin of the lower jaw oedematous – arms and back slightly – The Labia, where they are in contact with the thighs, were excoriated from great distension. Incisions made into several of these parts gave issue to an abundant discharge of serosity without swell and almost without color. Thorax – The Pericardium and Heart occupied two-thirds of the thorax in breadth and stretched proportionally upwards on the left, the lung of which side being compressed and diminished is a fourth of its size compared with the capacity of the same side. The right lung was also pushed some way upwards and towards the ribs. Both lungs were farther compressed, by a considerable quantity of serum, from two to three pounds in each cavity, slightly tinged with yellow, almost without swell and perfectly clear. The lungs contained a small quantity of serum, but did not appear to have undergone any change of structure from the pressure which they had suffered."

72 Robert Carswell to Council, London University; University College Archives MS 304.

73 Ibid.

74 University of London Council Minutes, *I*, 157–58, 164.

75 Robert Carswell to Leonard Horner, 25 April 1828; University of London, D. M. S. Watson Library, MS 673.

76 Robert Carswell to Leonard Horner, 14 June 1828, University of London (D. M. S. Watson Library) Archives, MS 674.

77 Ibid., MS 675.

78 University of London Council Minutes, *II*, pp. 49–50.

79 Robert Carswell MSS, ibid. (n. 75), P61–P64.

80 Ibid., P63.

81 Ibid.

82 University of London Council Minutes, *II*, p. 279 (26 May 1831).

83 Ibid. *II*, p. 291.

84 Robert Carswell MSS, ibid. (n. 75), MS 2093.

85 On a later expression of this tension see R. C. Maulitz, " 'Physician versus bacteriologist': the ideology of Science in clinical medicine," in Morris Vogel and Charles E. Rosenberg, eds., *The Therapeutic Revolution: Essays in the Social History of American Medicine* (Philadelphia: University of Pennsylvania Press, 1979), pp. 91–108.

86 Cf., e.g., Carswell MSS, ibid. (n. 75), MSS 4141, 4200.

87 Ibid., MS 2095.

88 J. F. Clarke, *Autobiographical Recollections* (n. 67), p. 322.

89 MSS, "Medical Classes, 1828/29–1830/31; 1831/32–1835/36," College Record Office, University College, London.

90 University of London *Annual Reports*, 1828–41.

91 Ibid., 1833: "Report of annual general meeting," appendix, p. 6.

92 Carswell's income did not suffer unduly, however, but remained apparently in the 250–350 range despite the problems of launching his specialty.

93 Compare his remarks in London Medical Gazette, 1828, ii (4 October 1828) pp. 565–68; the apothecaries' requirements extended to less than the surgeons' fifteen months.

94 University of London *Annual Report*, 1836 (London: Richard Taylor, 1836), p. 16.

95 University of London Council Minutes of Meetings, *II*, p. 442 (1 March 1834).

96 R. K. Merton, "The Matthew effect in science," *Science* (1968), *159:56–63*. Merton's original application of the principle based on this effect was that of explaining one result of the stratification of science. His concern was focused on why members of a scientific mandarinate may continue to contribute to the enterprise of science and draw disproportionately on its resources after their own productivity is on the wane. Hence, the rich get richer. The principle has come to be applied more generally and loosely to the notion that those who can maintain centrality may fare far better than those (like Carswell) who start out at the margins.

97 Clarke, *Autobiographical Recollections* (n. 68), p. 322.

98 "Robert Carswell," *Dictionary of National Biography IX*, 191.

99 See R. C. Maulitz, "Pathology," in Ronald Numbers, ed., *The Education of the American Physician* (Berkeley: University of California Press, 1979), pp. 122–42.

100 Richard Quain, *Observations on Medical Education* (London: Walton and Maberly, 1865), pp. 16–17.

CONCLUSION

1 See chapter 7, "Experimental pharmacology," pp. 145–65 in John E. Lesch, *Science and Medicine in France: the Emergence of Experimental Physiology, 1790–1855* (Cambridge, Massachusetts: Harvard University Press, 1984). Judiciously, Lesch does not attempt to make sweeping statements about the impact of the newly available alkaloids and other poisons, though he does draw attention to the barebones fact of their recent discovery in the late 1810s.

2 The point is made nicely, in terms of "the sheer indeterminacy of the past," in L. S. Jacyna's provocative essay, "Images of John Hunter in the nineteenth century," *History of Science* (1983), *21:* 85–108; at p. 105.

3 Caroline Hannaway, [review of] Toby Gelfand, *Professionalizing Modern Medicine* (ch. I, n. 2), *Bull. Hist. Med.* (1984) *58:*596–98.

4 Again I emphasize that these perceptions were not wholly mutually exclusive. Surgeons could be heard to adduce humoral explanations and, less frequently, physicians to adduce localistic ones. They were, after all, dealing with the same phenomenon, the human organism, and it was not then any more than it is now a natural object that could be perceived in infinitely plastic ways. Thus purists might rightly claim that what the surgical and medical subcultures of the late eighteenth and early nineteenth centuries were promoting were not different languages, but different codes or dialects within the same language.

5 William Coleman, "The cognitive basis of the discipline: Claude Bernard on physiology," *Isis* (1985), *76:*49–70.

6 Laurence Veysey, "Intellectual history and the new social history," pp. 3–26 in John Higham and Paul Conklin, eds., *New Directions in American Intellectual History* (Baltimore: Johns Hopkins University Press, 1979).

Selected bibliography

Ackerknecht, Erwin H. *Medicine at the Paris Hospital* (Baltimore: Johns Hopkins University Press, 1967).

Ackerknecht, Erwin H. "Laennec und sein Vorlesungsmanuskript von 1822," *Gesnerus 21* (1964), 142–54.

Ackerknecht, Erwin H. "Recurrent themes in medical thought," *Sci. Monthly 49* (1949) 80–83.

Albury, W. R. "Experimentation and explanation in the physiology of Bichat and Magendie," *Stud. Hist. Biol. I* (1977) 47–131.

Albury, W. R. "Magendie's physiological manifesto of 1809," *Bull. Hist. Med. 48* (1974). 90–99.

Alcock, Thomas. "An Essay on the education and duties of the general practitioner in medicine and surgery," *Transactions of the Associated Apothecaries and Apothecary–Surgeons* (1823), pp. 57–133.

Allen, David. *The Naturalist in Britain* (London: Allen Lane, 1976).

Amerio, Adriana. " 'Sensibilita' e 'irritabilita' nella dottrina vitalistica di Anthelme Richerand," *Medicina Nei Secoli 9* (1972) 23–28.

Arène, A. "Essai sur la philosophie de Xavier Bichat," *Arch. d'Anthropol. Crim. 26* (1911) 753–825.

Bailey, James D. "The medical societies of London," *British Medical Journal 2* (1895) 25.

Bayle, G. L. "Considérations générales sur les secours que l'anatomie pathologique peut fournir à la médecine," in: Adelon et al., *Dictionnaire des Sciences Médicales* (Paris: Panckoucke, 1812–22), pp. 61–79.

Bayle, G. L. *Recherches sur la phthisie pulmonaire* (Paris: Gabon, 1810).

Béclard, Pierre. *Anatomie pathologique: dernier cours de Xavier Bichat* (Paris: Baillière, 1825).

Behrman, Simon. "John Farre (1775–1862) and other nineteenth century physicians at Moorfields," *Med. Hist. 6* (1962) 73–76.

Bellot, H. Hale. *University College London: 1828–1926* (London: University of London Press, 1929).

Bichat, Xavier. *Anatomie générale, appliquée à la physiologie et à la Médecine* (Paris: Mequignon, an IX [1801]).

Bichat, Xavier. "Mémoire sur la membrane synoviale des articulations," *Mém. Soc. méd. d'Em. 2* (an VII [1799]) 350–70.

Bichat, Xavier, ed. *Oeuvres chirurgicales, ou exposé de la doctrine et de la pratique de P.-J. Desault* (Paris: Citoyenne veuve Desault – Mequignon l'ainé, an VI [1799]).

Bichat, Xavier. *Traité des membranes en général et de diverses membranes en particulier* (Paris: Richard, Caille et Ravier, an VIII [1799]).

Bichat, Xavier, ed. *Oeuvres chirurgicales de Desault*, 3 vols. (Paris, 1798–99; 3rd ed. Paris: J.-B. Baillière, 1830).

Bichat, Xavier. "Discours preliminaire," *Mém. Soc. méd. d'Em. 1* (an V [1797]) iv–v.

Bordeu, Théophile de. *Recherches sur le tissu muqueux, ou l'organe cellulaire* (Paris: Didot le jeune, 1767).

Boulle, Lydie, Grmek, Mirko D., and Samion-Contet, Janine, eds. *Laennec: catalogue des manuscrits scientifiques* (Paris: Masson, 1982).

Bud, Robert F. "The Discipline of Chemistry: The Origins and Early Years of the Chemical Society of London." (Ph.D. diss., Univ. of Pennsylvania, 1980).

Bynum, William, and Porter, Roy, eds. *William Hunter and the Eighteenth Century Medical World* (Cambridge: Cambridge Univ. Press, 1985).

Bynum, William, ed. *Theories of Fever from Antiquity to the Enlightenment. Med. Hist. Suppl.* No. 1, (London: Wellcome Institute for the History of Medicine, 1981).

Campbell, J. M. H. "The history of the Physical Society," *Guy's Hospital Gazette* (1925) 107–19.

Canguilhem, Georges. *On the Normal and the Pathological,* trans. C. R. Fawcett ([orig. ed. Paris: Presses Universitaires de France, 1966] Dordrecht, Holland: D. Reidel, 1978).

Carswell, Robert. *Pathological Anatomy* (London, 1838).

Cawadias, A. "Théophile de Bordeu: an eighteenth century pioneer in endocrinology," *Proc. Roy. Soc. Med.* 43 (1950) 93–98.

Chitnis, Anand. "Medical education in Edinburgh, 1790–1826, and some Victorian social consequences," *Med. Hist.* 17 (1973) 173–85.

Clarke, J. F. *Autobiographical Recollections of the Medical Profession* (London: Churchill, 1874).

Cobb, Richard. *Death in Paris: 1795–1801* (Oxford: Oxford Univ. Press, 1978).

Coleman, William. "The cognitive basis of the discipline: Claude Bernard on physiology," *Isis* 76 (1985) 49–70.

Coleman, William. *Georges Cuvier: Zoologist* (Cambridge, Mass.: Harvard Univ. Press, 1964).

Collins, Treacher. *The History and Traditions of the Moorfields Eye Hospital* (London, 1929).

Comrie, J. D. *History of Scottish Medicine to 1860,* 2nd ed. (London: Wellcome Research Institution, 1932).

Cope, Zachary. "Dr. Charles T. Haden (1786–1824), a friend of Jane Austin," *British Medical Journal,* i, 9 April 1966, 974.

Cope, Zachary. *The History of the Royal College of Surgeons of England* (London: Anthony Blond, 1959).

Coquerelle, J. *Xavier Bichat (1771–1802): ses ancêtres et ses arrière-neveux* (Paris: Maloine, 1902).

Cornil, V., ed. *Traité inédit sur l'anatomie pathologique . . . [de Bichat]* (Paris: Felix Alcan, 1884).

Coury, Charles. "La méthode anatomo-clinique et ses promoteurs en France: Corvisart, Bayle, Laennec," *Médecine de France,* no. 224 (1971) 13–22.

Coury, Charles. *L'Hôtel-Dieu de Paris* (Paris: Palais de la Découverte, 1969).

Coury, Charles, and Billion, M. "Registre du personnel de l'Hôtel-Dieu pour la période 1795–1820," *Histoire des Sciences Médicales 1* (1967) 123–31.

Cruveilhier, Jean. *Vie de Dupuytren* (Paris: Bechet Jeune et Labe, 1841).

Cruveilhier, Jean. *Anatomie pathologique du corps humain* (Paris, 1830–42).

Cruveilhier, Jean. "Anatomie pathologique, considérée dans ses applications pratiques," in: G. Andral et al., eds., *Dictionnaire de médecine et de chirurgie pratiques,* II (Paris: Gabon, Méquignon-Marvis, J.-B. Baillière, 1829), pp. 346–72.

Cruveilhier, Jean. *Médecine eclairée par l'anatomie et la phisiologie pathologique* (Paris, 1821).

Cunningham, Andrew. "The kinds of anatomy," *Med. Hist.* 19 (1975) 1–19.

Dalrymple, John. *Pathology of the Eye* (London, 1852).

Daremberg, Charles. *Histoire des Sciences Médicales,* 2 vols. (Paris: Baillière, 1870).

Daremberg, Charles. *Les grands médecins du XIXᵉ siècle* (Paris: Masson, 1907).

De Montaigu. *Obervations des médecins de l'Hôtel-Dieu de Paris sur une réclamation.* (Paris: Egron, 1818).

Delaunay, Paul. *D'une révolution à l'autre, 1789–1848: l'évolution des théories et de la pratique médicales* (Paris: Editions Hippocrate, 1949).

Delaunay, Paul. *Le monde médicale Parisien au dix-huitième siècle.* 2ème ed. (Paris: Rousset, 1906).

De Mercy, F.-C.-F., *Demande du rétablissement d'un chair d'Hippocrate, année 1821: mémoire pour la Commission de l'Instruction Publique.* (Paris: n.d.).

De Mercy, F.-C.-F., *Plan d'organisation de l'art médical* (Paris, 1815).

Dulieu, Louis. "Bordeu." *Dictionary of Scientific Biography,* II, 301–2.

Dupuytren, Guillaume. "Nouvelles observations de M. Dupuytren sur la Note de M. Laennec," *J. Méd. 10* (1804) 96–102.

Dupuytren, René. "Observations sur la note relative aux altérations organiques, publiée par M. Laennec dans le dernier numéro du Journal de Médecine," *J. Méd. 9* (1804) 441–46.

Dupuytren, René. Extrait d'un mémoire sur l'anatomie pathologique, lu à l'Ecole de Médecine de Paris, par le citoyen Dupuytren," *J. Méd. 4* (1802) 575–83.

Durey, M. J. "Medical elites, the general practitioner and patient power in Britain during the cholera epidemic of 1831–32," in: Ian Inkster and Jack Morrell, eds., *Metropolis and Province: Science in British Culture, 1780–1850* (Philadelphia: Univ. of Pennsylvania Press, 1983) pp. 257–78.

Durey, M. J. "Bodysnatchers and Benthamites: the implications of the dead body bill for the London schools of anatomy, 1820–42," *London Journal*, 1976, 2: 200–25.

Edwards, W. F. *De l'influence des agens physiques sur la vie* (Paris: Crochard, 1824). Engl. trans. Thomas Hodgkin (London: S. Highley, 1832).

Elaut, Leon. "La théorie des membranes de F. X. Bichat et ses antecédents." *Sudhoffs Archiv 53* (1969) 68–76.

Faber, Knud. *Nosography in Modern Internal Medicine* (New York: Hoeber, 1923).

Farre, John Rihard. "Introductory and leading article," *Journal of Morbid Anatomy 1* (1828) x.

Farre, John Richard. *An Apology for British Anatomy, and an Incitement to the Study of Morbid Anatomy* (London, 1827).

Farre, John Richard. *Pathological Researches. Essay 1. On Malformations of the Human Heart: Illustrated by Numerous Cases, and Five Plates . . . and Preceded by Some Observations on the Method of Improving the Diagnostic Part of Medicine* (London, 1814).

Farre, John Richard. *The Morbid Anatomy of the Liver* (London: Longman, Hurst, Rees, Orne, and Brown, 1812).

Fearing, F. *Reflex Action.* (Baltimore: Williams & Wilkins, 1930), pp. 74–107.

Fleck, Ludwik. *Genesis and Development of a Scientific Fact* (Basel, 1935 [English ed.: Chicago: Univ. of Chicago Press, 1979]).

Foucault, Michel. *Naissance de la clinique.* 2nd ed. (Paris: Presses Universitaires de France, 1972); trans. *Birth of the Clinic* (New York: Pantheon, 1973).

Fourcroy, Antoine et al. *Plan générale de l'enseignement dans l'école de santé de Paris* (Paris: Ballard fils, an III).

Fourcroy, Antoine. *Rapport et projet de décret sur l'établissement d'une Ecole centrale de Santé à Paris, fait à la Convention nationale au nom des comités de salut public et d'instruction publique.* (Paris: Imprimerie nationale, an III).

Fox, Celina. "The engravers' battle for professional recognition in early nineteenth century London," *London Journal 2* (1976) 325.

Fox, Robert, and Weisz, George, "The institutional basis of French science in the nineteenth century." in: *idem, The organization of science and technology in France, 1808–1914* (Cambridge: Cambridge Univ. Press, 1980), pp. 1–28.

Franklin, Rachel E. "Medical Education and the Rise of the General practitioner, 1760 to 1860," Ph.D. diss., Faculty of Medicine, Univ. of Birmingham (England), 1950.

Gaskell, Eric. "Early American English translations of European medical works," *Med. Hist. 14* (1970) 300–7.

Geison, Gerald, ed. *Professions and the French State, 1700–1900* (Philadelphia: Univ. of Pennsylvania Press, 1984).

Geison, Gerald. *Michael Foster and the Cambridge School of Physiology* (Princeton, N.J.: Princeton Univ. Press, 1978).

Gelfand, Toby. "A 'monarchical profession' in the Old Regime: surgeons, ordinary practitioners, and medical professionalization in eighteenth-century France," in: Gerald Geison, ed., *Professions and the French State, 1700–1900* (Philadelphia: Univ. of Pennsylvania Press, 1984), pp. 149–80.

Gelfand, Toby. *Professionalizing Modern Medicine* (Westport, Conn.: Greenwood Press, 1980).

Gelfand, Toby. "A confrontation over clinical instruction at the Hôtel-Dieu of Paris during the French Revolution," *J. Hist. Med. 28* (1973) 268–82.

Genty, Maurice. "Bichat," in Pierre Huard, ed., *Biographies médicales et scientifiques* (Paris: Dacosta, 1972).
Gierlich, Hugo. "Zur Frühgeschichte der Paracentesis pericardii," *Sudhoffs Archiv für Geschichte der Medizin und der Naturwissenschaften 40* (1956) 119–55.
Gillispie, C. C. *Science and Polity in France at the End of the Old Regime* (Princeton, N.J.: Princeton Univ. Press, 1980).
Gley, E. "Xavier Bichat et son oeuvre biologique," *Bull. Soc. Fr. d'Hist. de la Méd.* 1 (1902, repr. 1967) 285–92.
Granville, A. B. *Autobiography of A. B. Granville, M.D., F.R.S., – Being Eighty-Eight Years of the Life of a Physician, II* (London: Henry S. King, 1874).
Great Britain, Parliament, House of Commons, Report from the Select Committee on Medical Education (London: 1834), Appendix 24.
Great Britain, Parliament, House of Commons, Report from the Select Committee on the Matter of Obtaining Subjects for Dissection in the Schools of Anatomy, and into the Laws Affecting Persons Employed in Obtaining or Dissecting Bodies (Session 1828). Volume 7, pp. 1–550.
Grmek, Mirko D. "L'invention de l'auscultation médiate, retouches à un cliché historique," in A. J. Rose, ed., *Commemoration du Bicentenaire de la Naissance de Laennec, 1781–1826: Colloque Organisé au Collège de France les 18 et 19 février 1981, Revue de Palais de la Découverte,* N° spécial 22, 1981, pp. 107–16.
Gross, Michael. "The lessened locus of feelings: a transformation in French physiology in the early nineteenth century," *J. Hist. Biol.* 12 (1979) 231–71.
Gross, Michael. "Function and Structure in Nineteenth Century French Physiology." (Ph.D. diss., Princeton Univ., 1974).
Guttmacher, Alan F. "Bootlegging bodies: a history of body snatching," *Bull. Soc. Med. Hist. Chicago* 4 (1935) 353–402.
Haden, Charles T. *Practical Observations on the Management and Diseases of Children* (London: Burgess and Hill, 1827).
Haden, Charles. "Introductory essay," *Transactions of the Associated Apothecaries and Apothecary–Surgeons* (1823), pp. i–cxl.
Hahn, Roger. *The Anatomy of a Scientific Institution: the Paris Academy of Sciences, 1666–1803* (Berkeley: Univ. of California Press, 1971).
Hahn, Andre. "Laennec à la faculté de Médecine," *Hist. de la Méd.* 8 (1958) 17–31.
Haigh, Elizabeth. *Xavier Bichat and the Medical Theory of the Eighteenth Century. Medical History Supplement* No. 4 (London: Wellcome Institute, 1984).
Hall, T.S. *Ideas of Life and Matter.* 2 vols. (Chicago: Univ. of Chicago Press, 1969).
Hall, T.S. "On biological analogs of Newtonian paradigms," *Phil. of Sci. 35* (1968) 6–27.
Heller, Robert. "*Officiers de santé:* the second-class doctors of nineteenth century France," *Med. Hist.* 22 (1978) 25–43.
Hodgkin, Thomas, *Lectures on the Morbid Anatomy of the Serous and Mucous Membranes* (London: Sherwood, Gilbert, and Piper, 1836–40).
Hodgkin, Thomas. *Lectures on the Means of Promoting Health, delivered at the Mechanics' Institute, Spitalfields, 12mo 1835* (London: Arch, 1835, repr. London: Simkin, Marshall, 1841).
Hodgkin, Thomas. "On some morbid appearances of the absorbent glands and spleen," *Medico-Chirurgical Transactions* 17 (1832) 68–114.
Hodgkin, Thomas. *An Essay on Medical Education, Read before the Physical Society of Guy's Hospital, at the First Meeting of the Session 1827–28* (London: William Phillips, 1828).
Hodgkin, Thomas. *Dissertatio physiologica inauguralis de absorbendi functione* (Edinburgh: J. Pillans and Son, 1823).
Holloway, S. W. F. "The Apothecaries Act, 1815: a reinterpretation," *Med. Hist.* 10 (1966) 107–29, 221–36.
Huard, Pierre. "Quelques idées sur la structure de la matière vivante au XIXème siècle; leur incidence sur la pratique médicale," *Clio Med.* 9 (1974) 57–64.
Huard, Pierre, "Bichat anatomiste," *Histoire des Science Médicales* 6 (1972) 98–106.
Huard, Pierre, and Grmek, Mirko D. "Les élèves étrangers de Laennec," *Rev. d'Hist. Sciences* 26 (1973) 315–37.

Huard, Pierre, and Imbault-Huart, M.-J. "La formation de l'oeuvre scientifique de Dupuytren (1777–1835)," *Histoire des Sciences Médicales 12* (1978) 217–31.

Huard, Pierre, and Imbault-Huart, M.-J. "La clinique Parisienne avant et après 1802," *Clio Méd. 10* (1975) 173–82.

Huard, Pierre, and Imbault-Huart, M.-J. "La vie et l'oeuvre de Jean Cruveilhier, anatomiste et clinicien," *Episteme 8* (1974) 46–57.

Hunter, John. *The Works of John Hunter, F.R.S., with Notes,* ed. James F. Palmer (London: Longman, Rees, 1837). 4 vols.

Hunter, John. *A treatise on the Blood, Inflammation, and Gunshot Wounds* (London, 1794).

Husson, [Henri-Marie]. "Premier mémoire historique sur l'Ecole de médecine de Paris," *J. Méd. I* (1800–1) 65–73.

Imbault-Huart, M.-J. "Bayle, Laennec, et le méthode anatomoclinique," in A. J. Rose, ed., *Commemoration du Bicentenaire de la Naissance de Laennec, 1781–1826: Colloque Organisé au Collège de France les 18 et 19 février 1981, Revue de Palais de la Découverte,* N° spécial 22, 1981, pp. 79–90.

Imbault-Huart, M.-J. *L'Ecole pratique de dissection de Paris de 1750 à 1822, ou l'influence du concept de médecine pratique et de médecine d'observation dans l'enseignement médico-chirurgical au XVIIIème siècle et au début du XIXème siècle.* Thèse, Univ. de Paris I, 1973 (Lille: Service de Reproduction des Thèses, 1975).

Inkster, Ian, and Morrell, Jack, eds., *Metropolis and Province: Science in British Culture, 1780–1850* (Philadelphia: Univ. of Pennsylvania Press, 1983).

Inkster, Ian. "Science and society in the metropolis: a preliminary examination of the social and institutional context of the Askesian Society of London, 1796–1807," *Annals of Science 34* (1977) 1–32.

Isichei, Elizabeth. *Victorian Quakers* (London: Oxford Univ. Press, 1970).

Ivins, William M., Jr. *Prints and Visual Communications* (London, 1953).

Jacyna, L. S. "Images of John Hunter in the nineteenth century," *Hist. Sci. 21* (1983) 85–108.

Jarcho, Saul. "An early mention of the stethoscope (Locock 1821)," *Bull. New York Acad. Med. 41* (1965) 374–77.

Jarcho, Saul. "Henry I. Bowditch on pleuritic effusion and thoracentesis (1852)," *American Journal of Cardiology 15* (1965) 832–36.

Jarcho, Saul. "The differentiation of the diagnosis of pericarditis (Bouiller, 1812)," *American Journal of Cardiology 12* (1963) 853–59.

Jarcho, Saul. "The difficulty of the diagnosis of pericarditis," *Amer. J. Cardiol. 12* (1963) 539–43.

Jarcho, Saul. "The review of John Forbe's translation of Laennec," *Amer. J. Cardiol. 10* (1962) 859–63.

Jarcho, Saul. "Early mentions of the endocardium by Bouillaud (1835) and Bichat (1800)," *Amer. J. Cardiol. 2* (1958) 767–69.

Jolly, J. "Les sciences biologiques au Collège de France," ch. VIII, pp. 133–45 in: A. Lefranc et al., *Le Collège de France (1530–1930)* (Paris: Presses Universitaires de France, 1932).

Jones, R. M. *The Parisian Education of an American Surgeon* (Philadelphia: American Philosophical Society, 1978).

Kass, Edward H., and Bartlett, A. H. "Thomas Hodgkin, M.D. (1798–1866): an annotated bibliography," *Bull. Hist. Med. 43* (1969) 138–77.

Kass, Edward H., Carey, Anne B., and Kass, Amalie M. "Thomas Hodgkin and Benjamin Harrison: crisis and promotion in academia," *Med. Hist. 24* (1980) 197–208.

Keel, Othmar. "The politics of health and the institutionalisation of clinical practices in Europe in the second half of the eighteenth century," pp. 207–56 in: W. F. Bynum and Roy Porter, eds, *William Hunter and the Eighteenth Century Medical World* (Cambridge: Cambridge Univ. Press, 1985).

Keel, Othmar. *La généalogie de l'histopathologie, une révision déchirante: Philippe Pinel, lecteur discret de J.-C. Smyth (1741–1821)* (Paris: Vrin, 1979).

Kerrison, Robert Masters. *Observations and Reflections on the Bill Now in Progress through the*

House of Commons, for 'Better Regulating the Medical Profession as Far as Regards Apothecaries' (London, 1815).

Kervran, Roger. *Laennec: His Life and Times* (New York: Pergamon, 1960).

King, Lester, and Meehan, Marjorie C. "The history of the autopsy," *Amer. J. Path. 73* (1973) 514–44.

King, Lester. *The Medical World of the Eighteenth Century.* (Chicago: Univ. of Chicago Press, 1958).

Kondratas, Ramunas. "Joseph Frank (1771–1842) and the Development of Clinical Medicine: A Study of the Transformation of Medical Thought and Practice at the End of the 18th and the Beginning of the 19th Centuries" (Ph.D. diss., Harvard Univ., 1977).

Laennec, R. T. H. *Traité d'Auscultation Médiate, ou Traité du Diagnostic des Maladies des Poumons et du Coeur* (2 vols., Paris: Brosson & Chaude, 1819).

Laennec, R. T. H. "Anatomie pathologique," Adelon et al., eds., *Dictionnaire des Sciences Médicales* (Paris: Panckoucke, 1812–22), *II*, pp. 46–61.

Laennec, R. T. H. "Note sur l'anatomie pathologique," *J. Méd. 9* (1804) 360–78.

Laennec, R. T. H. "Réponse aux observations, etc., de M. Dupuytren," *J. Méd. 10 (1804) 89–95.*

Laennec, R. T. H. "Sur des tuniques qui enveloppent certains viscères, et fournissent des gaines membraneuses à leurs vaisseaux," *J. Méd. 5* (1802–3), 539–75.

Laennec, R. T. H. "D'inflammation du péritoine, recueillies à la clinique interne de l'école de médecine de Paris, sous les yeux des professeurs Corvisart et J. J. Leroux," *J. Méd. 4* (1802) 499–547.

Lain-Entralgo, Pedro. "Sensualism and vitalism in Bichat's anatomie générale," *J. Hist. Med. 3* (1948) 47–64.

Laporte, Yves. "Allocution d'ouverture," in *Laennec, 1781–1826: colloque organisé au Collège de France les 18 et 19 février 1981, revue du Palais de la Découverte,* N° spécial 22, Août 1981, pp. 12–21.

Launois, P.-E. *Xavier Bichat: sa vie, son oeuvre, son influence sur les sciences biologiques* (Paris: Naud, 1943).

Lawrence, Christopher. "Ornate physicians and learned artisans: Edinburgh medical men, 1726–76," pp. 153–76 in: W. F. Bynum and Roy Porter, eds., *William Hunter and the Eighteenth Century Medical World* (Cambridge: Cambridge Univ. Press, 1985).

Lawrence, Susan. "Science and medicine at the London Hospitals: the Development of Teaching and Research, 1750–1815" (Ph.D. diss., Univ. of Toronto, 1985).

Lefanu, W. R. "British periodicals of medicine: A chronological list," *Bull. Hist. Med. 5* (1937) 735–61.

Legée, Georgette. "La participation de Georges et de Frederic Cuvier à l'organisation de l'instruction publique (1802–38)," *Histoire et Nature* No. 4 (Nouv. ser.) fasc. 2 (1974) 47–72.

Léonard, Jacques. *Les médecins de l'ouest au XIXème siècle.* Thèse, Univ. de Paris IV, 1976 (Paris: [Diffusion] Librairie Honoré Champion, 1978).

Léonard, Jacques. *La France médicale: médecins et malades au XIXe siècle* (Paris: Gallimard, 1978).

Léonard, Jacques. *La vie quotidienne du médecin de province au XIXe siècle* (Paris: Hachette, 1977).

Leroux, J. J., and Süe, P. Séance publique de la faculté de médecine de Paris, tenue le 14 novembre 1810, pour la rentrée des écoles, et discours prononcés par M. J. J. LeRoux et par M. Süe" (Paris: Didot le jeune, 1810).

Leroux, J. J. et al. "Consitution médicale observée à Paris, depuis le mois de Novembre 1805, jusqu'au mois de Juin 1806, inclusivement," *J. Méd. 12* (1806) 30–39.

Lesch, John. *Science and Medicine in France: The Emergence of Experimental Physiology, 1790–1855* (Cambridge, Mass.: Harvard Univ. Press, 1984).

Levache de la Feutrie, A. F. T. "Eloge de Marie-Francois-Xavier Bichat," *Mém. Soc. méd. d'Émo. 5* (1803) xxvii–lxiv.

Leveille, M. *Mémoire sur l'état actuel de l'enseignement de la médecine et la chirurgie en France, et sur les modifications dont il est susceptible* (Paris: Dentu, 1816).

Liard, Louis. *L'Université de Paris* (Paris: Renouard, 1909).

Liard, Louis. *L'enseignement supérieur en France, 1789–1889* (Paris: Colin, 1888).

Loudon, Irvine S. L., and Stevens, Rosemary. "Primary care and the hospital," in: John Fry, ed., *Primary Care* (London: Heinemann, 1980), pp. 139–75.

Maulitz, Russell. "Metropolitan medicine and the man–midwife: the early life and letters of Charles Locock," *Med. Hist.* 26 (1982) 25–46.

Maulitz, Russell. "Pathology," in Ronald L. Numbers, ed., *The Education of American Physicians* (Berkeley: Univ. of California Press, 1980), pp. 122–42.

Maulitz, Russell. " 'Physician versus bacteriologist': the ideology of science in clinical medicine," in: Morris Vogel and Charles E. Rosenberg, eds., *The Therapeutic Revolution: Essays in the Social History of American Medicine* (Philadelphia: Univ. of Pennsylvania Press, 1979), pp. 91–108.

Maulitz, Russell. "Rudolf Virchow, Julius Cohnheim, and the program of pathology," *Bull. Hist. Med.* 52 (1978) 162–82.

Maulitz, Russell. "A Treatise on Membranes: Concepts of Tissue Structure, Function, and Dysfunction from Xavier Bichat to Julius Cohnheim," (Ph.D. diss., Duke Univ., 1973).

McMenemey, W. H. *The Life and Times of Charles Hastings* (Edinburgh and London: Livingstone, 1959).

Meding, Henri, *Paris Médical: Vade-Mecum des médecins étrangers* (Paris: Baillière, 1853).

Merrington, W. R. *University College Hospital and Its Medical School: A History* (London: Heinemann, 1976).

Merton, R. K. "The Matthew effect in science," *Science* 159 (1968) 56–63.

Miciotto, Robert. "Carl Rokitansky: a reassessment of the hematohumoral theory of disease," *Bull. Hist. Med.* 52 (1978) 183–99.

Mondor, Henri. "Laennec," *Histoire de la Médecine* 8 (1958) 7–17.

Monteil, Jean. *Le cours d'anatomie pathologique de Bichat: un nouveau manuscrit* (Grenoble: Guirimand, 1960).

Moore, Norman, and Paget, Stephen. *The Royal Medical and Chirurgical Society of London Centenary, 1805 to 1905* (Aberdeen: Aberdeen University Press, 1905).

Moreau de la Sarthe, J.-L. "[Extrait et analyse du] Traité des membranes en général et des diverses membranes en particulier," *Rec. pér. Soc. méd. Paris* 7 (an VIII [1800]) 321–42, 457–62.

Muehry, Adolph. *Observations on the Comparative State of Medicine in France, England, and Germany, during a Journey into These Countries in the Year 1835* (Philadelphia, 1838).

Mulkay, Michael. "The mediating role of the scientific elite," *Social Studies of Science* 6 (1976) 445–70.

Murphy, Terence D. "The French medical profession's perception of its social function between 1776 and 1830," *Med. Hist.* 23 (1979) 259–78.

Newman, Charles. *The Evolution of Medical Education in the Nineteenth Century* (London: Oxford Univ. Press, 1957).

Nicole-Genty, N. "Bichat: médecin du grand hospice d'humanité" (Thèse, Faculté de médecine de Paris, 1943).

Outram, Dorinda. *Georges Cuvier: Vocation, Science and Authority in Post-Revolutionary France* (Manchester: Manchester Univ. Press, 1984).

Parry, Noël, and Parry, Jose. *The Rise of the Medical Profession: A Study of Collective Social Mobility* (London: Croom Helm, 1976).

Peitzman, Steven. "Bright's disease and generation: toward exact medicine at Guy's Hospital," *Bull. Hist. Med.* 55 (1981) 307–21.

Peterson, M. Jeanne. "Specialist journals and professional rivalries in Victorian medicine," *Victorian Periodicals Review* 12 (1979) 25–33.

Peterson, M. Jeanne. *The Medical Profession in Mid-Victorian London* (Berkeley: Univ. of California Press, 1978).

Pickstone, John, "Bureaucracy, liberalism and the body in post-revolutionary France: Bichat's physiology and the Paris school of medicine," *Hist. Sci.* 19 (1981) 115–42.

Pons, Giorgio. "Essai de sociologie des malades dans les hôpitaux de Paris pendant les années 1815 à 1848," *Züricher medizingesch. Abhndlgn.*, N.R., No. 63 (Zürich: Juris, 1969).

Ponteil, Félix. *Histoire de l'enseignement en France, 1789–1964* (Paris: Sirey, 1966).

Ponteil, Félix. *Les institutions de la France de 1814 à 1870* (Paris: Presses Universitaires de France, 1966).

Ponteil, Félix. *Napoléon Ier et l'organisation autoritaire de la France* (Paris: Colin, 1956).

Power, D'Arcy, ed. *British Medical Societies* (London: The Medical Press and Circular, 1939).

Prost, A. *Histoire de l'enseignement en France, 1800–1967* (Paris: Colin, 1968).

Quain, Richard. *Observations on Medical Education* (London: Walton and Maberly, 1865).

Ramsay, Matthew. "The politics of professional monopoly in nineteenth-century medicine: the French model and its rivals," in: Gerald Geison, ed., *Professions and the French State, 1700–1900* (Philadelphia: Univ. of Pennsylvania Press, 1984), pp. 225–305.

Rather, L. J. *The Genesis of Cancer* (Baltimore: Johns Hopkins Univ. Press, 1978).

Reiser, S. J. *Medicine and the Reign of Technology* (Cambridge: Cambridge Univ. Press, 1978).

Reiser, S. J. "Aspects of the role of the stethoscope in the introduction of auscultation to Great Britain and the United States," *Proceedings 23rd International Congress of the History of Medicine, [London, 1972]* (London, 1974).

Richerand, B. A. "Réflexions critiques sur un ouvrage ayant pour titre, traité des membranes," *Mag. Encycl.* 5 (an VIII [1799]) 260–72.

Richmond, P. A. "The Hôtel-Dieu on the eve of the Revolution," *J. Hist. Med.* 16 (1961) 335–53.

Risse, Guenter, *Hospital Life in Enlightenment Scotland* (Cambridge: Cambridge Univ. Press, 1986).

Rodin, Alvin. *The Influence of Matthew Baillie's "Morbid Anatomy"; Biography, Evaluation, and Reprint* (Springfield: Thomas, 1973).

Rolleston, Humphrey. "The early history of the teaching of I. Human Anatomy in London. II. Morbid anatomy and pathology in Great Britain," *Annals of Medical History* 1 (1939) 203–38.

Rosen, George. "The philosophy of ideology and the emergence of modern medicine in France," *Bull. Hist. Med.* 20 (1946) 328–39.

Rosen, George. "A note on the reception of the stethoscope in England," *Bull. Hist. Med.* 7 (1939) 93–94.

Rouxeau, Alfred. *Laennec après 1806: 1806–26, d'après des documents inédits* (Paris: Baillière, 1920).

Royer-Collard, A.-A. *L'institut de médecine de Paris* (Paris, 1810).

Rudwick, M. J. "The emergence of a visual language for geological science, 1760–1840," *History of Science* 14 (1976) 149–95.

Saucerotte, Constant. *Les médecins pendant la révolution, 1879* (Paris: Perrin, 1887).

Saunders, John Cunningham. *A Treatise on Some Practical Points Relating to Diseases of the Eye . . . to Which Are Added, a Short Account of the Author's Life, and His Method of Curing the congenital Cataract, by J. R. Farre.* New [2nd] ed. (London, 1816).

Schiller, Joseph. "Henri Dutrochet et la terminologie scientifique." *97ème Cong. Soc. des Savants* (1972).

Sellers, Ian. *Nineteenth-Century Nonconformity* (London: Edward Arnold, 1977).

Shapin, Steven. "The politics of observation: cerebral anatomy and social interests in the Edinburgh phrenology disputes," in: *On the Margins of Science: The Social Construction of Rejected Knowledge, Sociol. Rev. Monograph* No. 27 (March 1979), pp. 139–78.

Shapin, Steven, and Barnes, Barry. "Science, nature and control: interpreting the mechanics' institutes," *Social Studies of Science* 7 (1977) 31–74.

Sprengel, Kurt. "De l'opération de l'empyème," pp. 1–90 in: *Histoire de la médecine*, IX. Trans. A. J. L. Jourdan (Paris: Baillière, 1815–32).

Staum, Martin. *Cabanis: Enlightenment and Medical Philosophy in the French Revolution.* (Princeton, N.J.: Princeton Univ. Press, 1980).

Suleiman, Ezra. *Elites in French Society: The Politics of Survival* (Princeton: Princeton Univ. Press, 1978).

Suleiman, Ezra. *Politics, Power, and Bureaucracy in France* (Princeton: Princeton Univ. Press, 1974).

Temkin, Owsei. "The role of surgery in the rise of modern medical thought," *Bull. Hist. Med.* 25 (1951) 248–59.

Temkin, Owsei. "The philosophical background of Magendie's physiology," *Bull. Hist. Med.* 20 (1946) 10–35.

Thomson, John. *Lectures on Inflammation, Exhibiting a View of the General Doctrines, Pathological and Practical, of Medical Surgery* (Edinburgh: Blackwood, 1818).

Thouret, Michel. *De l'état actuel de l'Ecole de santé de Paris* (Paris: Didot le jeune, an VI [1798]).

Tröhler, Ulrich. "Quantification in British Medicine and Surgery, 1750–1830" (Ph.D. diss., London 1978).

Vaughan, M. and Archer, M. S. *Social Conflict and Educational Change in England and France, 1789–1848* (Cambridge: Cambridge Univ. Press, 1971).

Vess, David. *Medical Revolution in France, 1789–1796* (Gainesville: Florida State Univ. Press, 1975).

Veysey, Laurence. "Intellectual history and the new social history," in: John Higham and Paul Conklin, eds., *New Directions in American Intellectual History* (Baltimore: Johns Hopkins Univ. Press, 1979) pp. 3–26.

Wall, J. R. "The Guy's Hospital Physical Society," *Guy's Hospital Reports 123* (1974) 159–70.

Warner, John. *The Therapeutic Perspective: Medical Practice, Knowledge, and Identity in America, 1820–1885* (Cambridge, Mass: Harvard Univ. Press, 1986).

Weiner, Dora, ed. *The Clinical Training of Doctors: An Essay of 1793, by Philippe Pinel* (Baltimore: Johns Hopkins Univ. Press, 1980).

Weiner, Dora. "French doctors face war, 1792–1815," in: C. K. Warner, ed., *From the Ancien Regime to the Popular Front: Essays in the History of Modern France in Honor of Shepard B. Clough* (New York: Columbia Univ. Press, 1969).

Weisz, George. "The medical elite in France in the early nineteenth century," *Minerva 25* (1987) 150–70.

Weisz, George. "Constructing the medical elite in France: the creation of the Royal Academy of Medicine 1814–20," *Med. Hist.* 30 (1986) 419–43.

Whitley, Richard. "Umbrella and polytheistic scientific disciplines and their elites," *Social Studies of Science 6* (1976) 471–97.

Wilks, Samuel, and Bettany, G. T. *A Biographical History of Guy's Hospital* (London: Ward, Lock, Bowden and Co., 1892).

Wilks, Samuel. "Cases of enlargement of the Lymphatic Glands and Spleen, or Hodgkin's Disease, with remarks," *Guy's Hospital Reports 22* (1877, ser. 3) 259–74.

Williams, Charles J. B. *Memoirs of Life and Work* (London: Smith, Elder, 1884).

Wilson, J. W. "Cellular tissue and the dawn of the cell theory," *Isis 35* (1944) 168–73.

Wiriot, Mireille. *L'enseignement clinique dans les hôpitaux de Paris entre 1794 et 1848* (Paris, 1970).

Wright, Peter, and Treacher, Andrew, eds. *The Problem of Medical Knowledge: Examining the Social Construction of Medicine.* (Edinburgh: Edinburgh Univ. Press, 1982).

Zeldin, Theodore. *France: 1848–1945*, 2 vols. (Oxford: Oxford Univ. Press, 1973).

Index

surgeon–apothecaries, 118–25, 170–74
surgical mentality, 12, 227–28
sympathies, doctrine of, 16–17, 32
synovial membranes, 27, 28; *see also* membranes

Thomson, John, 143–46
Thomson, William, 146
thoracentesis, 101
Thouret, Michel, 10, 38, 46
  gatekeeper role, 64
  1798 report, 43
tissu cellulaire, 16
tissue pathology, 21; *see also* pathology
  Bichat's theory, 31; *see also* Bichat
  English variant, 133

Transactions of the Associated Apothecaries,
  173
Treatise on Membranes (Bichat), 30

unification of medicine and surgery, 11,
  83–85, 226
University College; *see* London University
University of London; *see* London University

vitalism, 14

Wakley, Thomas, 130, 155
Williams, Charles, J. B., 146–47

Young, George W., 131–32

Printed in the United States
By Bookmasters